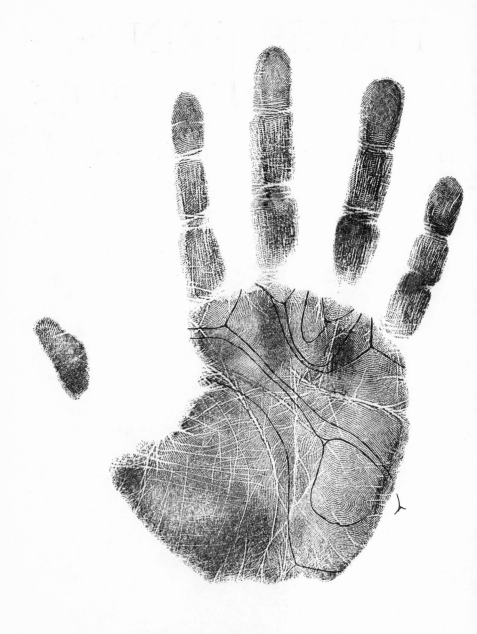

PRINT OF THE RIGHT HAND OF HARRIS HAWTHORNE WILDER

FINGER PRINTS, PALMS AND SOLES

AN INTRODUCTION TO DERMATOGLYPHICS

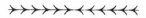

by

HAROLD CUMMINS, PH.D.
Professor of Anatomy and Assistant Dean,
School of Medicine, Tulane University

and

CHARLES MIDLO, M.D.
Formerly Associate Professor of Microscopic Anatomy
Tulane University

DOVER PUBLICATIONS, INC.
NEW YORK

This Dover edition, first published in 1961, is an
unabridged and corrected republication of the work
first published by The Blakiston Company in 1943.
A supplementary chapter on "Identification in Action" has been especially prepared by the authors
for this Dover edition.

Standard Book Number: 486-20778-1
Library of Congress Catalog Card Number: 61-66240

Manufactured in the United States of America
Dover Publications, Inc.
180 Varick Street
New York, N.Y. 10014

To the memory of

Harris Hawthorne Wilder (1864-1928)

Pioneer investigator of dermatoglyphics

>>>>>>>>>>>>>>>>>>>>>>> <<<<<<<<<<<<<<<<<<<<<<

PREFACE

THERE is a prevalent but mistaken notion that dermatoglyphics have no importance beyond their use in personal identification. Perhaps because the publications of research are scattered, and the generalizations seemingly hidden in complexities of descriptive method, it is not generally appreciated that the patternings of epidermal ridges on fingers, palms, toes and soles have broader and more fundamental significance. The configurations are formed in the early fetus and they persist unchanged. Their variants exhibit differential trends among races, between the sexes and among constitutional types. Dermatoglyphics also elucidate various morphological principles, including bodily symmetry. Some traits of the dermatoglyphics are heritable, hence they are useful in recognizing the types of twins and have promise of application in cases of questioned paternity. With these and related topics forming its central theme, the present volume is designed to fill the want of a comprehensive treatise on dermatoglyphics. For those of a biological turn—especially anatomists, physical anthropologists, physicians interested in constitution, geneticists and zoölogists—the book is intended as a means of acquaintance with a relatively neglected aspect of human biology. Though aiming to bring the biological phases of the field also to the attention of workers in identification, this *Introduction to Dermatoglyphics* does not purport to be an account of routine methods for finger-print men, who already have available several excellent manuals of practice.

The text is arranged in three parts, and a representative working bibliography is appended. Part I supplies historical background and a general orientation of the field. Part II deals with methods and description. Part III is devoted to the more fundamental biological phases of dermatoglyphics. It is suggested that the reader might pass from Part I to Part III, referring to Part II as questions on methodology and description arise.

Several colleagues in research—Norma Ford, G. Tyler Mairs, D. C. Rife, and, now deceased, Heinrich Poll, Inez Whipple Wilder and Harris H.

Wilder—have furthered indirectly the preparation of the book. Debts to them for benefits gained from personal discussions and correspondence have accumulated since 1922, when our interest in dermatoglyphics had its beginning. For reading parts of the manuscript we are indebted to: Beverly Blood, Edwin A. Ohler and H. M. Johnson, all of Tulane University; G. Tyler Mairs of the Finger Print Bureau of the City Magistrates' Courts, New York; D. C. Rife of Ohio State University. They have read critically and their comments have been helpful. Any errors of omission or commission which remain are our own. Genevieve Lee made drawings and graphs for most of the new illustrations. Sarah Dyson typed several drafts of the manuscript in successive revisions. Sources of borrowed illustrations are indicated in legends of individual figures; additional courtesies in connection with illustrations are here acknowledged. Figures credited to H. H. Wilder and I. W. Wilder are mostly printed from blocks originally used in publications by these authors, their collection of cuts having been placed at our disposal by authorities of Smith College. For the gift of cuts previously used in our own publications we are indebted to The Wistar Institute of Anatomy, to The Scientific Monthly and to the Journal of Criminal Law and Criminology.

HAROLD CUMMINS,
CHARLES MIDLO.

NEW ORLEANS
August 9, 1943

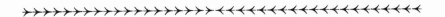

CONTENTS

Part Three — BIOLOGY

Part I

ORIENTATION

HISTORY

Primitive Knowledge of Dermatoglyphics

THE patterned traceries of fine ridges on fingers, palms and soles must have aroused interest long ago, though when it was that men first noticed them never can be known. There exist records that indicate acquaintance with these traceries, or dermatoglyphics, long prior to the period of scientific study. One of the most telling fragments of this unwritten history is an aboriginal Indian carving found at the edge of Kejimkoojik Lake in Nova Scotia. Within the outline of a human hand, scratched in stone, are lines roughly representing dermatoglyphics and flexion creases (Fig. 1). The thumb, the most faithfully pictured region, bears a spiral whorl. This petroglyph is generally credited with an age of at least several hundreds of years, and it may be older. Its significance lies

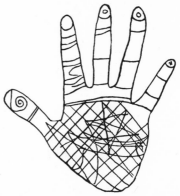

Fig. 1.—An aboriginal Indian petroglyph (Nova Scotia), representing dermatoglyphics and flexion creases of the human hand. (*From Mallery.*)

in the fact that the maker, though living under primitive conditions, had become familiar with the dermatoglyphics and flexion creases and was inspired to engrave a picture of them.

Had the maker of this petroglyph drawn the whorl of the thumb as a design isolated from the outline of a hand or digit, there would have been no clue to its identity as a skin pattern. Such is exactly the status of many ancient stone carvings resembling dermatoglyphics, discovered in widespread parts of the globe. In a Utah Basketmaker pictograph,[1] for exam-

---

[1] Douglas, F. H., and R. d'Harnoncourt. *Indian Art of the United States.* New York, The Museum of Modern Art, 1941.

ple, there are several human figures accompanied by designs of questionable significance, including four isolated concentric and spiral patterns
resembling the whorls of finger prints. The monumental work by Mallery,
Picture-writing of the American Indians,[2] illustrates numerous examples of
similar designs drawn as independent pictures. It seems unlikely that they
were intended to represent finger-print patterns, though Mallery makes
this comment suggesting the possibility:

> The frequency with which partial representations of the eye are met
> with appeared to me so striking that I requested Mr. Jacobsen to ask
> the Bella Coola Indians whether they had any special idea in employ-
> ing the eye so frequently. To my great surprise the person addressed
> pointed to the palmar surface of his finger tips and to the fine linea-
> ments which the skin there presents; in his opinion a rounded or
> longitudinal field, such as appears between the converging or parallel
> lines, also means an eye, and the reason of this is that originally each
> part of the body terminated in an organ of sense, particularly an eye,
> and was only afterward made to retrovert into such rudimentary
> conditions.

Probably the most famous of ancient "finger-print" designs are
carvings (4) on the walls of a Neolithic burial passage, or dolmen, situated

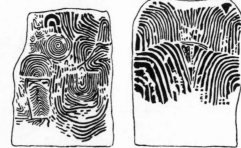

FIG. 2.—Carvings, which resemble dermatoglyphics, on granite wall slabs in the Neolithic
dolmen of L'Ile de Gavr'inis. (*From Stockis.*)

on an island off Brittany, L'Ile de Gavr'inis. The dolmen, constructed of
slabs of stone, is a gallery leading into an enlarged chamber, the structure
being imbedded in a low mound of earth. Its inner walls are covered with
incised designs—systems of horse-shoe form, more or less circular concentric figures, spirals, arching lines, sinuous and straight lines and other
markings, occurring in various combinations (Fig. 2). It is claimed by
some writers, notably Stockis and Bridges, that the carvings represent

---

[2] Tenth Annual Report, Bureau of Ethnology, 1893.

dermatoglyphics. A note published anonymously in France ventures even the fantastic suggestion that they are reproductions of finger prints of chieftains, graved in the dolmen as an identification register. Stockis' publication illustrates the whole series of carvings, many of them accompanied by figures of corresponding patterns in actual finger prints. The likeness of some of the carvings to dermatoglyphic configurations is striking, but in others there is no similarity whatsoever. Several authors offer quite different explanations of the origins of the Gavr'inis designs. Faure[3] sees in the carvings of this dolmen "moving lines on the surface of low water, undulations or the tremblings of seaweed, which must be signs of conjuring or magic."

Under the circumstances it is incautious, to say the least, to make a specific attribution of the designs on the walls of the Gavr'inis dolmen. Certainly indeed, the argument of resemblance, upon which the claim of finger-print origin rests, has insecure support. Neither this dolmen nor any other similar series of gravings on stone furnishes intrinsic evidence of the use of dermatoglyphics as models, since clues comparable to the hand outline in the Nova Scotian petroglyph are wanting. Many designs in nature resemble dermatoglyphics, and they might have served as models. Then, too, the symbolisms which may enter into man-made designs render interpretation of their sources a venturesome undertaking, perhaps even for those versed in a subject "which contains so many pitfalls for the unwary."[4]

The worker in clay has especially favorable opportunities for observation of skin patterns, impressed in the plastic mass (5). It is not impossible that pottery-making peoples, even in remote time, were by this means prompted to an interest in finger prints. Such prints are often conspicuous, and the patterns may be more compelling of attention in the clay than on the skin.

In figure 3 there is shown a clear finger print dating to the fourth or fifth century of the Christian era. The fragment of a clay lamp on which it is impressed was excavated in Palestine by the late Doctor Badè. Numerous objects recovered at the site bear prints of the same potter. Other examples of prints in ancient clay objects are known, but all except the one next to be mentioned lack signs supporting the contention of some writers that such prints were applied for personal identification. Recognition of their identifying value, for which there is no convincing proof, would signify familiarity with finger-print characteristics. Besides,

---

[3] Faure, Elie. *History of Art*, vol. 1, *Ancient Art*. (Translated from the French by W. Pach.) Garden City, Garden City Publishing Co., Inc., 1937.

[4] Haddon, Alfred C. *Evolution in Art*. Scribner's, 1895.

there are indications that the imprints are most often merely marks of the fingers used as tools, though it is conceivable that finger prints in some

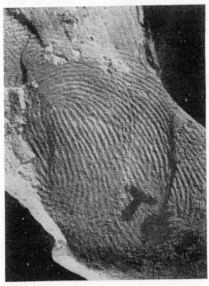

Fig. 3.—An identifiable print on a fragment of a Palestinian lamp of the fourth or fifth century A.D. (*From Badè. Courtesy of the Palestine Institute, Pacific School of Religion.*)

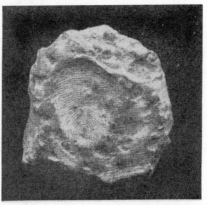

Fig. 4.—A clear thumb print on a Chinese clay seal, made not later than the third century B.C. (*From Laufer. Courtesy of the Field Museum of Natural History.*)

instances may have figured in symbolic identification, as a token expressing a relationship of the individual to an object or to an act concerning it.

The argument for purposeful recording of an identifying finger print in clay is stronger in the case of the Chinese seal illustrated in figure 4.

This seal, made not later than the third century B.C., is a pat of clay which would have been attached to some document, letter or package. On one surface it bears a name impressed by a personal seal, and on the other there is a clearly defined thumb print. The provenience of this print suggests its nature as a personal mark, but whether the mark was made with a purpose equivalent to that of current finger-print identification is a debatable question.

The significance of prints on old documents of the East, where the practice of imprinting fingers extended over centuries, is equally open to unlike interpretations.

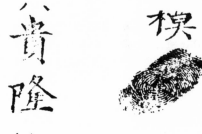

Figure 5 reproduces part of a Chinese deed of sale of a plot of land, executed in the year 1839.

Receipt of payment is acknowledged in the deed by the woman heading the family which disposed of the property.

FIG. 5.—A Chinese deed of sale, 1839, signed with a finger print. (*From Laufer. Courtesy of the Field Museum of Natural History.*)

As is true of many other Chinese documents, this deed bears a finger print with an accompanying inscription denoting that the print is a form of signature. The inscription reads: "Impression of the finger of the mother, born Ch'en."

A Chinese contract of loan executed nearly twelve hundred years ago closes with a formula, which is in substance like some other examples: "The two parties have found this just and clear, and have affixed the impressions of their fingers to serve as a mark." The prints of witnesses are added. Like the print on the Chinese seal and deed, and like the finger-nail indentions on Assyrian clay tablets, prints such as these might only signify that the persons intended to leave a tangible sign of their participation in an act. That sign would have served its object, as conceived by the participants, without the introduction of any principle concerned in modern finger-print identification.

The whole palm and sole also may have figured in the history of Chinese knowledge of dermatoglyphics. In his work *Asia*, published in 1563, de Barros (cited by de Pina), records a custom prevailing in 16th-century China in connection with the sale of children. Prints of the palm and sole were impressed in ink on the deeds of sale. De Barros states that these prints provide against false personation. The practice, however, may have been independent of any conception of the individuality of dermatoglyphics.

More acceptable evidence of an appreciation of finger-print characteristics is the personal mark of Thomas Bewick, 1753–1828, English
engraver, author and naturalist. Bewick made wood engravings of patterns of his own fingers (Fig. 6), and printed them as vignettes or colophons
in the books which he wrote. The engravings demonstrate familiarity
with the construction of skin patterns, including the details of branching
and interruption of the skin ridges. It has been stated (7) that Bewick
also stamped receipts with an engraved finger print. Bewick possibly
understood the individuality of finger prints, though neither the marks
themselves nor his custom of using them proves it. It is evident, however,

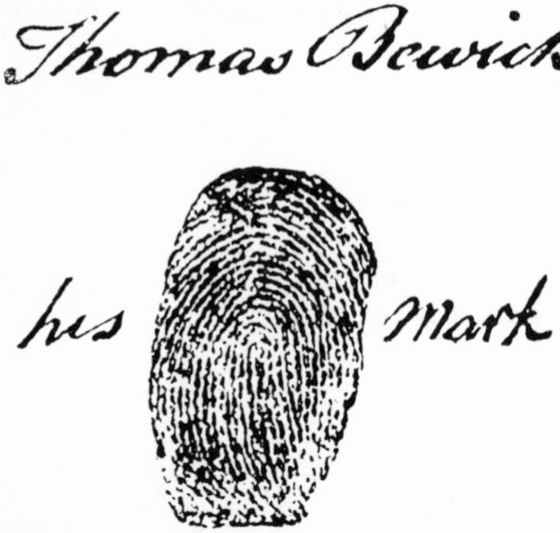

FIG. 6.—A Bewick finger print, engraved on wood: Thomas Bewick, engraver and autho r
of works on natural history, 1753–1828. (*From Wentworth and Wilder. Courtesy of the Finger
Print Publishing Association.*)

that he was among the few persons of his time who are known to have had
exact knowledge of dermatoglyphics, and it is to be supposed that familiarity gained through engraving them would have been intimate,
though perhaps not very comprehensive. Another personal mark of present
interest is the finger print and signature of Henry P. de Forest (Fig. 7),
published as a colophon in his brochure on finger-print history. Doctor de
Forest himself figures in this history, having made in 1902 the first prints
officially recorded for personal identification in the United States. In this
instance, unlike that of Bewick, it is certain that "his mark" was impressed
with knowledge of its uniqueness.

Consideration of the elements of symbolism, magic and superstition
which may have motivated early attention to finger prints lies outside
the province of this work. It suffices to emphasize that the outlook of the

peoples who made earliest use of finger prints should not be reconstructed solely on the basis of our own point of view. Be that as it may, dermatoglyphics had attracted notice long before the period of scientific record. Even folk-lore has incorporated a rudimentary cognizance of finger prints, as shown in the following Chinese formula for fortune-telling, in which the

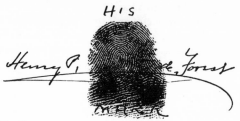

FIG. 7.—A print of Dr. Henry P. de Forest. Compare with figure 6, the similar mark of Thomas Bewick, made a century and a quarter earlier. (*Courtesy of Dr. de Forest.*)

future of the individual is predicted in accord with the number of whorls and loops borne on his fingers.

> One whorl, poor; two whorls, rich;
> Three whorls, four whorls, open a pawnshop;
> Five whorls, be a go-between;
> Six whorls, be a thief;
> Seven whorls, meet calamities;
> Eight whorls, eat chaff;
> Nine whorls and one loop, no work to do—
> eat till you are old.[5]

Dactylomancy, strangely enough, is practiced even now and in this country, though it does not rank with palmistry in popularity. One of the present authors was the subject of a reading, in 1935, made by a fingerprint expert who professes ability in dactylomancy. Though the reader was supplied with finger prints alone and had never seen the subject, the identity was known to him. The report is quoted in full, to illustrate the scope of characteristics which purportedly are revealed in the prints of this subject.

> I believe this, as much as I believe anything, that your fingerprints tell you what you are. Regardless of what you think, or want to be, the fingerprint tells the truth. Let us look at your own: this is the hand of the thinker, as opposed to the manual and physical. The whorl indicates a degree of tenacity, stamina, stick-to-it-iveness; on the other hand you

---

[5] Rearranged, from A. H. Smith, *Proverbs and Common Sayings of the Chinese*, Shanghai. 1902—quoted by Laufer.

would have double these virtues if you had two whorls (in the thumbs). You will be shorter-lived than your co-workers who have all whorls. Persons with ten whorls tend to longevity. I judge you to be a man aged about 45 to 47 years. You are a mental worker; not a physical type at all. You entered your profession after a long deliberation—due to uncertainty—and then decided to be a professor. In stature you are close to 6 feet in height and you are not physically robust. You weigh about 165 lbs. It would not surprise me but what you were a frail child. You are a tireless worker and do not spare yourself. The intro-vert type of hand is very desirable as it represents a sort of balance wheel; it is far more impetuous than the ten-whorl type. The whorl type of hand (extrovert) is one that reasons and weighs all sides and angles to a problem before making a decision. Were it not for the ten-whorl hand, the world would constantly run amuck.

Early Scientific Records

It is difficult to set a dividing line between what may be rightly con-sidered scientific knowledge of dermatoglyphics as distinguished from

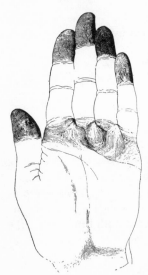

FIG. 8.—Dermatoglyph-ics drawn by Grew, 1684. *(From Wentworth and Wilder. Courtesy of the Finger Print Publishing Association.)*

primitive knowledge. The distinction is arbi-trary, and as made here it is only a definition of convenience. Beginning of the scientific period is arbitrarily set with the first records which conform to the prevailing notion of what constitutes a scientific record. As moderns, we are inclined to think of manuscripts, books and journals as media, forgetting that primitive conditions of life restrict the modes of recording ideas. After all, the aboriginal who carved the hand on a rock in Nova Scotia may have been as truly scientific in spirit and method as the author of a technical article or book. Bewick was at least an observer of finger prints, and he might have been also a practitioner of scientific personal identification. Perhaps the Chinese who impressed his thumb in a clay seal, more than two thousand years ago, was likewise following a scientific practice then recognized. The facts in these and similar cases are obscured by time and the lack of validating records. In spite of a conviction that there was a scientific recognition of derma-toglyphics long before the first written records concerning them, these records are at least a definite milepost of advance.

The old writings of the East, China in particular, have been considered at length by historians of finger-print science.

It is probable that the identifying value of finger prints had been appreciated many centuries before the appearance of the published notice (Faulds, 1880) which inaugurated the now extensive literature on finger-print identification. Some of the ancient writings, however, are of extremely doubtful bearing on the question at issue. Relating as they do to finger-printing customs, and neglecting explanation of rationale, these writings are no more convincing than the finger-print signatures themselves, which witness only that the prints were made.

The works of Grew, 1684, Bidloo, 1685, and Malpighi, 1686, are among the earliest scientific descriptions of dermatoglyphics. Grew presented before the Royal Society in London a report of his observations on

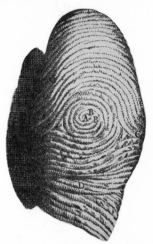

FIG. 9.—One of the earliest scientific records of the anatomy of dermatoglyphics—Bidloo, 1685. (*From Dankmeijer, after the 1728 edition of Bidloo.*)

patternings of the fingers and palm. He describes the sweat pores, the epidermal ridges and their arrangements, and presents a drawing of

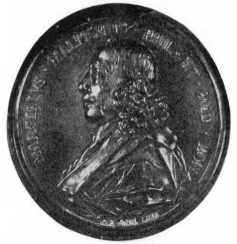

FIG. 10.—Marcello Malpighi, 1628–1694. (*A medallion issued on the occasion of the fourth International Congress of Anatomy, Milan, 1936.*)

the configurations of one hand (Fig. 8). Bidloo's book on human anatomy includes a drawing of a thumb (Fig. 9) and a description of the detailed arrangement of the ridges in this one digit. Though breadths of individual ridges are exaggerated in the drawing, perhaps to emphasize details, the illustration gives evidence of a careful attempt to portray the characteris-

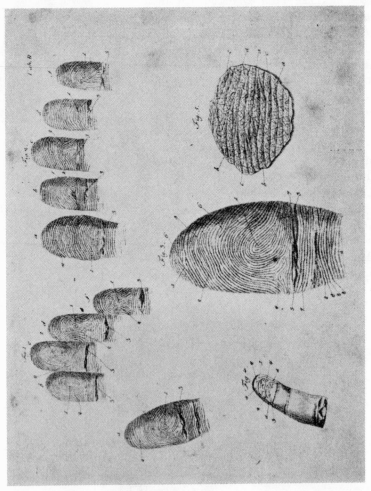

FIG. 11.—Mayer's drawings of finger prints, 1788.

tics of the ridged surface. It was but one year later that Malpighi (Fig. 10) briefly described the configurations:

> The hand presents for examination, on its palmar surface, elevated ridges which course in diverse designs. On the terminal segments of the digits they are drawn into spirals; if examined microscopically they show the mouths of sweat glands along their middles.

The eighteenth century was marked by the appearance of several anatomical works in which dermatoglyphics receive mention, among them: Hintze, 1747, Albinus, 1764, and Mayer, 1788. Mayer's contribution has escaped previous notice by commentators on the history of finger-print science. His book is an atlas of anatomical illustrations, accompanied by brief explanations. The plate of finger prints is here copied in figure 11. His explanation of the plate contains the following statement, which opens with the first clear enunciation of a basic principle of finger-print identification:

> Although the arrangement of skin ridges is never duplicated in two persons, nevertheless the similarities are closer among some individuals. In others the differences are marked, yet in spite of their peculiarities of arrangement all have a certain likeness.

In the early nineteenth century several authors made contributions to the literature on dermatoglyphics. Schröter, 1814, in dealing with the

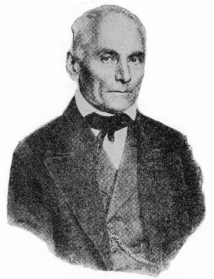

FIG. 12.—J. E. Purkinje, 1787–1869. (*From Wentworth and Wilder, after Locy. Courtesy of the Finger Print Publishing Association.*)

sense of touch, presents a discussion of the morphology of the palmar skin and illustrates the arrangement of ridges and pores. The work of Purkinje (Fig. 12) is a more important landmark in history, for it was he who in 1823 first classified systematically the varieties of patterns of the fingers. He distinguishes "nine principal configurations of the rugae and sulci serving the sense of touch on the terminal phalanges of the human hand" (Fig. 13). He mentions briefly also the patternings of the human palm, of the hands of monkeys and of the prehensile tail of the spider monkey. A sense of the high variability of dermatoglyphics is implicit in his writing, though at no point does Purkinje suggest that this variability might be utilized in personal identification. His interest was confined to physiological processes and the structures which serve them.

Another writer of the early nineteenth century, Bell, has a place in the history of dermatoglyphics. In 1833 Bell contributed one of the volumes in the series of Bridgewater Treatises on *The Power, Wisdom, and Goodness of God, as Manifested in the Creation*, the title of his work being *The Hand:*

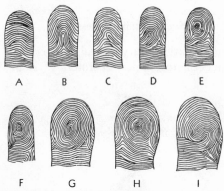

FIG. 13.—Purkinje's nine types of finger patterns, 1823. *A*, the transverse curves [plain arch]; *B*, the central longitudinal stria [tented arch]; *C*, the oblique stripe [loop, ulnar or radial]; *D*, the oblique loop [loop, ulnar or radial]; *E*, the almond [whorl]; *F*, the spiral [whorl]; *G*, the ellipse—elliptical whorl [whorl]; *H*, the circle—circular whorl [whorl]; *I*, the double whorl [composite, twin loop].

Its Mechanism and Vital Endowments as Evincing Design. As an anatomist, Bell made a searching analysis of the structural and functional adaptations of the hand. He described, just as they are recognized now, the two functional advantages mediated by the epidermal ridges. Following a consideration of "the fulness and elasticity of the ends of the fingers," he writes:

> But to return—on a nearer inspection, we see a more particular provision in the points of the fingers. Wherever the sense of feeling is most exquisite, there are minute spiral ridges of cuticle. These ridges have, corresponding with them, depressed lines on the inner surface of the cuticle; and these again give lodgment to a soft pulpy matter, in which lie the extremities of the sentient nerves. . . . Had the cuticle been finely polished on its surface, it would have been illsuited to touch; on the contrary, it has a very peculiar roughness which adapts it to feeling.

A provision for friction, as opposed to smoothness, is a necessary quality of some parts of the skin; thus the roughness of the cuticle has the advantage of giving us a firmer grasp, and a steadier footing. Nothing is so little apt to slip as the thickened cuticle of the hand or foot.

Purkinje remarks in 1823 that some mention of the epidermal rugae and sulci "occurs in every physiological or anatomical epitome." Through the nineteenth century and even later such books continued to include casual notice of the dermatoglyphic features. With the advent of finger-print identification, books and articles specially devoted to the subject multiplied.

PRACTICAL APPLICATION IN IDENTIFICATION

The possibility of early use of prints for personal identification, in the East, has been suggested. The publication in 1880 by Faulds (Fig. 14) is the first item in modern literature relating to finger-print identification. It is a brief note appearing in the English journal, *Nature*. Faulds, on the basis of his own observations, points out that chance prints left at the scene of crime would provide for positive identification of offenders when apprehended. The article was followed promptly by a letter written by Herschel and published in the same journal. In it Herschel asserts that he had been actually using this method of identification in India for about twenty years. Thus while to Faulds is due credit for having first published on the method, Herschel was the first European of the modern period actually to practice finger-print identification. These two men had different points of view as to practical

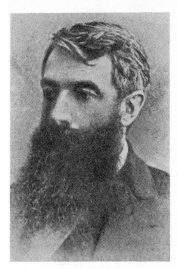

FIG. 14.—Henry Faulds, 1843–1930. *(Courtesy of Dr. Henry P. de Forest.)*

applications of finger prints. Faulds envisioned their service especially in establishing the identities of persons leaving chance prints at the scene of crime, and Herschel conceived a broader usefulness, the registration of prints as a measure against false personation.

The latter part of the nineteenth century is notable also for the publications of Galton, Henry and Vucetich, who with Faulds and Herschel were concerned in developing practical methods of finger-print identification. Henry (Fig. 15) established the scheme of classification which is the most widely adopted of all the numerous systems. There are several others, however, who figure in the history of this formative period.

First mentioned by Galton in 1892, and since then frequently quoted in discussions of finger-print history, is the device used by Gilbert Thompson. While at the head of a surveying party in 1882, Thompson paid its members by written orders to the camp sutler. The inscription of the amount on the order was surcharged by his own thumb print. It seems

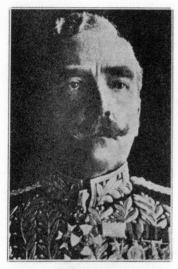

FIG. 15.—Edward Richard Henry, 1850–1931. (*Courtesy of Dr. Henry P. de Forest.*)

to be clear that the thumb print was intended not as an identification of Mr. Thompson but as a means of preventing alteration of the written figures. When it is noted that the duplicate order which Thompson presented to Galton was drawn in favor of one "Lying Bob," the precaution is understandable.

At about the same time Tabor, a photographer in San Francisco, chanced to notice the pattern impressed by his own inked finger on paper. After carrying out some experiments with finger prints, he proposed that the method be adopted for the registration of Chinese immigrants, where the difficulties in ordinary identification had been a vexing problem. Neither this proposal nor the one made in 1885 by an unknown resident of Cincinnati for the use of identifying

prints on railroad tickets was carried out, but the fact that the suggestions were made demonstrates early recognition of promise of the finger-print method. A European parallel (8) is that of Wilhelm Eber, a veterinarian in Berlin who was convinced of the practical usefulness of finger prints and who formally reported his conclusions to the Ministry in 1888; the Ministry was not impressed.

Mark Twain did much to further popular interest in finger prints through two of his books, *Life on the Mississippi* and *Pudd'nhead Wilson*. In *Life on the Mississippi* the character Karl Ritter is made to say that he had read a fortune from a thumb print, and that he had known an old French prison keeper who insisted that the lines in the ball of the thumb are never exactly alike in any two human beings and that they do not change from the cradle to the grave. These basic ideas are amplified in

Pudd'nhead Wilson. Pudd'nhead's address to the jury has been characterized as "one of the finest explanations of the logical basis of finger-print
identification ever given either in fiction or in life" (48).

The source of Mark Twain's finger-print plot is not known, though
doubtless he received the idea second-hand, as did Galton, Henry or any
one of many others who built on foundations already laid. Herschel states
that his interest in finger prints probably originated by inspection of
Bewick's mark. Faulds was an originator, and it appears that some others,
Tabor for example, were also original. Laufer takes the position that
original ideas are so rare that "it is most unlikely that a complex series
of ideas as presented by the finger-print process was several times evolved
by different nations [or individuals] independently." However, and notwithstanding the antiquity of the use of finger prints in China, there is
no need to assume that all ideas about finger-print identification must have
stemmed from that source.

Finger-print identification was introduced on a large scale only after a
period of probation extending through several decades. The method now
is in universal use, and has been extended from its original criminal
limitations to varied applications in civilian and military life. So many have
participated in this expanding use and in developing details of method that
the listing of names and individual contributions would encumber what
is intended to be only a sketch of the main historical framework.

Current Popular Interest in Finger-printing

The use of prints in identification has attracted widespread interest.
Mark Twain's example of using a finger-print plot has been followed by
many a writer of fiction. More effectively, accounts in the press have
brought constantly to the attention of readers the operation of the finger-
print method, through reports of cases of identification of criminals, the
unknown dead, victims of amnesia and the like. Feature stories, addresses
and radio talks are active outlets of information on the subject. The foot-
printing or palm-printing of newborn infants, the finger-printing of
soldiers, sailors and certain classes of employees, as well as widespread
finger-printing of civilians in the war emergency have broadened first-
hand familiarity with the objectives of personal identification.

The fruits of this dissemination of interest in finger prints are apparent.
It is not uncommon to read about a troop of Boy Scouts engaged in a
finger-printing project, or of the members of a club or the citizens of a
community responding enthusiastically in a finger-printing campaign.
The Federal Bureau of Investigation and other agencies of law enforcement have extended to civilians invitations to be finger-printed, and the

favorable reception is measured by the large number of finger-print cards now deposited in official files.

For several years the toy stores have carried simple finger-print kits, and it may be taken for granted that the youngster who possesses the kit will acquire some knowledge of the character of finger prints and of their individual differences as revealed among his relatives and friends. But a boy need not await the ownership of this equipment to learn something about the subject. Comic strips and cartoons often feature finger prints in identification. "Tarzan of the Apes" was proved to be the son of Lord and Lady Greystoke, by means of finger prints which as an infant he had made in touching with inky fingers a page of the father's diary. The youth's interest also might be aroused by a puzzle in which a name is hidden in a labyrinth of lines, a purported finger print. Quite recently there has been patented a finger-print game,[6] "Fingo Printo," which is played on the principle of "Bingo." Each player is supplied with a large card bearing the outline of a hand and designs of finger-print types. The chips are small cards each bearing a single print. On successive deals the players endeavor to fill all five finger bulbs with specified prints.

Popular notice is gained even through advertising writers, who sometimes turn to finger-print science for ideas toward their copy. This copy in turn carries its influence farther, and in a way that is bound to instil an appreciation of some of the principles of finger-print identification. The clothier tells his prospective customers that "A finger print is an unquestioned means of identification. So is ——'s label."[7] A garment maker who wishes to emphasize the distinctiveness of his wares claims that the garment has "personality," and is "as individual as your finger print." Even the qualities of latent prints are not neglected. The producer of a brand of tobacco advertises: "Wanted—the 123,232 missing pipe smokers whose thumb prints are on the wrong packages of tobacco." The publishers of a popular magazine also based recent advertising on latent prints, on copies of the magazine collected from homes: "Inside the covers of —— Magazine we found an average of 407.8 clear fingerprints per copy. . . . We found the thumbprints of 3.26 different persons on each typical copy."

With all these signs pointing to broad popularization of finger prints, it is apparent that the day is soon coming when there will be no longer a significant objection to finger-printing. The feeling against it is on the wane, though there are still some who regard finger-printing as a stigma because they associate it with the police records of criminals. It is not too

---

[6] The game was devised by E. Reichert, a finger-print expert of New York City.

[7] The quotations in this paragraph are from actual advertisements.

much to hope that universal registration of prints will be eventually realized (Chap. 8). Objections can be based only on misconceptions, namely that the method is tainted by its criminal application and that compulsory registration would violate principles of personal liberty.

BIOLOGICAL PHASES

Certain biological principles are basic in finger-print identification. (a) Individual epidermal ridges are so highly variable that their charac-

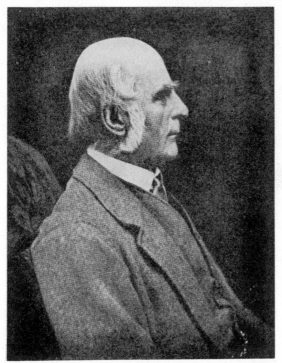

FIG. 16.—Francis Galton, 1822–1916. (*From Wentworth and Wilder, after Locy. Courtesy of the Finger Print Publishing Association.*)

teristics, even in a small area of a finger, palm or sole, are not duplicated either in another region or in a different individual. (b) The configurations and details of individual ridges are permanent and unchanging. (c) The configuration types are individually variable, but they vary within limits which allow for systematic classification.

How these principles came to be established in the minds of those who first recognized them remains unknown, though it may be assumed that the process would have been essentially no different from the recorded experience of Faulds. Faulds relates that he first became attracted to the study of finger prints by the finding of impressions on ancient Japanese pottery. This led to an examination of "the characters of the skin-furrows in human fingers generally," which convinced him of the high degree of variability of patterns and of their "for-ever-unchangeable" character. The observations prompted his proposal of the use of prints in identifica-

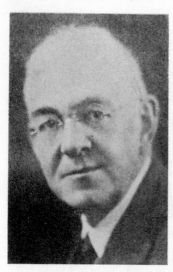

tion and stimulated his further investigations of dermatoglyphics in different races and in monkeys. Others before and after Faulds, perhaps directed by some observation as casual, might easily have been led into independent studies of finger prints. Workers primarily engaged in personal identification, anatomy, physical anthropology, zoölogy and genetics have turned to studies of various phases of dermatoglyphics. Their contributions form a body of living history, since they are a part of the working literature of current studies. It would be pointless to name all these authors and to indicate their individual studies, but there are some whose pioneer work is so highly significant as to merit special mention even if it must be brief.

FIG. 17.—Harris Hawthorne Wilder, 1864–1928.

Galton (Fig. 16) pioneered in fundamental finger-print studies concerned with morphology, classification, inheritance and racial variation.[8]

Wilder (Fig. 17) inaugurated a program of biological investigations with a study of comparative dermatoglyphics. His first paper on the subject was published in 1897, and in the following three decades he continued with studies devoted to morphology, the methodology of plantar and palmar dermatoglyphics, inheritance and racial differences.[9]

[8] There is at the University of London a Galton Room which houses memorabilia of this great biologist—photographs, letters, finger-print material, and many instruments of which some were specially designed for his studies of finger prints.

[9] It may be of interest to note the stimulus which prompted Wilder's studies in the field of dermatoglyphics. On first meeting one of the present authors (Cummins) Wilder held out his right hand and said: "Notice how the hypothenar pattern resembles that of the monkeys. Long ago my attention was directed to this similarity, and the speculation aroused by it was the stimulus for my later work." (See frontispiece.)

Inez Whipple (Fig. 18), a student and later the wife of Wilder, began her study of dermatoglyphics with a comparative survey which is a classic in the field (147). Early during the period of Mrs. Wilder's study, two other pioneer workers were engaged in research on comparative dermatoglyphics—Schlaginhaufen and Kidd.

Kristine Bonnevie has accomplished more than any other person in analyzing the inheritance of finger-print characteristics. Her first major contribution (44) was followed by a succession of important studies on

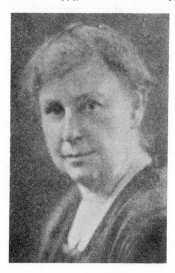 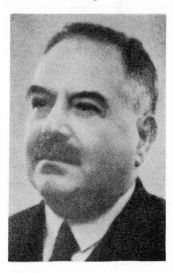

FIG. 18.—Inez Whipple Wilder, 1871–1929. FIG. 19.—Heinrich Poll, 1877–1939.

various aspects of inheritance and on the embryological processes leading to the expression of particular configurations.

Heinrich Poll (Fig. 19) devised novel and revealing methods for the analysis of finger prints. He investigated racial differences, geographic variation within races, constitution and symmetry.

From the work of these and other investigators, whose interests have been centered on biological problems, the substance of Part 3 in this volume is drawn, and their contributions figure largely in Part 2 also.

GENERAL CONSIDERATIONS

RIDGED SKIN

THE palmar and plantar surfaces of the human hand and foot are clothed by skin which is different from that covering other parts of the body. The skin here is continuously corrugated with narrow ridges, and there are neither hairs nor sebaceous (oil) glands. Sweat glands are abundant and of relatively large size. Further distinctions, of thickness and of histological structure, are observable by dissection and by microscopical examination. Ridged skin is not strictly confined to the palmar and plantar surfaces. Ridges occur over the tips of digits, and on the digital margins, where as along the margins of the palm and sole they extend about halfway to the dorsal surface. The extent of ridged skin is emphasized in the Negro by reduced pigmentation throughout the areas of dermatoglyphic specialization.

The palms and soles of all primates bear ridged skin, and the tails of certain monkeys and the paws in some mammals other than primates also are thus characterized (Chap. 9). In no group other than primates, however, is this volar specialization consistently present.

Prior to 1926, when the word *dermatoglyphics* was proposed (276), there had been no satisfactory term embracing the skin patternings of fingers, toes, palms and soles. Dermatoglyphics (*derma*, skin + *glyphē*, carve) is a collective name for all these integumentary features, within the limits to be defined, and it applies also to the division of anatomy which embraces their study. The word is literally descriptive of the delicately sculptured skin surface, inclusive of single ridges and their configurational arrangements. Flexion creases and other secondary folds are not elements of dermatoglyphics. Though the term has come to be generally adopted among biological investigators, the practical finger-print man has had no reason to substitute it for his own useful and familiar terms. Most commonly, he needs only to refer to finger prints, or patterns, and his field is adequately designated by any one of several names, such as dactyloscopy.

The structural specializations of palmar and plantar skin are advantageous in the functioning of contact surfaces. Corrugation of the surface, moistening by sweat and absence of hair counteract slipping, this adaptation being recognized in the term *friction skin*. Like the milling on the handle of a tool or the tread on an automobile tire, the ridging serves as an anti-slipping device. The drag against a surface as the skin is passed over it may be increased by imbrication of the epidermal ridges. Imbrication is detectable (133) when the end-on profiles of ridges are examined under a lens, and it is evident also in sections cut vertically to the surface of the skin and across the ridges (Fig. 20). Varying among regions and individuals in its presence, imbrication is evident as skewing of the contour of the

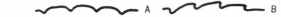

FIG. 20.—*A*. Diagrammatic profile of ridges without imbrication. *B*. Actual profiles of imbricated ridges, traced from a histological section. (*Kidd.*)

ridge. Ridges within a limited area all have their skewed margins facing the same direction.

Abundant nerve endings in the skin of the palmar and plantar surfaces serve the sense of touch. Their functioning is aided by corrugation of the skin. In testing the texture of a surface the fingers or palm are rubbed back and forth over it. The drag against the ridges heightens the intensity of stimulation of the nerve endings. Galton (57) supplies a vivid description of the process:

> It is interesting to ask a person who is ignorant of the real intention, to shut his eyes and to ascertain as well as he can by the sense of touch alone, the material of which any object is made that is afterwards put into his hands. He will be observed to explore it very carefully by rubbing its surface in many directions, and with many degrees of pressure. The ridges engage themselves with the roughness of the surface, and greatly help in calling forth the required sensation, which is that of a thrill; usually faint, but always to be perceived when the sensation is analysed, and which becomes very distinct when the indentations are at equal distances apart, as in a file or in velvet.

The effectiveness of epidermal ridges in heightening frictional resistance is increased by the arrangements of ridges in patterns. As Whipple (147) emphasizes, the pattern arrangements counteract slipping regardless of the direction of drag because the designs are formed by ridges coursing in different directions. Tactile acuity also is favored by the patterned arrangements of ridges. In experiments on tactile acuity Schlaginhaufen (144) makes use of two-point discrimination, the subjects being tested for ability to recognize the duality of stimulation when the skin is touched at two points simultaneously. A measure of the refinement of this ability is afforded by the distance separating the two points of a compass esthesiometer. The findings indicate that two-point discrimination is more acute when the points of the compass are applied in a line at right angles to the ridges than when they are aligned with the ridges. From this it follows that the patterns multiply the opportunities for contacts most favorable for tactile acuteness.

Ridge breadth, according to Galton (57), does not afford a proportionate index of discriminative ability in different areas of the same hand. Though ridges in the palm are but 18% broader than on fingers (24), the compass points, to be recognized as a double stimulation, must be more than four times farther apart in some regions of the palm than on the fingers.

PRINTS OF DERMATOGLYPHICS

Accustomed as we are to examining contact prints rather than the features themselves, no awkwardness is sensed in the use of "finger print" to signify the actual pattern of the distal phalanx.[1] Other regions may be similarly described in terms of their prints. The indirection in such a phrase as "individual differences of finger prints" somehow has become less unseemly than would be the case if one were to refer, for example, to "individual differences of photographs of fingers."

The impressions left in ordinary contacts with objects are termed *chance prints* or finger-print *traces*. Chance prints may be clearly visible, transferred from smearings of the hand with ink, paint, blood or other substances, or impressed in a plastic mass, such as clay. Chance prints usually are *latent*, invisible or only faintly visible, being formed by a film of natural skin secretions or of colorless foreign matter adhering to the skin. Latent prints may be rendered visible by various methods of development. The impressions which remain after ordinary contacts of the hands are exemplified in figure 21, which illustrates a sheet of bank checks carelessly handled by investigators searching for evidence in a case of forgery.

A unique self-developing variety of latent prints (31) is illustrated in figure 22. These "prints" are formed in growths of bacteria seeded by the touch of a thumb on the surface of a solid culture medium. Though it is quite unlikely that such prints would assume an importance in personal identification, this demonstration is a novel addition to the list of materials composing latent prints, aside from its significance bacteriologically.

---

[1] The word "finger" is commonly used to include the thumb as well as fingers in the strict sense.

Plastic materials of suitable consistency and texture yield impressions which may be either chance prints or purposefully made. Impressions in clay are discussed in Chapter 1 in connection with the history of dermatoglyphics. Only rarely are such prints presented to the identification worker or chosen by the biological investigator as a form of record. In some

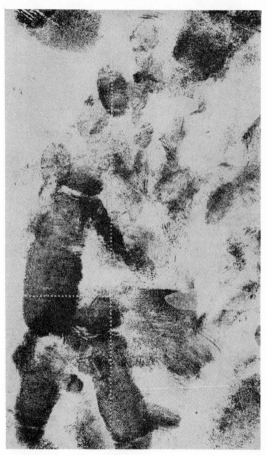

FIG. 21.—Latent prints on paper, developed with silver nitrate. (*Courtesy of M. Edwin O'Neill and the Journal of Criminal Law and Criminology.*)

materials these negative imprints are registered with fine detail, as in the slab of dental impression compound illustrated in figure 23. This print, incidentally, is one of numerous identical finger prints produced in the seances of the medium "Margery," purportedly impressed by the phantom thumb of the medium's deceased brother (50). It will be obvious that a print rendered in the negative, in clay, wax, plaster or any other material allowing for registration of the skin details, would be a suitable mold for a positive cast showing the true reliefs of the dermatoglyphics. Such casts

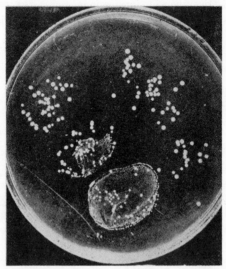

FIG. 22.—Prints formed by growth of bacterial colonies, the organisms having been seeded in the culture medium by contact of a thumb. (*Courtesy of M. Edwin O'Neill and the Journal of Criminal Law and Criminology.*)

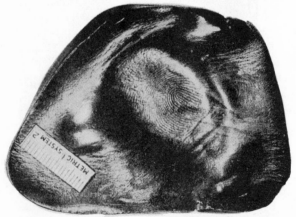

FIG. 23.—A thumb print in dental impression compound.

are sometimes useful. The method does not yield a record which is literally a print, but it is not unfitting to refer to these positive impressions as prints.

The term "print" is applied popularly and in a loose sense to any contact impression of the skin, even if it is a mere blob or smudge (Fig. 24). The prints made by the biological investigator or by the identification worker are clearly decipherable impressions, usually in ink, corresponding in quality to that shown as a companion to the blob in figure 24.

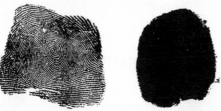

FIG. 24.—A clear finger print contrasted with a featureless blob.

CHARACTERISTICS OF SINGLE RIDGES

Even without magnification the skin ridges (epidermal ridges or rugae) are evident as slightly elevated ribbings of the surface, separated by narrow grooves (sulci). The surface might be compared to the appearance of corduroy, but with the important difference that epidermal ridges do not course uninterruptedly like the ribs of corduroy, nor are they straight except over areas of limited expanse.

The detailed superficial construction of individual ridges may be made out by examining the skin with a magnification of several diameters (Fig. 25). Individual ridges present numerous interruptions, branchings and other irregularities; these details, as they appear in prints, will be considered later. On the ridge summits are the orifices of sweat-gland ducts, each ridge having a single row of these pores, spaced at fairly regular intervals. The ridges frequently show transverse constrictions (Fig. 39) suggesting a segmentation into units, each unit being associated with one sweat pore (21). These individual segments are sometimes completely disjoined, forming "islands." The distances between successive sweat pores on a ridge are usually about equal to the width of the ridge.

Largely through the efforts of Locard, methods have been devised for the study of sweat pores from the standpoint of their variations and usefulness in personal identification. The pores are commonly evident in prints made by other methods, but Locard's process of developing with lead carbonate, or other metallic salts, is specially adapted to demonstrate them. The variations embrace the number of pores in a unit area, their pattern of distribution, the spacing between successive pores, alignment with reference to the axis of the ridge, and conformation of the pore outlines as registered in prints. The characteristics of sweat pores are as individual as the minute details of ridges. The individuality expressed in dermatoglyphics is evidenced on an extensive scale, the pores within any area being many times more numerous than ridge details. Even if a small patch of skin is devoid of other significant ridge characteristics, the pore details are sufficient to establish identification of an individual.

Ridge breadth over the hand as a whole averages 0.48 mm. in young male adults (24). With an average of 0.43 mm. in young adults, women have narrower ridges than men (30). Regional differences in the hand are

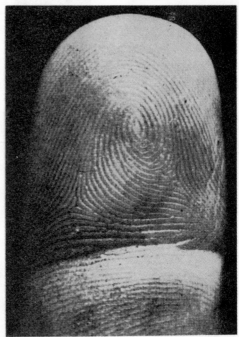

FIG. 25.—Photograph (×3) of the terminal phalanx of a left index finger.

marked (Chap. 11). Inspection indicates that the sole is distinguished by coarser ridges, but quantitative data for the comparison are not available. Ridges are extremely narrow in the infant, and they gradually broaden as the child grows, but there are no changes in their original characteristics of branching, ending and other details. A. F. Hecht supplies the following breadth measurements calculated from counts: in three prematurely born infants, examined at ages of 1½–2½ months, the breadth in each case is 0.15 mm.; in seven term newborns the breadth averages 0.18 mm., the range being 0.10–0.22 mm.; in an unstated number of children at ten years the values are 0.30–0.35 mm.

The details of ridge construction may be best described on the basis of their appearance in prints, since but rarely are they examined directly on the skin. Figure 26 is an ink print of the same digit shown in figure 25. In making this enlarged reproduction the photographic negative was reversed, so that the print might be directly compared with the photograph of the finger itself. Contact prints, it will be obvious, present the features of the skin in a mirrored relationship. In the relation which it

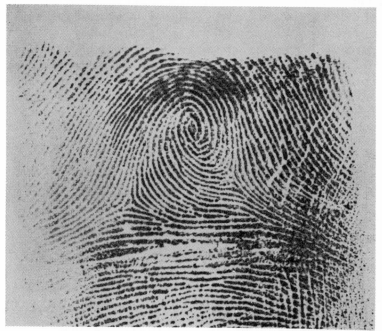

Fig. 26.—Ink print of the finger shown in figure 25, enlarged to the same scale and reversed photographically to facilitate comparison with the actual skin surface.

bears to the actual skin the print of a finger may be likened to a printed page, the mirrored impression of the type faces.

As in printing from type, the printing of a finger (or any dermatoglyphic area) involves the transfer of a film of ink from raised lines and points. In a print made with an optimum amount of ink and proper control of pressure, the sweat pores appear as uninked dots within the inked lines which mark the contacts of ridge summits. Like a rubber stamp, the finger ball and ridges are yielding. The pressures applied in making repeated prints of a finger can never be exactly the same in degree and distribution, hence two prints of the same digit are bound to exhibit differences of technical origin. Variations in pressure, as well as lack of uniformity in inking, may introduce discrepancies in the breadth of a ridge or in the appearance of a ridge detail. A bifurcation, for instance, might be completely registered in one impression, and in another the point of branching might not be recorded. In pronouncing two finger prints identical, the identification expert means that there are no material differences between them, and that they are imprints from the same pattern. He knows that they can not be strictly duplicates, since the mechanics of printing are such that immaterial unlikenesses of two impressions from a finger are inevitable. Such purely technical discrepancies between two prints made from the same finger are readily recognized as such.

Excessive pressure may squeeze ink into the sulci, which then will be printed darker than the ridges. A print of this character is in a sense a negative impression inasmuch as attention is directed to the sulci, here made more conspicuous than the ridges. The sulci obviously present a

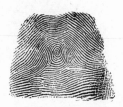
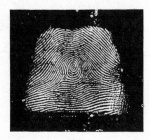

Fig. 27.—Two prints of the same finger, one in the form of an ordinary ink print and the other (with black background) a negative.

negative counterpart of the ridges, though with the usual exclusive emphasis on ridges little thought is given to the configuration of the intervening sulci. The two reproductions of the same finger print shown in figure 27 are made with the purpose of emphasizing the mutual relationship of ridges and sulci. One of these prints is an ordinary contact print. The same print in negative form is shown with a black background, the black lines being sulci and the uninked intervals between them representing the ridges.

Epidermal ridges are compared earlier to the ribs of corduroy, but contrasted in having irregularities of direction, discontinuities and branchings. Such characters are collectively termed *minutiae* or *ridge characteristics*. The occasional *incipient, rudimentary* or *nascent ridges*, though not usually grouped among the minutiae, have a logical place in the consideration of ridge characteristics. Incipient ridges lie in the sulci; they are very narrow and frequently interrupted. Such ridges are illustrated not only in the diagram of minutiae (Fig. 28) but also in the enlarged actual prints (Figs. 26 and 53). They differ from typical epidermal ridges in the characteristic absence of pores as well as in position and morphology. Several standard types of minutiae are illustrated in figure 28. An *island* in strict usage is the ultimate abbreviation of ridge structure, a unit bearing but one sweat pore. Two, three or several such ridge units, consolidated to form a short ridge, were originally also called islands by Galton, though it is preferable to designate them as *short ridges* and to reserve the name island for the ultimate ridge unit. An abrupt stop in the course of a ridge is an *end* or *termination*. Occasionally a ridge may branch, forming a *bifurcation* or *fork;* if the two ridges were considered as coursing from the opposite direction they might be described as fusing, but the common designation is based on the consideration of one ridge branching rather than of two ridges joining. Two such branches, however, may

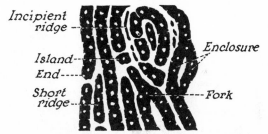

FIG. 28.—Characteristic minutiae of individual ridges.

rejoin after a short course, forming an *enclosure* or *eyelet*. Some special variants of ridges are named in systems of classifying and filing single finger prints.

RIDGE CONFIGURATIONS

The epidermal ridges form definite local designs on the terminal segments of digits and in consistent sites on the palm and sole. The high variability of these configurations makes them useful in personal identification, studies of inheritance, racial variation and other biological aspects of dermatoglyphics.

The distal phalanges of fingers and toes present configurations which according to their general construction are classed (by Galton) as arches, loops and whorls, an example of each being illustrated in figure 29. All configuration types except plain arches appear as designs composed of abruptly curved ridges. For convenience, plain arches are often termed patterns. Actually they do not conform to the definition of a true *pattern*, which, as in a whorl or loop, is composed of sharply recurved ridges. The plain arch, being a succession of ridges coursing across the digit transversely in a gentle curve, is actually patternless and is a special form of *open field*.

Patternless configurations in some regions of the palm and sole may have an arched form, though frequently they lack arciform courses and are termed *open fields*. The middle and proximal segments of digits rarely

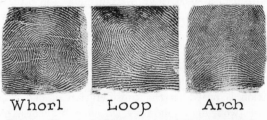

Whorl   Loop   Arch

FIG. 29.—Three typical finger prints: whorl, loop and arch.

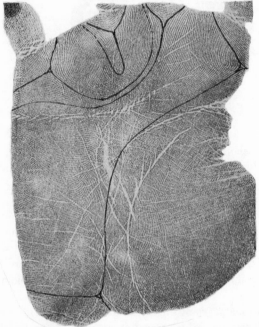

FIG. 30.—Print of a left palm. The traced lines are lines of interpretation. (*From Wilder.*)

show true patterns, their configurations being open fields or erratic local disarrangements of ridge direction, designated as "*vestiges.*"

In the palm there are six configurational zones. In each of these the configuration may appear as a true pattern of one or another type, an open field or a vestige. Figure 30 is a palm print in which only two of these areas are patterned: the fourth interdigital area, lying in proximal relation to the interval between the ring finger and little finger, and the hypothenar area appearing in the lower part of the illustration. Both patterns are constructed as loops. The remaining four zones of the palm are patternless.

The sole has eight regions in which local patterns may occur. The territories of six of these areas are included in the print reproduced in

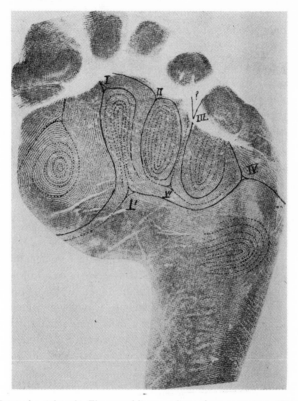

FIG. 31.—Print of a right sole. The traced lines are lines of interpretation. (*From Wilder.*)

figure 31. The configuration in the lower part of the illustration is an open field, while the other five areas have true patterns—whorls and loops.

The configurations of palms and soles, like finger prints, are highly variable among individuals, the variability expressing itself not only in the details of ridges but also in the presence or absence of definite patterns and in the types of patterns which occur.

A consolidation of ridges in triangular formation lies at the conjunction of three ridge systems of opposed courses. Variable in detail of construction, these consolidations may conform to Galton's original conception of *deltas*, but even in the absence of a true delta formation a triradiate structure is apparent, giving the name *triradius* to these features. They have been likened to three-pointed stars, each point being extended as a *radiant*. Whorls on digits are each associated with two triradii, and loops have one (Fig. 29). The palm and sole present triradii (Figs. 30 and 31) which are placed in fairly consistent positions in different individuals. In palm and sole, as well as in patterns of the digits, the radiants are the origins of lines of interpretation which are significant morphologically.

OTHER PATTERNINGS IN NATURE

There are numerous parallelisms in nature of dermatoglyphic configurations and of minutiae of individual ridges. The analysis of what might be termed the geometry of biology is a field in itself.[2]

One of the most striking illustrations of dermatoglyphic parallelism is

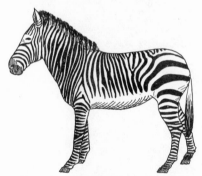

FIG. 32.—Configurations and "minutiae" of stripes in a zebra. (*Traced from a photograph.*)

the form and arrangement of stripes in some animals, the zebra being a familiar instance (Fig. 32). The bands of pigmentation in the zebra, and in a negative fashion the light stripes separating them, show remarkable resemblance to the configurations and minutiae of epidermal ridges. The stripes have ends and forkings which simulate minutiae, and there are triangular consolidations of stripes which resemble triradii. The several areas presenting unlike directions of stripes might be likened to configurational areas in a palm or sole. In some zebras there are regional organizations of stripes that may be likened to dermatoglyphic patterns and vestiges.

Hair arrangement also is suggestively similar to dermatoglyphic configurations. Hairs are projected at a slant from the skin. In a restricted region of the body the hairs slant in a common direction (Fig. 33), but adjoining regions may present quite different slants, as exemplified by the "parting" of the hair of the scalp and the occurrence of one or two whorls on the crown. Other regions of the body likewise present local

---

[2] Cook, Theodore A. *The Curves of Life*. New York, Henry Holt and Co., 1914; Thompson, D. W., *Growth and Form*. Cambridge, University Press, 1917 (2nd ed., 1942).

distinctions of hair arrangement, and though that arrangement accords with a common general topography, there are individual differences. The areas in which the hairs point uniformly in one direction may be compared to open fields of the dermatoglyphics. The crown whorl and similar configurations elsewhere are patterns, and the irregularities localized at the

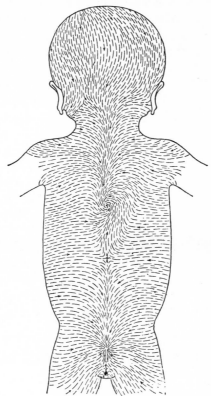

FIG. 33.—Hair streams on the back of a human fetus, the pointing of the hairs being indicated by arrows. (*From Ludwig.*)

points of juncture of three or four areas of different hair slants correspond to triradii.

Like bands of pigmentation in the zebra, the ridged elevations formed on the shell of the argonaut and on the giant cactus of the West present bifurcations and ends resembling the minutiae of epidermal ridges. Inanimate nature is not lacking in similar illustrations. Sand, whipped by wind or waves, may show ridges conforming with surprising exactness to the characteristics of epidermal ridges, with forkings, enclosures and ends (Fig. 34). Similarly, some cloud formations exhibit bands with ends and forkings. Periodic precipitates (Liesegang rings), resulting from diffusion into a gel of a substance reactive with another substance contained in the gel, behave under some conditions like the lines of cellular proliferation

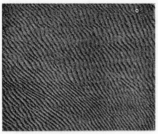

which produce epidermal ridges. If the gel is contained in a capillary tube of uniform bore and no disturbing factors modify the reaction, the passage of the diffusing solution is marked by a succession of regularly spaced discs of precipitate, which on edge view are seen to be perfectly plane. Variations in caliber of the tube or sudden changes in temperature produce warping and other irregularities of these discs[3] which, as shown in figure 35, are in edge view curiously like the irregularities of epidermal ridges.

FIG. 34.—Ridges and "minutiae" in wind-blown sand.

The physical principles responsible for the configuration of wind-swept sand, banded clouds, or of periodic precipitates are probably simpler in their operation than the factors which underlie the production of dermatoglyphic configurations and ridge minutiae. Nevertheless, the forces con-

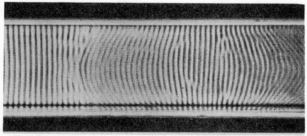

FIG. 35.—Periodic precipitates in a capillary tube containing 0.5% sodium iodide in 5% gelatin, the reaction being produced by diffusion of 10% silver nitrate through the gel. The irregularities of the precipitation discs in the right-hand section of the tube are the result of a sudden elevation of temperature, from 20° C. to 40° C. (*Courtesy of Dr. Eben J. Carey.*)

cerned may prove to have more in common than mere outward resemblance of their effects.

SKIN CREASES

Flexion creases are not components of dermatoglyphics, but they are significant because of peculiarities of epidermal ridges coursing in them. The flexion creases of the palm are the "lines" of the palmist. Several

---

[3] Carey, E. J. Comparative morphology of muscle striations and of periodic precipitates in capillary tubes. Biodynamica, vol. 3, pp. 251–321, 1941.

major creases cross the palm. Other creases occur at the wrist, at the junctions of digits with the palm, and in relation to the joints between the phalanges of digits. Flexion creases are present also on the sole, though with the exception of those associated with the toes they are not conspicuous after early childhood. Flexion creases represent the location of firmer attachment of the skin to underlying structures, and they are regions which remain relatively fixed during move-

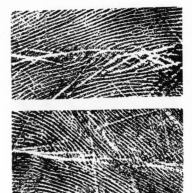

FIG. 37.—Parts of two palm prints, enlarged, showing ridge irregularities in flexion creases.

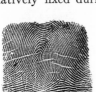

FIG. 36.—A finger print showing "white lines."

ment of the parts. There occur also, and more frequently in later life, certain groovings produced by buckling of the skin rather than by motion in flexion. From their appearance in prints, such furrows are known as *white lines* (Fig. 36).

Flexion creases are associated with localized deficiencies of ridge formation (Figs. 26 and 37). A series of ridges transected by a very narrow crease may appear sharply incised. Within the wider flexion creases ridges may be abruptly turned in their courses, and typically they are broad, low and frequently interrupted. Their suppression is sometimes so extreme that ridge structures are not apparent, either in direct examination of the skin or in prints. The deficient ridge formation noted in a flexion crease evidently is developmentally dependent upon factors associated with the crease. A case suggesting this dependence is illustrated in figure 38. The proximal interphalangeal flexion creases of this finger are normally present, but in the area where the distal creases would be expected the print shows no sign of them. The ridges in this region are typical in structure and course. The distal interphalangeal joint is congenitally not movable, though the X-ray shows the joint to be present.

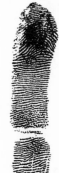

FIG. 38.— Print of the left ring finger of a negro boy, showing absence of the distal interphalangeal flexion creases. Note the lack of ridge disturbances in their expected position.

HISTOLOGY

The skin of the volar regions, like skin everywhere, is composed of two main layers, *epidermis* and *dermis*, or *corium* (Fig. 39). The epidermis, the superficial layer, is subdivided into several strata having different structural characteristics. Its outermost layer is the *stratum corneum*, composed of an accumulation of dead, cornified cells that constantly

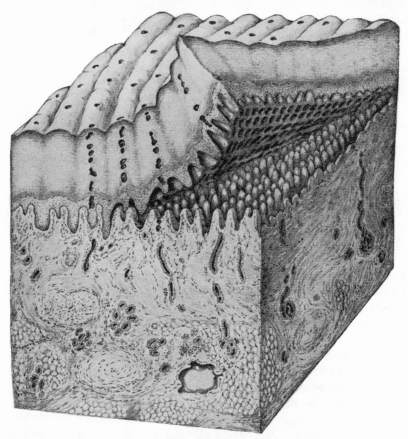

FIG. 39.—A three-dimensional representation of the structure of ridged skin. The epidermis is partly lifted from the dermis, to expose the dermal papillae.

slough as scales from the exposed surface. In the volar skin this layer is thick and is molded on the surface as ridges and sulci. The deepest layers of the epidermis consist of living cells, cells which are constantly multiplying to replace the dead scales lost from the surface of the stratum corneum.

In the intermediate strata the cells undergo progressive cornification as they approach the stratum corneum. Every epidermal cell begins its life history in the deepest part of the epidermis and is gradually shifted to the surface, the cornification occurring in the course of its migration.

The plane of junction of epidermis and dermis is not smooth. It presents closely dovetailed irregularities of the two layers. The irregularities of the dermis are blunt pegs, *dermal papillae*, composed of more delicate connective tissue than that of the main thickness of the dermis. In addition to its framework of connective tissue, a papilla enlodges tufts of capillaries which are brought into close functional relation with the epidermis. It is thus that the epidermal cells receive their oxygen and food supply and deliver their wastes to the blood and lymph. Other dermal papillae possess nerve endings which serve the sense of touch, such endings being more numerous in the volar skin than in other regions.

The dermal papillae are arranged in double rows. Each double row lies deep to a ridge of the surface, and presents the same variations of direction and minutiae. The presence and characteristics of epidermal ridges are determined, from their first formation in the fetus, by proliferations of cells in the zone of epidermis which is invaded and molded by the dermal papillae. If a wound or disease process destroys the skin within the level of this zone the original ridge characteristics can not be restored. When the damage is more shallow the effacement of ridges in the involved area is only temporary.

The thicker portion of the dermis beneath the level of papillae is composed chiefly of a densely woven feltwork of connective-tissue fibers. Its composition and density may be best appreciated by recalling that dermis is the source of leather. Vessels and nerves penetrate this layer of the dermis, and the secreting parts of sweat glands, which mainly lie in the still deeper subcutaneous layer, have their ducts extended through it to enter the epidermis.

The thickness of the skin and of its component layers varies in different regions of the volar surfaces, and different individuals present variations of thickness in corresponding areas. An idea of the dimensions involved may be gained from the following measurements, made in a thin section prepared for microscopical study. This section, selected at random, is from the ball of a finger of an adult male. The skin is 1.8 mm. thick, measured from the summits of the epidermal ridges to the plane of junction of dermis and subcutaneous tissue. The epidermis and dermis are of approximately equal thickness, if the measurement is made from the ridge summits to the limit of the deepest extensions between dermal papillae; the heights of the dermal papillae measure about 0.2 mm. The superficial layers of córnified cells in the epidermis are 0.6 mm. in thickness, accounting for about two thirds of the depth of the epidermis as a whole.

Beneath the skin there is a layer of loose connective tissue and fat. The looseness of this subcutaneous layer admits mobility of the skin, though mobility is restricted in the palmar and plantar areas as compared with most regions. The layer serves as a padding, and it contains the secreting parts of sweat glands, sensory nerve endings of a special type, and vessels and nerves which are on their way to the skin.

The secretion produced by sweat glands is mainly water. It carries in solution sodium chloride, varying in concentration from 0.2% to 0.5%, with traces of urea and other salts. Some methods of developing latent prints depend upon the presence of chloride, which is concentrated on the skin by evaporation; in the silver nitrate method the reaction is the formation of visible silver chloride.

CONSTANCY OF RIDGES AND THEIR CONFIGURATIONS

Epidermal ridges are developed in the fetus in what may be accepted as their fixed and permanent character (Chap. 10). This differentiation takes place in the third and fourth months of the fetal period, hence it is impossible actually to observe the earliest continuity of the configurational features. However, the processes of ridge development are such that any change subsequent to differentiation is highly improbable. Observation of ridges in the same individual over long periods of time make it certain that in postnatal life there is no significant alteration in the details of ridges or in their configurational arrangements. During the period of growth of the body the ridges enlarge, keeping pace with the growth of the hand and foot. Wentworth and Wilder (79) illustrate a series of six prints of the right thumb of a child, taken at intervals beginning at an age of nearly five years, the last print being made at 14½ years. During this period of rapid bodily growth the ridges grew, as did the pattern as a whole, but without changing morphologically. With the widespread use of sole prints and palm prints in registration of the newborn, observations more extended in time ultimately may be available. Abundant illustrations of the permanency of dermatoglyphic features through later life are on record, and the experience of finger-print identification workers would add many more cases now unrecorded in the literature. Galton (57) made repeated printings of several individuals after the passing of years, but none of his time intervals approaches those to be mentioned. Herschel first made his own finger prints in 1859, at the age of 26. He made them again at the age of 44 years, and for the last time at 83. The successive prints show no alterations of ridges and patterns. A similar demonstration was presented by Welcker in prints of his own fingers and palms, first made in 1856 at the age of 34, and repeated in 1897. Another case is that of Jennings (19), who made prints of his palm in 1887, when he was 27 years old; prints repeated 50 years later display no alterations.

These and other like records give sufficient proof of the unchangeability of dermatoglyphic characteristics. This permanency is one of the basic premises in the use of prints for identification. Permanency furthermore is a keystone in various biological investigations of dermatoglyphics, including studies of inheritance, constitution and race. The investigator may be confident that he is dealing with morphological characteristics which appear in the individuals always exactly as they had been from the first.

The permanency ascribed to dermatoglyphics terminates, under usual circumstances, only with complete post-mortem decomposition of the skin. There are, however, some conditions in which the dermatoglyphics of a living individual may suffer temporary or permanent disorganization.

The prints of dish-washers, scrub-women and workers in lime, plaster and similar substances usually show effects of prolonged exposure of the hands to alkali and water. The ridges appear only faintly and are discontinuously printed, yet the pattern type may be recognized by direct inspection of a finger, and clearly defined impressions may be made after these occupations are abandoned. Comparison with earlier prints shows that no alteration of the pattern or of ridge details has resulted.

Leprosy may produce cutaneous disintegration of greater or lesser degree (36). When the damage is slight and superficial the original characteristics of the skin may be restored. Deeper invasion of the disease process permanently effaces dermatoglyphics in the region involved. Excessive exposure of the hand to the action of X-rays may lead to similar damage of the skin.

Burns, caustic agents and wounds produce no permanent effect if the injury is not deep enough to destroy the papillae. Cuts and abrasions lead to varying degrees of damage to the ridges. An extremely shallow linear cut may leave no perceptible permanent defect. Should a wound be deep and extensive, or should active infection occur, the ridges exhibit permanent interruptions and distortions associated with scarring (Fig. 40). As a rule even slight injuries may be readily distinguished from the skin creases which in prints appear as "white lines."

Total destruction of finger prints obviously would result in loss of their identifying characteristics. The loss may not be total even when an individual tries to destroy these evidences of identity. Several notorious gangsters have made such attempts by searing the fingers with acid or by cutting them (23). In these instances only small areas of the patterns are involved, and each digit retains sufficient ridged skin to provide for its positive identification. From the description of the thicknesses of the skin layers it will be clear that if ridges are to be permanently destroyed the skin must be damaged to a depth of about one millimeter. More superficial injury leaves unimpaired the regenerative deep portion of the epidermis and associated dermal papillae.

A patch of ridged skin may be removed and successfully grafted in the same individual. In a skin graft of sufficient thickness to include the epidermis and at least the more superficial portion of the dermis the ridges retain all their original qualities. The first recorded case (25) is that of a man who inadvertently sliced off a patch of skin from the thenar eminence. Immediately he restored this piece to the raw surface and applied a bandage. The slip of skin engrafted itself and the ridges were preserved. A more remarkable case (37) is that of a patient in whom

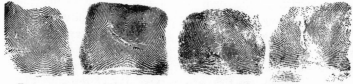

FIG. 40.—A series of finger prints showing characteristic effects of scarring.

grafts were made to correct distortions and contraction of a hand, following severe burns. The surgeon interchanged patches of skin of a finger tip and an area on the palm. Both grafts "took," and in consequence the distal phalanx of the finger now bears a pattern which originally had been on the palm, and the palm carries the finger pattern, both unchanged except in the marginal zones of scar.

Another instance, made public through Ripley's press feature, *Believe It or Not*, was thus described: "Has 10 finger prints but only 9 fingers—He lost his thumb in an accident and the thumb print was grafted back on the palm of his hand." Investigation of this case proved its authenticity.[4]

Perhaps the most spectacular case (20) of finger-print grafting is one in which the skin of all ten fingers was replaced by skin from the sides of the chest. The operation, designed for removal of the finger prints, was successful insofar as concerned the grafting of ridgeless skin in their place—but its object was frustrated, since the man was identified by means of ridge characteristics in portions of the middle segments of the fingers.

---

[4] The Ripley feature appeared on May 27, 1941. The surgeon who performed the operation states, in response to a query from the authors, that the case was an emergency, and that his only object was to preserve the usefulness of the hand. The skin of the thumb was used in this repair because of its availability rather than with any aim to test the preservation of the thumb print.

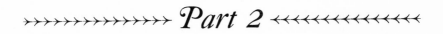

Part 2

METHODOLOGY AND DESCRIPTION

METHODS OF PRINTING

THIS chapter provides an introduction to methods, but only routine procedures of making prints for identification and for biological studies are to be described. Every worker finds that experience suggests details of procedure which serve to advantage.

EQUIPMENT AND SUPPLIES

The materials necessary for making ink prints are few and simple. Several dealers handle equipment and supplies specially made for finger-print workers. Though equipment may be purchased at little expense, satisfactory results may be obtained with largely improvised facilities. The essentials are: ink, cards or paper, roller, inking slab and a pressure pad for palm and sole prints. Other equipment, suggested later, may be added for the convenience of the operator.

Before and after printing, the skin may be washed with soap and water, or the necessary cleaning may be done by wiping with a cloth moistened in gasoline, kerosene, benzine or alcohol. The same fluids may be used to remove ink from the equipment, but in cleaning the roller their prolonged action should be avoided.

The *ink* best suited is printer's ink, the "job black" of the trade. It yields a dead-black print, and the mixing oils ensure almost instantaneous drying. Mimeograph ink may be used instead, but it is hardly as satisfactory. Neither writing ink nor stamp-pad ink is suitable for the purpose.

For finger-print identification files, standard *cards* (Fig. 41) measuring 8 × 8 inches have been generally adopted. The cards are printed with spaces for registration of the prints in a fixed order and for written entries, uniformity being an obvious requisite in identification files. Fingers, as well as palms and soles, may be printed on *paper* of the size most convenient to the individual worker. In selecting paper both durability and quality of surface are to be considered. The paper should have enough body to be durable, and at least one surface should be slightly glazed.

It should not be too stiff to conform to the irregular contours of the palm and sole in printing. In the authors' collection, assembled for biological studies, the sheets measure 8½ × 11 inches. The entire hand is printed on a sheet, which carries also along the lower margin rolled prints of the fingers, arranged in the natural order. The digital sequence is verifiable by the plain prints registered in the impressions of the whole hand. The sole prints in this collection are not similarly accompanied by toe prints,

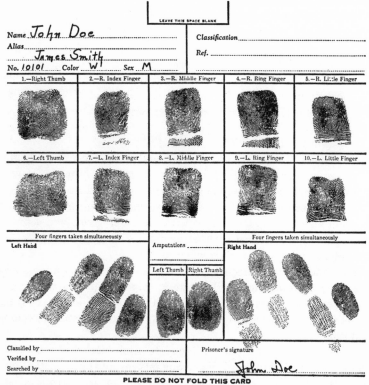

FIG. 41.—A finger-print card of the type used by the Federal Bureau of Investigation. (*Courtesy of J. Edgar Hoover.*)

for reasons to be explained. Schlaginhaufen uses printed sheets measuring 24 × 24 inches, ruled into sections for registration of all areas of each subject. In addition to spaces for whole prints of both hands and both feet, he provides for separate impressions of several of the more critical regions of the palm and sole. Spaces are ruled on the form for the complete series of fingers and toes, but the toe patterns are sketched rather than printed. Elimination of the multiple sheets which are otherwise required seems too small an advantage to compensate for the awkwardness of so large a form.

A *roller* is necessary for spreading ink. Rollers specially designed for finger-printing are obtainable, but the soft rollers used by printers and engravers also have the desired qualities. The firm rubber rollers used in photographic work will serve, though they are not as satisfactory.

An *inking slab* is a plane surface on which ink is rolled into a thin film. The slab may be of glass, preferably plate glass, or a sheet of polished metal (e.g., copper or brass) solidly backed with wood. The size of the slab will vary according to individual needs and preferences. Those in most common use are from 4 to 6 inches in width and from 10 to 14 inches in length.

A *rigid plane surface* upon which the card or paper is laid during the process of printing is indispensable. A smooth table top or sheet of glass meets most requirements. In finger-print offices a part of the equipment is a special card holder, which provides a rigid surface and exposes only that portion of the card in immediate use.

A *pressure pad* instead of a rigid surface is recommended for printing palms and soles. The pad may be cut from a chair-cushion or "kneeling pad" made of sponge rubber. Because the pad is yielding it secures full contact of the hollow of the palm in printing. Some other devices advocated for the same purpose make use of a rigid surface, a cylinder or a convex platform.

For printing fingers and palms, a *table* of a height best suited to the standing of both subject and operator should be provided. Such a table might be either an independent piece of furniture, 42 to 45 inches in height, or a small platform giving this elevation when set on an ordinary table. If much printing of toes and soles is to be done, the operator may place a chair for the subject on a platform raised to a height affording convenience in printing.

Procedures in Making Ink Prints

General Directions. The use in identification offices of a standard finger-print card, with spaces for entries of name and other information, makes almost automatic the routine of recording data for each subject. For biological studies, where procedures are not thus standardized, the worker plans his own system of recording. Whatever the details of such a plan may be, it is imperative that every sheet for one subject be properly identified with that subject, perhaps with an accession number referring to a catalog of the collection. When separate slips of paper are used for printing areas singly (e.g., toes) each slip must be marked also with an identification of the digit or region.

Many biological studies are immediately concerned with some limited region of the dermatoglyphics, frequently finger prints alone. However, the worker might profitably record the prints of all areas. There are many biological problems which remain to be studied, and, since all ultimate needs of records are not foreseen, future disappointments may be obviated by completely printing the subjects while they are available.

The skin of the parts to be recorded should be cleansed and dried before printing. The intervals of cleaning the roller and inking slab will depend upon whether the equipment is in use continuously or only occasionally. In any case, their cleaning must be timed so that the ink will neither thicken on the equipment nor accumulate dust and lint. Such deposits interfere with the making of good prints.

A small daub of ink is placed on the inking slab and spread with the roller into a thin, even film. The requisite amount of ink can be determined only by practice. After a few trials the operator will have learned to use the optimum quantity, and will be able to gauge the amount needed for preparation of the slab and for replenishment during continued printing.

In printing some regions, especially the fingers, the part is applied to the ink film directly. Ink clings to the ridge summits, the corresponding lines of depleted ink being apparent on the slab. Unless unmarked film surface is available for successive impressions the slab must be rolled again, for if two impressions are taken from the same area the second print will be discontinuously inked.

The subject should remain relaxed and passive, giving the operator complete freedom in the manipulations.

The prime objective is complete and clearly decipherable prints. Improper inking, poorly controlled pressures, and dragging across the paper are the common sources of imperfection. The prints should be inspected as they are made, to check for possible technical defects. While the subject is accessible an imperfect record may be replaced, and steps may be taken to correct faults of technique.

FINGERS. A *plain*, or *dab*, print is made by contact of the ball of the finger without rotation of the digit. A *rolled* print involves rotation of the finger both in inking and in printing, to obtain a complete impression of the ball of the finger. On a standard finger-print card the rolled prints are recorded within labeled squares, one for each of the ten digits (Fig. 41). In other sections of the card the plain prints are added to validate the sequence of the separate rolled prints. The plain prints are useful also as duplicate impressions, sometimes presenting details more clearly and truly than the rolled prints. In plain prints, however, the patterns usually are incompletely registered, and in some pattern types this incompleteness might lead to erroneous classification (Fig. 42).

In making a rolled print the finger is first placed edge down on the ink film and then rolled until the opposite margin is in contact. With this one roll the inking is completed. The inking should extend from near the end of the finger to a level slightly proximal to the flexion creases of the distal interphalangeal joint. The finger is next pressed edge down on the card or paper and rolled to its opposite edge with the same motion as in inking. Certain of these manipulations will be least awkward if the operator takes advantage of the anatomical adaptations to rotation of the hand and arm. Thus a thumb would be placed ulnar edge downward

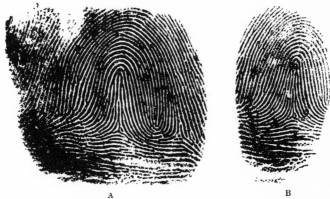

A   B

Fig. 42.—Two prints of the same finger: *A*, rolled; *B*, plain. Note that the plain print, if alone available, might be erroneously classed as a tented arch. (*Courtesy of J. Edgar Hoover.*)

and rolled toward the body, and other digits are placed radial edge downward and rolled away from the body.

The making of plain prints calls for no description, since the illustration of a finger-print card (Fig. 41) is sufficiently explanatory of the imprinting of the four fingers of each hand together in one contact, and of the two thumbs in another.

PALMS. An impression may be made of the palm alone or of the palm and fingers, according to the chosen system of record. Of several suggested methods for inking, the simplest is passing the inked roller repeatedly over the whole area to be printed. The following areas require special attention: the zone of flexion creases at the wrist, the ulnar margin, the flexion creases where the fingers join the palm, the central "hollow" of the palm. Unless these areas are inked and printed the palmar impression will lack critical features.

After the inking is completed a sheet of paper is laid on the pressure pad, and the operator brings the ulnar margin of the subject's hand against it. The hand is then rolled palm downward, and pressed firmly against the pressure pad. Pressure is exerted particularly over the central region of the hand and over the knuckles, to ensure printing of the hollow of the palm and the distal border. Should the central region escape printing, the blank area in the print will obstruct the tracing of lines of interpretation through this region. If the distal palmar zone is incompletely printed the tracing of these lines is impossible, since their starting points are the triradii lying near the distal margin. Imprinting the ulnar border of the hand is important, because of an occasional relation of hypothenar patterns on this border. A frequent pattern of the hypothenar region is a loop with its head, or enclosed extremity, directed toward the ulnar margin (Fig. 63). The head of such a pattern may lie on the ulnar border instead of on the flat of the palm, and a print of the flat of the palm alone would display no evidence of the existence of this pattern. A complete palm print is comparable to a rolled print of a finger.

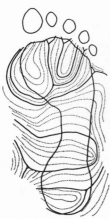

Fig. 43.—Tracing from a sole print, with tread area outlined to emphasize the extent beyond it of important elements of the configurations.

SOLES. The plain print formed by the foot in the ordinary weight-bearing contact is a print of the tread area. There are individual variations in the extent of the tread area, associated with differences of the plantar arch and general conformation of the foot, but almost never is a tread-area print a complete dermatoglyphic record. Figure 43 is a tracing of a sole print, with the tread area outlined to demonstrate the extent beyond it of the area of ridged skin and the occurrence, in this instance, of significant configurations along the tibial and fibular borders. An ideal print of the sole, in which the ridged skin is completely recorded, corresponds to a rolled print of a finger.

The sole is inked by passing the roller over it as described in palm-printing. Care must be taken to secure complete inking of the digito-plantar zone (where there are digital triradii as in the palm) and of the tibial and fibular borders. The pressure pad is used to advantage in printing, though other devices may give equally good results. With the paper lying on the pad, the fibular border of the foot is brought into contact, and then the sole is rolled downward on the paper; to complete the impression of the tibial border, it may be necessary to manipulate the pad and paper against it. Even with these precautions the sole print may be incomplete. The worker must then employ some expedient to secure impressions of the inadequately printed regions. It is possible, for example, to reconstruct a total print from several regional prints of successive transverse zones, the individual zones being printed independently on strips which are pressed around the inked foot.

TOES. Toes are more difficult to print than fingers, palms or soles. Even when the toes are not compressed and distorted, as they usually are, their shortness and limited mobility are a decided handicap in printing. Consequently, toe prints are lacking in most collections of dermatoglyphics. A set of toe prints is not likely to be technically perfect, but impressions adequate for study may be secured.

The toes are inked and printed one by one on small slips of paper. A separate slip for each print is most convenient, but care must be taken to mark it for identification of the digit. Ink may be applied with a small roller or by swabbing with an inked rubber paddle. The slip of paper is first loosely wrapped around the ball of the toe and then pressed against it, thus obtaining an impression equivalent to a rolled print. Some of the devices used for making finger prints of the dead might be applicable in toe-printing. These devices are "spoons," shaped to receive the finger and to hold the paper strip for printing. The plain toe prints which are registered in the impression of the sole, except for the big toe, are usually too incomplete to be of any use. Often the pattern area makes no contact in printing, and sometimes no part of the toe is printed, owing to displacements associated with compression in shoes.

SPECIAL CASES. In many hospitals the soles or palms of newborn *infants* are printed as a supplement to other more immediately serviceable identifying devices such as labels or necklaces of lettered beads. The need to print infants arises occasionally also in biological investigations and in cases of questioned paternity. Successful finger-printing before the fifth or sixth month is practically impossible, and difficult from that time to the close of the first year (204). Palms and soles are managed with less difficulty.

According to Pond (91), wiping with dry gauze is usually sufficient to prepare the palms of newborn infants for printing. He advises that when a persistent greasy paste remains it may be removed by a swab moistened with hydrogen peroxide. The ink film must be spread thin since the ridges in infants are delicate. With the infant placed on a table, the operator straightens its fingers and then applies the inking slab against the extended palm. The card or paper, backed by a supporting board, is then pressed against the inked palm. Printing of soles is simpler, since they are accessible without manipulation of digits.

Identification workers are familiar with various *kits* designed to hold equipment for printing, several types being supplied by dealers. The biological investigator also may have need of a portable outfit for work in homes, institutions or elsewhere away from the conveniences of his laboratory. It is unnecessary to detail the design and content of such a kit, since the requirements for printing are the same as those outlined above and the only further need is convenient portability. The operator will most likely wish to transport no more than the bare essentials for printing.

The occasion may arise for securing prints of a subject who is not accessible to the investigator. If some person, perhaps the subject himself, is willing to make the prints the necessary materials may be easily supplied. Ink may be rolled on waxed paper, two such sheets being placed with their inked surfaces together. An adequate number of these inked sheets, paper, brief directions and sample prints for guidance are all that the amateur collaborator will need.

INKLESS METHODS OF PRINTING

Inkless printing may be carried out either with commercially available equipment (e.g., the Faurot or the Kuhne outfit) or with materials assembled by the operator himself. The advantages of the inkless methods are their tidiness and avoidance of offending the sensibilities of subjects who object to being smeared with ink. The outstanding disadvantage of these methods is lessened control of the operations in printing.

In the photo-paper method (85) a stock solution is prepared: sodium sulphide, 25 grams; sodium hydroxide (sticks), 5 grams; soluble starch, 2 grams; distilled water, 100 cc. The sodium sulphide and sodium hydroxide are dissolved in part of the water; the remainder of the water is boiled and the starch dissolved in it. The starch solution is then added slowly to the first mixture, and the material is stirred vigorously and allowed to cool. The working solution is made by adding one part of the stock solution to four or five parts of distilled water. A blotter moistened with this mixture serves as the "inking slab." The part to be printed is first pressed against the moist blotter for a few seconds, and is then applied against a sheet of photographic paper. For permanence the prints must be fixed in hypo, washed and dried as in the usual photographic process. The fixing may be done immediately or delayed for several days if the paper is protected from light. One user of the method has reported it to be superior to the ink method, especially in dealing with infants.

Some investigators make prints in latent form. In Bauder's procedure, blotting paper soaked with a light machine oil serves as the "inking slab," and the finger or other part is applied to it in the manner of the ink method. The paper on which the impression is made is dusted with the black powder commonly used in treating latent prints, and then sprayed with a fixing solution (alcohol, 20 parts; white shellac, 2 parts; sandarac gum, 1 part). A similar method is employed by MacArthur and Ford (216), who describe it as follows:

> The first step consists of rubbing a hand lotion into the skin surface; a face cream is preferable if the skin is particularly dry. The moist hand is then pressed lightly upon kimeograph paper [kymograph paper, which has a glazed surface] laid on a rubber pad; two or three impressions may be made after a single moistening. A generous amount of very finely powdered and sifted lampblack rolled back and forth repeatedly over the face of the paper with a rocking motion develops very clearly the invisible ridge and sweat pore impressions. The bulk of the excess powder is poured off and the remainder removed by a vigorous shaking, after which the print is fixed from the back in a shallow tray containing a small amount of a solution of 30 gms. of resin to one liter of 95% alcohol. The chief merits of this method are that it affords no inconvenience to the subject, since it avoids completely any staining or even a temporary discoloration of the hands, and it brings out details possibly better than does ink with young children whose fine ridges flatten with the least pressure.

A method involving use of photographic film is reported by Schött, whose experience with Lapplanders convinced him of the need of an inkless method when dealing with peoples who shy from being smeared with ink. Lanolin is rolled on a glass plate, as ink is rolled in the ordinary method, and the impression from it is applied to photographic film. The film is then processed and prints made therefrom as in ordinary photography. The lanolin is removed from the film by wiping during fixing. Both the original impression and the processing may be done in daylight, though Schött recommends storing the film in a light-proof container until processing.

The X-ray is of occasional value in finger-print identification. It is useful when other possibilities of finger-printing fail, as when prints are to be made from a body in an advanced state of decomposition. The method has possibilities of application in biological studies. Several workers supply accounts of methods, which are reviewed by Castellanos (122). Briefly, Beclere's procedure in dealing with a living subject is to smear the skin with lanolin; the X-ray opaque medium, bismuth carbonate, is then applied and distributed by gentle massage. The excess is wiped off and the shadowgraph taken by the usual X-ray procedure. Other substances opaque to the X-ray, such as white lead, may be employed. The X-ray shadowgraph (Fig. 44) shows, in addition to bones and soft parts, the finer details of the skin surface, the opaque medium having been retained in the sulci and sweat pores.

Valsik (99) utilizes an indirect form of X-ray record in correlating the positions of triradii with the hand skeleton. He affixes a small lead pellet

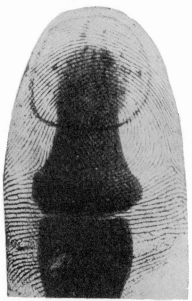

FIG. 44.—An X-ray "finger print." (*Courtesy of Dr. Israel Castellanos.*)

with adhesive at the point of a triradius, and the X-ray shadow of the pellet marks the location of the triradius for reference to bony landmarks

Equipment for the Examination of Prints

For examinations requiring a large working field, as in studies of palms and soles, a reading glass or a loupe which is worn as spectacles will be useful, though the low magnifying power of such lenses limits their effectiveness. A lens magnifying from four to five diameters is necessary for the inspection of print details. The selection of a particular form of lens mounting may be guided by the character of the work to be done. For examination of finger prints there are several commonly used forms of mountings. An excellent style (Fig. 45), designed especially for finger-print work, is in a threaded mount for focusing. It has a horse-shoe base, slotted to receive the ruled glass discs which serve special purposes in some finger-print methods. Rulings are available for coding pattern details as prescribed in certain single-finger-print systems. Another ruling, a straight line crossing the entire disc through its middle, is designed as an aid in counting ridges. (Special rulings fitted for particular purposes might be supplied by the manufacturers. One of the American manufacturers of

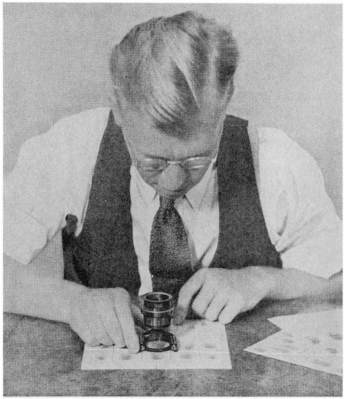

FIG. 45.—A recommended style of finger-print magnifier, shown in use with a disc in place. (*Courtesy of Bausch and Lomb Optical Company.*)

optical instruments has supplied on special order a ruling for a study of breadth of epidermal ridges, the ruling in this instance being a one-centi-meter line engraved in the center of the disc.)

In counting ridges, whether with or without a ruled disc, an indispensable accessory is a needle with its head inserted in a convenient holder. This is used as a pointer in following from one ridge to another. The tip of the needle must be sharp, since this pointer as well as the print is magnified.

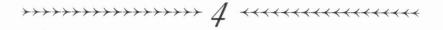

FINGERS

ARRANGED according to the amount of available information concerning them, the dermatoglyphic areas rank in this descending order: fingers, palms, soles, toes. It is not surprising that finger prints, in view of their wide application in personal identification, stand first in the list. The fingers, moreover, are printed easily, and even investigators whose interests are not confined to identification have tended to neglect regions more difficult to record.

FUNDAMENTALS OF FINGER-PRINT CONSTRUCTION

FINGER-PRINT TOPOGRAPHY. The finger print of conventional description is a print of the configuration of the ball of the finger. The configura-

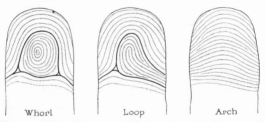

| Whorl | Loop | Arch |

FIG. 46.—Three basic types of finger prints: whorl, loop, arch.

tion is incompletely registered since the rolling process is not designed to secure the imprint of the extreme tip of the finger. To introduce the principles of finger-print construction, attention may be devoted first to the three basic pattern types distinguished by Galton—the whorl, loop and arch (Fig. 46), choosing an example of each which represents the type in ideally simple form.

The typical *whorl* is a generalized pattern which may be used to advantage as a standard of reference. It is distinguished by concentric design. The majority of the ridges make circuits around the *core*, a pivotal feature in the interior of the pattern. The whorl in figure 46 is completely and continuously circumscribed by the *type lines*, here drawn as solid lines for emphasis.[1] These type lines, traced on the print according to conventions which are to be defined, are the radiants extended from the two triradii. The area enclosed by the type lines (but continuously enclosed only in the meet whorl, to be characterized later) is the *pattern area*. The type lines are appropriately termed the *skeleton* of the pattern. The form and design of the pattern are suggested by the skeleton, much as the bony framework of an animal gives a clue to the form of that animal in the flesh. If one were to lift away the type lines and examine them without access to the remainder of the configuration, it would be possible still to recognize the general character of the design. The pattern area represents only a part of the whole finger print. The region distal to the pattern area is the *distal transverse system*, and the territory proximal to the pattern area is the *proximal transverse system*.

The *loop* (Fig. 46) is simpler in construction than the whorl. It possesses only one triradius. Instead of coursing in complete circuits as in the whorl, the ridges curve around only one extremity of the pattern, forming the *head* of the loop. From the opposite extremity of the pattern, ridges flow to the margin of the digit; this extremity of the pattern thus may be described as *open*. If the loop opens to the ulnar margin it is an *ulnar* loop, and if to the radial margin it is a *radial* loop.

The finger print with a loop pattern has the same topographic zones described in connection with the whorl: pattern area, distal and proximal transverse systems. These zones are not delimited on the open side of the loop because there is no triradius with which to establish boundaries.

The *arch* here illustrated (Fig. 46) is a plain arch, the simplest of all finger-print configurations. Though usually loosely referred to as a "pattern," the plain arch is actually patternless. The ridges pass from one margin of the digit to the other with a gentle, distally bowed sweep which gives the name to the pattern type. There is no triradius, and the three topographic zones of other finger-print types are not distinguishable.

TRIRADII. A triradius is located at the meeting point of three opposing ridge systems. In a typical whorl or loop such a meeting occurs at the conjunction of the three topographic zones—the pattern area, the distal transverse system and the proximal transverse system.

---

[1] The style of drawing in figure 46 is that commonly adopted for illustrating configurations under conditions in which ridge details are unimportant. The type lines of finger prints and the corresponding lines of interpretation traced on a palm or sole are reproduced accurately and emphasized in the drawing, while courses of other ridges are filled in only sufficiently to portray the general aspect of the configuration. This method of drawing has the advantage of representing the configuration stripped to its skeletal features.

The term delta is often used as a synonym for triradius, but a distinction may be made between them on the basis of the arrangement of minutiae (71). A delta in the strict sense is a triangular plot, and the triradius is represented by ridges forming its boundary. A triradius, however, may be present when there is no delta in the strict sense, being formed in this instance by three ridges radiating from a common point. In the usage here adopted no discrimination is made between these two main forms of structural organization. Since a triradius is present even when there is no true delta, the term triradius is used throughout this work. This requires substitution of the term *triradial point* (point of triradius) for the more generally familiar *point of delta*, a term which would be inappropriate for triradii not associated with deltas.

The triradius has a double importance in finger-print analysis. First, the ridges extended from it are the three *radiants*, the type lines above described; they aid in interpreting the configuration because they consti-

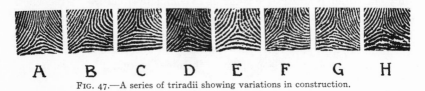

A   B   C   D   E   F   G   H

FIG. 47.—A series of triradii showing variations in construction.

tute the skeletal framework. The other significance of the triradius is that it provides a landmark (triradial point) for ridge counting and tracing.

All triradii are associated with abutment of three ridge systems coursing in different directions. The organization of ridge elements composing triradii is variable. One of the more common types of construction is that shown in figure 47,A–C, where three ridges radiate from a common point, the angles separating them being nearly equal. Other varieties of construction are illustrated in figure 47.

In its service as a landmark for ridge counting, a specific feature of the triradius is singled out as the *triradial point*. This point forms the *outer terminus* of the line along which ridges are counted. In triradii constructed as in figure 47,A–C, the meeting point of the three ridges is the triradial point. If there are two or more bifurcations, the triradial point is located on the one nearest the core. If an island forms a central structure (Fig. 47,E), that island is the triradial point. The corresponding locus in less orderly formations (Fig. 47,G–H) may be ordinarily identified under comparison with the simpler constructions.

A pattern may be so expanded that its margins encroach into the zone of junction of ridged skin and the generalized skin of the dorsum of the finger. In such cases triradii do not occur in the expected relation to patterns, for the reason that their potential sites are devoid of ridges. Though triradii are not actually present, their potential formation is predicated by the character of the pattern, and they may be described as *extralimital,* i.e., beyond the limit of ridged skin. (Common examples are afforded by patterns of the palmar hypothenar area and the hallucal area of the distal sole; less frequently is a pattern on a finger or toe thus characterized.)

RADIANTS. The three *radiants* of a triradius are traced (though not necessarily marked) on the print by following the ridges which issue from the triradius. In some triradii (Fig. 47,A–C), three rays are easily defined as the starting points for tracing. Otherwise, the starting points are the ridges which form the angles of the delta. In following a radiant beyond an interruption of a traced ridge, the tracing is continued on the ridge which is in end-to-end relation, or, if there is no such ridge, the tracing line is transferred to the next ridge on the side *away* from the interior of the pattern area;[2] similarly, in meeting a bifurcation the tracing is followed on the peripheral branch of the fork.

From their typical association with patterns the three radiants (Fig. 46) are named according to their relations with the finger and with the pattern: the *marginal radiant,* passing to the digital border; the *distal pattern radiant,* in marginal and distal relation to the pattern area; the *proximal pattern radiant,* in proximal relation to the pattern area. The two *pattern radiants* may define a complete boundary of the pattern area, as they do in a whorl around which the proximal and distal radiants meet (Fig. 48—patterns 1, 4, 5, 6). The pattern radiants may invade the pattern area (Fig. 48—patterns 7, 8, 13, 14, 15). When invading radiants become involved in the pattern design, the tracing is discontinued with the recognition of this relationship; if carried further, the tracing would only build a more nearly complete skeleton.

CORES. The *core* is an internal feature of a pattern. In a typical whorl the core, or hub of the encircling system, may appear as an island, a short straight ridge, a hook-shaped ridge or staple, or as a circle or ellipse. Some whorls have duplex cores. In a typical loop the core may be a single straight ridge (rod), a series of two to several such parallel rods, or,

---

[2] This direction to "step outward" in the tracing of radiants is in accord with the procedure prescribed by Henry. In presenting a numerical system for indexing finger prints, wherein the courses of radiants assume a special significance, Mairs (69) modifies the prescriptions for tracing. According to his modification, the rule to "step outward" applies only to radiants forming outermost boundaries of patterns, while in tracing radiants which lie within the pattern area there is a "step inward" instead of outward.

among other common arrangements, it may be a ridge formed as a hairpin loop (staple). Characteristics of the core area are of special importance in single-finger-print systems of identification, since classification of the single impressions must be based upon the minutiae which are most likely to be available in chance prints.

The *point of core* is a landmark for ridge counting. It is not the core as a whole, but only a centrally located core element, subject to a fixed, though sometimes arbitrary, definition. In a loop having a single rod core, the distal tip of the rod is the point of core (Fig. 53). If there are two rods, the one farther from the triradius is the point of core; with three or any uneven number of rods, it is the tip of the central one, and if there are four or six rods the central pair is treated as described for a two-rod core. In a staple core the point lies on the limb opposite the delta, at the junction with the distal recurvature of the staple. The cores of other pattern types are analyzed according to the same general principles. Ridge counts, as will be explained, do not include the triradial point and point of core, their service being limited to the orientation of the line of counting.

PATTERN TYPES

In the arch-loop-whorl classification of Galton any pattern having two or more triradii would be assigned to the class of whorls. This broad sense of the term "whorl" is still the standard in those biological problems which can be most satisfactorily analyzed by employing gross classes rather than refinements of classification. For personal identification and for some biological investigations finer groupings are necessary. The two usages of the term "whorl" are distinguished here by qualifying as "true whorls" those patterns of the Henry classification characterized by concentricity. When the term is applied without this qualification it is used in the sense of Galton, to include composites as well as true whorls.

Various workers have proposed schemes of classification of pattern types. The principle of classification is similar to that of all branches of the natural sciences. The main groups are each composed of forms alike in some character or characters, but with differences which allow for subdivision of the group. For the present purpose it suffices to present the essentials of the Henry classification and nomenclature. The Henry system is more widely used than any other, and it is moreover the foundation of the modified systems (47, 60).

In the Henry classification there are four main types of patterns: arches, loops, [true] whorls and composites. The composites, as will be shown, form a heterogeneous assemblage of patterns.

In characterizing pattern types frequent reference will be made to the sketches of 39 patterns assembled in figure 48. References to the figure number will be omitted in this section, the identifying numbers of the patterns being cited alone.

TRUE WHORLS. True whorls typically possess two triradii, and are patterns so constructed that the characteristic ridge courses follow circuits around the core. A frequent configuration is a succession of rings or ellipses (Patterns 1, 5). Another common arrangement is a spiral course (Pattern 2). The continuity and expanse of the spiral in reference to the pattern area are variable, and the direction of spiraling may be either clockwise or counter-clockwise. In some whorls a part of the pattern area may be truly concentric and another part spiral. The *shape* of the pattern area may be either essentially circular or elliptical. The periphery of the whorl determines the general shape of the pattern area. The shape of the central part of the whorl may differ, so that a circular conformation of ridges in the immediate neighborhood of the core may be associated with a generally elliptical periphery, or the reverse.

Cores are of various forms: an island, a short straight ridge, a small circle or ellipse, two interlocked hook-shaped ridges or staples, and other less common forms.

The four pattern *type lines* have variable relations: they all *meet* (Patterns 1, 5, 12) to circumscribe the whorl continuously; the two distal pattern radiants meet but the proximal ones do not (Patterns 11, 13); only the proximal radiants meet (Patterns 7, 8); there is no meeting of radiants.

The word "meet," as just used, applies to a literal joining of the traced type lines. In identification practice under the Henry system three classes of whorls are distinguished according to the relation of the proximal pattern radiants: inside whorl, meet whorl, outside whorl. Arbitrarily, the tracing is from the triradial point on the left side of the print, irrespective of whether the digit is of a right or left hand. The tracing is carried from this "left" triradial point toward the right. The whorl is described as a "meet" whorl if the traced line runs into the proximal pattern radiant on the opposite side (Patterns 1-8), or if the tracing is separated from it by not more than two ridges, either inside or outside the pattern radiant. When the tracing passes external to the opposite triradial point, separated from it by three or more ridges, the pattern is an "outside" whorl (Patterns 13-15). The pattern is an "inside" whorl if the tracing passes toward the interior of the pattern area, with three or more ridges between this line and the right triradial point (Patterns 9, 11). Ridge counts may be made between the traced line and the right triradial point as a means of subclassification.

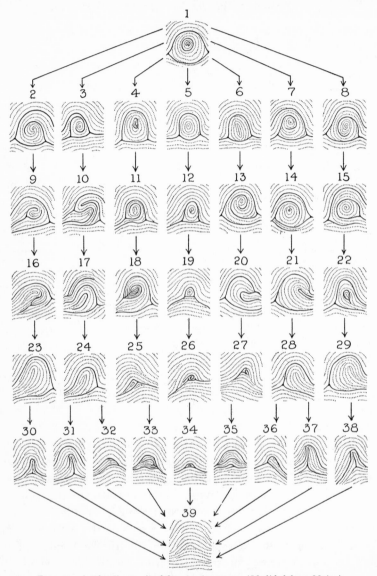

FIG. 48.—A "family tree" of finger-print types. (*Modified from Mairs.*)

For biological analyses some of these procedures, designed for identification routine, call for modification. Practicable though it is in identification to ignore the true position of the "left" triradial point and of a non-meeting with respect to radial or ulnar side, any study involving asymmetries of patterns will of necessity distinguish the radial and ulnar directions. The same principle applies to the descriptive designations of non-meeting distal pattern radiants.

The *size* of a whorl may be described by its ridge count, the method to be detailed later. Inspection alone shows that there are wide differences in the expanse of the pattern area (Patterns 1, 5, 12, 19, 26).

COMPOSITES. Composites are compound patterns in which two or more designs, each conforming to the general aspect of one of the simpler types, are combined in one pattern area. Two or more triradii are present. There are four chief types of composites: central pocket loops, lateral pocket loops, twin loops, accidentals—all, as before noted, being members of Galton's class of whorls.

A *central pocket* in its characteristic form (Pattern 22) is essentially a whorl of reduced size lying in the interior of a pattern area which is constructed mainly as a loop. A central pocket is a pattern intermediate between a whorl and a pure loop (compare patterns 15, 22 and 29). Central pockets are classed as radial or ulnar according to the direction of the open extremity of the loop. They may be subclassified according to type lines, cores and ridge counts.

Lateral pocket loops (Pattern 10) and *twin loops* are closely allied morphologically, either type being composed of two interlocked loops. The distinction between them is of importance in identification, but is ordinarily negligible in biological studies. They differ with respect to the coursing of ridges traced from the cores of the two loops. When lines traced from the two cores emerge on the same digital margin (radial or ulnar) the configuration is a lateral pocket loop, while if the two lines course to opposite margins it is a twin loop.

Accidentals are complex patterns, formed by combination of two or more usually unrelated configuration types—a whorl and a loop, a tented arch and a loop (Fig. 42,A), triple loops and other bizarre configurations not assignable to the standard types.

LOOPS. Loops already have been characterized in the preliminary discussion of Galton's three basic types of patterns, and the distinction between radial and ulnar loops has been made. Attention may be directed now to other criteria of classification applying equally to the radial and ulnar varieties. First to be distinguished are *plain loops*, loops which show no disturbed configurations suggesting affinity with composites. The plain loop (Patterns 23, 29) is composed of a succession of ridges which regularly follow a looped course, while "transitional" loops present abortive expressions of more complex patterns. For instance, pattern 17 is a loop with signs of an accompanying degenerate loop; if this degenerate element were perfected the pattern as a whole would be a composite, a twin loop. Corresponding configurations, but simulating degenerate lateral pocket loops, are shown in patterns 20 and 21. A central pocket (Pattern 15) would be converted to a transitional form of loop in the absence of recurved ridges between the triradius and core (Pattern 22).

Loops also may be classified according to size (as determined by ridge count), core construction and form of the pattern area. Some loops are narrow in relation to their height while others are broad. The placing of the core with reference to the triradius and the type lines is variable, this variation being independent of differences in pattern size. The inclination of the pattern in reference to the digital axis also varies. Loops may be erect, in line with the digital axis, or aligned obliquely or transversely to the digital axis—the range of slant thus being 90°.

ARCHES. The *plain arch* (Pattern 39) is composed of ridges which pass across the finger with a slight bow distally. There is no triradius. The *tented arch* (Patterns 30, 31) has a triradius, located in or near the mid-axis of the digit. The erect distal radiant is associated with abrupt elevation of the transversely coursing ridges, forming the "tent" which gives the name to the pattern. Both proximal radiants pass directly to the digital margins, while the distal radiant usually terminates after a short, straight course, though sometimes it recurves sharply as a staple. There are still other forms of arches presenting triradii, arches which simulate diminutive loops (Patterns 32, 36) or much reduced whorls (Pattern 34). All such arches are distinguished from reduced loops and whorls by the lack of a ridge count.[3]

TRANSITIONS BETWEEN PATTERN TYPES

With infrequent exceptions a finger print is easily assignable to one of the chief types of patterns, and usually to a particular subgroup. Now and then, question may arise as to classification of a pattern—for example, whether it is a central pocket or a loop, or whether it is a loop or an arch. In finger-print identification most decisions on such questions rest on arbitrary definitions which place the pattern in one or the other category. Were it not for agreement on standards, classification files would be chaotic and the statistics of biological investigators could not be

---

[3] Mairs proposes a method of counting ridges in tented arches. The line of count is not equivalent to that applied in other patterns. Finger Print and Ident. Mag., vol. 16, no. 9, 1935.

utilized for comparisons.[4] Rigid definitions are essential to minimize erroneous classifications. In some biological studies. however, modifications of these standards may be desirable. For instance, in a genetic analysis (154) the standard distinction between an arch and a loop which has a count of but one or two ridges may be meaningless, and the worker may accordingly group these reduced loops with true arches. It is assumed that the investigator who does not conform in all respects to the customary criteria will define his altered standards.

From the beginning of serious investigation of finger prints, transitions between types have been recognized, and students of the subject have speculated on their significance. Whipple (147) was among the first to search for the underlying causes of pattern differences and to trace affinities among the types. She ascribes gross differences among patterns to variability in the lowering of the volar pads (Chap. 10). Whipple reproduces a series of nine finger prints illustrating progressive transition from a whorl, in which all pattern radiants meet, to a plain arch. The successive connecting steps are: whorls with disjoined type lines, central pockets, plain loops of progressively decreasing size, tented arches. Such a sequence must be selected from a number of finger prints. One pattern can not be converted into another, the series being composed merely of descriptive transitions among patterns. Falco (51) and Grüneberg (202) also devote attention to the principle of transitions, but the subject has been especially investigated by Mairs (69). His "finger-print family tree," composed of 39 prints, illustrates several lines of descent from the "alpha whorl" to the "omega arch" (Fig. 48), the lines of transition being indicated by arrows. For some of the prints (the middle vertical column), the configuration involves no reference to origin from right or left hands, since all these patterns are symmetrical. Most of the patterns grouped in the other vertical rows are asymmetrical, and for description it will be assumed that all prints are from right hands. With few exceptions the prints were so chosen that the general form of each of the asymmetrical patterns is matched in the opposite section of the figure by its mirror image of radial or ulnar asymmetry.

The more important sequences shown in figure 48 are: (a) The middle vertical column (Patterns 1, 5, 12, 19, 26) is a series of five true whorls of different sizes, each with meeting pattern radiants. The smallest (Pattern 26) is indeed a whorl only by the last allowance of conventional

---

[4] Among the Heinrich Poll Papers there is a record of an agreement between Poll and Bonnevie with regard to their interpretation of pattern types. These two investigators used Windt and Kodicek's *Daktyloscopie* (Vienna, 1904) for reference and agreed on the classification of each of the finger prints illustrated in its numerous plates.

definition, being in its general aspect similar to the next print in the row (Pattern 34), which by definition is an arch. The plain arch (Pattern 39), with no sign of a triradius, concludes the sequence of pattern reduction. (b) The prints grouped to the right side of the middle vertical row show transitions from the whorl to the plain arch along another line, involving successively: whorls with non-meeting type lines, composites, transitional forms of loops, pure loops, arches with triradii. Having assumed that these prints are from right hands, the loops would be ulnar loops and other asymmetrical characteristics would correspond. (c) The prints to the left of the middle vertical row show the same interrelationships as those on the right, and, assuming that the prints are from right hands, the loops are radials.

From the descriptive standpoint alone the sequence just traced could be read also in the opposite direction, from the arch to the whorl. Comparative dermatoglyphics (Chap. 9) gives evidence that the sequence from whorl to arch corresponds to an actual evolutionary order from the primitive to specialized conditions (though it must be conceded that the deduction is based primarily upon palmar and plantar patterns, rather than those of the digits).

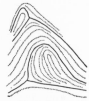

FIG. 49.—A supernumerary loop lying outside the pattern area of a thumb. (*Courtesy of Heinrich Poll.*)

Accidentals are omitted in the family tree (Fig. 48) because collection in numbers sufficient to establish connected series is hampered by their infrequency and diversity. Among the 50,000 finger prints compiled in table 1, accidentals occur only 64 times, a frequency of 0.13% of all patterns. Mairs (71), working with a collection of 411 accidental patterns, shows that they follow natural sequences which are no less orderly than those here illustrated for common pattern types.

It appears that patterns are interrelated descriptively because their formation depends upon an orderly system of developmental circumstances. An occasional pattern may be irreconcilable with this system. The thumb print reproduced in figure 49 is an example of such an aberrant configuration.[5] The pattern area presents an ulnar loop having a count of 19 ridges. There is nothing unusual in the configuration or position of this element of the print. The peculiar feature is the radial loop, with a count of four ridges, lying outside the normal pattern area. Because of the situation of this smaller loop, question might be raised as to the proper classification of this print.

---

[5] Both thumbs of this individual present the same type of configuration. The drawing was traced directly from a photographic enlargement of the print, loaned by Poll.

FREQUENCIES OF PATTERN TYPES AND DIGITAL DISTRIBUTIONS

The several pattern types display unlike total representations, unlike frequencies on different digits and on right and left hands, and differences of frequency in the sexes. Such differential trends are demonstrable only through statistical analysis of data from a series of individuals. As will be shown in later chapters, the trends are modified to some extent by race and other constitutional factors. The general trends are apparent in a series of 100 individuals or even less. Table 1 is a compilation of data

TABLE 1

PERCENT FREQUENCIES* OF FINGER PRINT TYPES IN 5,000 INDIVIDUALS—50,000 IMPRESSIONS
(*Data from Scotland Yard,* 1905)

Galton types:		Whorls				Loops		Arches		
Digit	Side	Whorls	Lat. pockets + twin loops	Central pockets	Acci-dentals	Ulnar	Radial	Tent-ed arches	Other arches	Indeter-min-able†
I	R	31.86	8.79	0.74	0.04	55.89	0.22	0.02	2.45	15
	L	19.19	9.84	0.36	0.00	65.90	0.20	0.00	4.51	12
	R + L	25.52	9.32	0.55	0.02	60.89	0.21	0.01	3.48	
II	R	25.03	2.94	2.40	0.42	32.30	26.03	2.30	8.57	41
	L	22.02	3.50	2.01	0.62	38.10	23.37	1.95	8.41	32
	R + L	23.52	3.22	2.21	0.52	35.20	24.70	2.13	8.49	
III	R	13.98	1.39	1.15	0.04	74.81	2.53	0.60	5.49	29
	L	13.21	2.11	0.80	0.06	73.32	2.51	0.86	7.12	26
	R + L	13.59	1.75	0.98	0.05	74.07	2.52	0.73	6.30	
IV	R	34.85	0.64	5.50	0.08	55.61	1.47	0.02	1.83	21
	L	22.11	1.07	4.64	0.00	68.92	0.50	0.08	2.67	25
	R + L	28.48	0.85	5.07	0.04	62.27	0.98	0.05	2.25	
V	R	11.41	0.38	2.01	0.00	85.46	0.20	0.00	0.54	22
	L	6.86	0.62	1.53	0.02	89.79	0.02	0.02	1.15	26
	R + L	9.13	0.50	1.77	0.01	87.62	0.11	0.01	0.84	
All digits	R	23.43	2.83	2.36	0.12	60.83	6.08	0.59	3.77	128
	L	16.68	3.43	1.87	0.14	67.21	5.31	0.58	4.77	121
	R + L	20.05	3.13	2.11	0.13	64.02	5.69	0.58	4.27	249
All digits, Galton types	R	28.74				66.91		4.36		
	L	22.12				72.53		5.35		
	R + L	25.43				69.72		4.86		

* Calculated on available totals, minus indeterminable impressions.

† Absolute numbers: digits amputated or prints indecipherable.

from 5000 individuals (mainly British). A collection of this size gives reasonably stable indications, for its particular racial and sexual composition, of frequencies of pattern types and their differential distribution on digits.

TOTAL FREQUENCIES OF PATTERN TYPES. The three Galton types are represented with widely different frequencies. In the Scotland Yard series (Table 1), loops are roughly 70% of all patterns, whorls 25% and arches 5%. With subdivision of these major classes, differences of frequency are disclosed also among the subtypes. Of the five classes of whorls, true whorls are nearly four times as frequent as lateral pockets, twin loops, central pockets and accidentals combined. In this series, true whorls have a frequency of 20% of all patterns, while lateral pockets and twin loops together amount only to 3%, central pockets 2%, and accidentals 0.1%. The frequency of ulnar loops, 64%, is about 11 times that of radial loops (5.7%). Arches, nearly 5% of all patterns, are comprised of tented arches and other arch types in the proportion 1:7.

The whorls exhibiting the character which Bonnevie (44) terms "twisting" merit separate attention, in view of the emphasis which they have received in studies of inheritance. They are all *double-cored patterns*— true whorls with two interlocked cores, lateral pocket loops, twin loops and accidentals. Bonnevie finds, in a series of 470 persons, that 43.6% of the individuals have at least one twisted pattern. Mueller (221) reports an incidence of 61.4% in 821 persons. Both comment on the high frequency of twisted patterns on thumbs (Table 2).

TABLE 2
FREQUENCIES OF DOUBLE-CORED PATTERNS (THE TENDENCY TO TWISTING, BONNEVIE) IN
821 PERSONS
(*Mueller*)

In individuals		In digits	
Number of double-cored patterns	Frequency	Digits	Frequency
0	38.6%	I R	18.9%
1	20.6	I L	17.4
2	14.4	II R	11.3
3	11.1	II L	12.0
4	5.8	III R	6.9
5	4.3	III L	6.4
6	3.0	IV R	7.7
7	1.1	IV L	7.5
8	0.6	V R	6.1
9	0.5	V L	6.0
10	0.0		

DISTRIBUTION OF PATTERN TYPES ON SINGLE DIGITS. In considering the digital distributions of pattern types corresponding digits of right and left hands are combined (Table 1 and Fig. 50). On every digit ulnar loops are the most abundant pattern, the frequency ranging downward from 88% in digit V, 74% in III, 62% and 61% respectively in IV and I, and 35% in II. Whorls, next in total frequency, are most numerous on I and IV, 35% and 34% respectively, while II is not much lower, 30%; III and V present a sharp reduction, 16% and 11% respectively. Of all pattern types, radial loops have the greatest relative range of frequency among the digits. They occur in 25% of index fingers, 3% in III, 1% in IV, and in I and V they are reduced to very small fractional percentages,

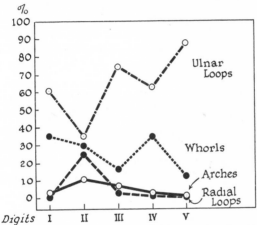

FIG. 50.—Frequencies of whorls, ulnar loops, radial loops and arches on individual digits. (*Based on Scotland Yard data for 5000 persons, table 1.*)

0.2% and 0.1%. Mairs' (71) data on the digital distribution of his series of 411 accidental patterns are more reliable than the data on 64 such patterns in table 1. They are accordingly substituted here, arranged in the order of descending frequencies: II, 70.3%; IV, 14.4%; III, 9.7%; I, 3.6%; V, 1.9% (frequencies based on percent of all accidentals rather than percent of all patterns). Arches likewise have a wide range of frequency among the digits, but a lesser range than those of accidentals and radial loops. Their frequencies for II, III, I, IV and V are 11%, 7%, 4%, 2% and 1% in order.

BIMANUAL DIFFERENCES. Whorls and radial loops are more frequent in right hands, while ulnar loops and arches are more common in left hands. The dextral excess of whorls is confined to true whorls, central pockets and accidentals; the greater frequency of lateral pockets and twin loops is in left hands. Since the trend of bimanual difference of double-loop patterns agrees with that of ulnar loops rather than that of true whorls and central pockets, the affinities of double loops to ulnar loops may be closer in other respects. (The occurrences of accidentals in Mairs' collection are: right, 54%; left, 46%. All digits except III, where there is a slight excess in left hands, show dextral excesses.)

To summarize the data on digital distribution (Fig. 50) and bilateral unlikenesses, the digits may be characterized singly. The term whorl will be used in the comprehensive sense of Galton.

Digit I presents the highest incidence of whorls. There is furthermore an extreme bimanual difference in whorl frequency, the right thumb bearing the larger number. The frequency of radial loops is reduced, in a proportion greater than the relative elevation of whorls in this digit.

Digit II bears more radial loops, arches and accidentals than any other digit. Of all radial loops, 86.6% occur here, and this digit bears 43.6% of the total number of arches and 70.3% of all accidentals (accidentals in Mairs' material; in table 1 the value is 81.3%).

Digit III has next to the greatest frequencies of ulnar loops, radial loops and arches, the abundance of these patterns being associated with a reduction of whorls.

Digit IV is similar to digit I with respect to high whorl frequency and large excess of these patterns on right hands.

Digit V presents the highest frequency of ulnar loops and minimum values for all other pattern types.

METHODS OF ANALYSIS

Data in a form such as that of table 1 may be restated in several indices and in the dactylodiagram. They do not meet the needs of biological studies which require analysis of pattern combinations in single individuals or in right and left hands separately. For these studies other forms of record are necessary. The following discussion is confined to simpler and more commonly used methods, and extensions of analysis of statistics comparable to those included in the table.

Useful in the interpretation of finger-print data, as indeed in all analyses of quantitative results, are the standard methods of statistics. The comparison of frequencies of pattern types in two populations, for example, is aided by determining the standard errors of the percent frequencies. By this means the investigator may judge the significance of an observed difference. Among other useful statistical determinations are means with their probable errors, standard deviations, coefficients of variation, coefficients of correlation and similar tests of association.

PATTERN-TYPE INDICES. Furuhata proposes the whorl/loop index for application in a mass sample. It is calculated by dividing the total frequency of whorls by the total frequency of loops (ulnar and radial combined), the quotient being multiplied by one hundred to give an index value in a whole number. Dankmeijer (280) prefers an index expressing the arch/whorl relationship. The arch/whorl index appears to be the more significant in comparative statistics. There is a reciprocal relationship in the frequencies of whorls and of arches. A rise in whorl frequency is associated with a drop in both loops and arches, but loop frequency is a less delicate indicator because these patterns are so numerous. In the Scotland Yard series (Table 1) the whorl/loop index is 36 and the arch/whorl index is 19.

Poll (15, 302) considers these indices inadequate for dealing with trifold pattern types. He uses the system of coördinates within an equilateral triangle and, by modification of the stereo-manuar method, the distribution may be represented also as a triangular pyramid.

PATTERN INTENSITY. Arches, loops and whorls form a sequence of increasing pattern complexity. This sequence has as its parallel an increase in the number of triradii—the plain arch having none, the loop one, and the whorl, two. The number of triradii accordingly is available for a simple quantitative statement of *pattern intensity* (279).

The value of pattern intensity may be stated either as the number of triradii per individual (279) or as the average number of triradii per finger (64). In either case the determination of the value in a mass sample may be made by compiling individual records of numbers of triradii or by translating the data of total frequencies of patterns (e.g., Table 1). In the latter procedure, the determination of pattern intensity ignores the fact that an arch other than a plain arch has a triradius, that occasional loops have two triradii, and that certain whorls (some composites) have more than two triradii. The number of triradii is approximated by adding the frequency of loops to twice the frequency of whorls, the total being divided by the number of individuals when the frequencies are in absolute numbers, or by ten for percent frequencies. The Scotland Yard data thus yield an index of 12.1 per individual, or 1.21 per digit.

When individuals are evaluated in terms of the index of pattern intensity the values range from 0, all arches, to 20, all whorls. Within a collected series the number of individuals in each index value is then determined. This procedure provides for more extended statistical analyses based upon frequencies of individual index values.

MANUARS. In some studies it is desirable to compile combinations of pattern types in single individuals and in single hands. The device best suited to this analysis and presentation of results is the *manuar*, developed by Poll (73). The manuar may represent pattern combinations on right and left hands separately (unimanuar) or on both hands of the individual (bimanuar). Kirchmair (348) originated the *ambimanuar*, combining the unimanuars of right and left hands in one diagram. Any of these manuars may be illustrated as a table or as a stereogram.

The following description of the method is confined to the bimanuar in its simpler form (Fig. 51), a table for the entry of all possible combinations of the numbers of whorls and arches in the finger-print sets of the individuals composing a series. The pattern combination represented by

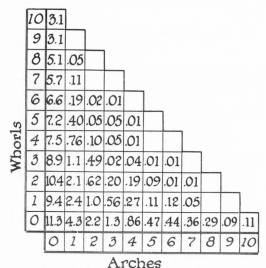

Whorls											
10	3.1										
9	3.1										
8	5.1	.05									
7	5.7	.11									
6	6.6	.19	.02	.01							
5	7.2	.40	.05	.05	.01						
4	7.5	.76	.10	.05	.01						
3	8.9	1.1	.49	.02	.04	.01	.01				
2	10.4	2.1	.62	.20	.19	.09	.01	.01			
1	9.4	2.4	1.0	.56	.27	.11	.12	.05			
0	11.3	4.3	2.2	1.3	.86	.47	.44	.36	.29	.09	.11
	0	1	2	3	4	5	6	7	8	9	10

Arches

FIG. 51.—A bimanuar, with the percent frequencies of finger-print pattern combinations in individuals. (*Data on* 8041 *Germans, from Poll.*)

each space is shown by the coordinate position of that space in reference to the indicated numbers of whorls and arches. The numbers of loops are implied in the remainders of these coordinate relations. Thus the space *o whorls-o arches* provides for ten-finger sets having loops only; the space *1 whorl-o arches* represents individuals with nine loops, and so on. The numbers inserted in this example (Fig. 51) are the frequencies observed in a series of 8041 Germans (15). The modal distribution of the pattern combinations is indicated by the concentration of frequencies at and near the lower left corner, since loops are the most frequent pattern type. Frequencies diminish toward the diagonal border of the manuar, and, so infrequent are the combinations which they designate, only in a much larger series would the spaces along this border be likely to contain entries. If it exists at all, the rarest of combinations would be that of five whorls and five arches. This combination would be expected, if chance alone determined the coexistence of arches and whorls, twice in about 500,000 individuals. Actually, the combination never has been recorded (73). The frequencies of combinations lying along the diagonal progressively diminish as the space *5 arches-5 whorls* is approached. Accordingly, it may be postulated that genetic factors determine mutual exclusiveness of increasingly larger numbers of whorls and arches in the same individual.

DACTYLODIAGRAM. Another analytic method devised by Poll is the dactylodiagram, the example illustrated (Fig. 52) representing the data from Scotland Yard (Table 1). The dactylodiagram is a five-point graph of whorl and arch frequencies in selected couplets of digits. The couplets, plotted in the usual order of increasing whorl frequencies are: V left and

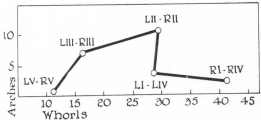

FIG. 52.—A dactylodiagram. (*Based on Scotland Yard data for 5000 persons, table 1.*)

right; III left and right; II left and right; I left and IV left; I right and IV right. Digits II, III and V are coupled as corresponding digits of right and left hands, but digits I and IV are treated differently because, with respect to whorl frequencies, I and IV of the same hand are closer to each other than is either of these digits to the corresponding one of the opposite hand. Poll (168) terms a couplet of corresponding digits a *pair*, while the couplet I and IV of the same hand is a *group;* the usual closer relation in the described pairs and groups is characterized as the *pair-group rule.* Some racial stocks are exceptions to the pair-group rule, digits I and IV being more closely related as pairs than as groups.

The general aspect of the dactylodiagram provides for various comparisons involving pattern-type frequencies on different digits. The scheme is useful in disclosing trends which differentiate racial stocks or other selected populations. Inspection of the graphs usually is sufficient to determine differences, but Poll favors measurements of certain angles of the dactylodiagram for more exact comparison.

RIDGE COUNTING

Ridge counts are made: (a) from triradial point to point of core; (b) from a traced radiant to a triradial point; (c) along a 1-cm. line placed at right angles to ridges, for indirect measurement of ridge breadth. End-points are prescribed in the first two applications.

GENERAL RULES. Accuracy in counting requires a magnification of about four or five diameters. All counts are made along a straight line,

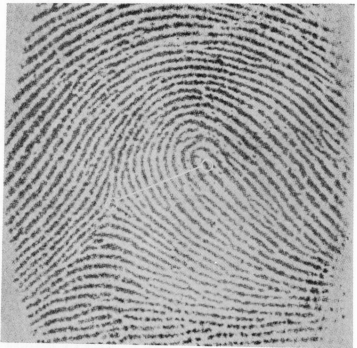

FIG. 53.—A loop with a count of eleven ridges. Ridges are counted along the indicated line which joins the point of triradius (outer terminus) and point of core (inner terminus).

and since the count extends in many instances along a considerable distance, an actual guiding line should be provided. This line is oriented according to the rule applying to the particular count. Though other straight-edge devices will serve, a convenient aid is the *Henry disc,* inserted in the base of the finger-print magnifier (Fig. 45). A fine pointer is used to pass from one ridge to the next along the line of count. Except nascent ridges, every ridge crossing the line is counted. A ridge termination which meets the line is included in the count, and on the same principle when the line cuts through a point of bifurcation two ridges are counted. A ridge which terminates short of touching the line is not included.

TRIRADIAL POINT TO POINT OF CORE. In finger-print identification this is a standard count for subclassifying loops, and in biological studies it is applied to various pattern types as a measure of pattern size (the *quantitative value* of Bonnevie). After locating the triradial point and point of core, as outer and inner termini of the count, the line is set in position to connect them. The triradial point and point of core are not included in the count. The line of count for a loop is illustrated in figure 53.

In true whorls and composites there are two lines of count instead of one, and the adjustment of these lines calls for special attention to the morphology of the configuration. Each line leads from a triradial point to the nearer point of core. Sometimes the determination of the point of core is difficult. Identification practice defines rules to guide ridge counts in these patterns (66). In biological analyses, where the object of the count is to secure a measure of pattern size, the safe rule in doubtful cases is to establish a line of count comparable to that applied in counting loops. When the core of a whorl is an island or a rod there is a common point of core for both counts, and if it is a circle, ellipse, or hook-shaped ridge the limbs of the figure often are so placed that the locations of two points of core are easily fixed according to the principles which govern counts in loops. The more complex cores of true whorls, and especially the cores of lateral pockets and twin loops, call for judgment in the individual case. It is seemingly impossible to construct generally applicable rules for specific problem cases beyond stating the guiding principle that the counts must aim to express pattern size on the same basis as that applying in loops and true whorls. In a double-looped pattern, for instance, it may be justifiable to create an inner terminus, locating it on a ridge which lies midway between the cores of the two loops; the selection of the point on that ridge will depend on the morphology of the two loops.

TRIRADII AND RADIANTS. Reference has been made to the tracing of a proximal pattern radiant of a whorl to determine whether the radiant courses into the opposite triradius, distal to it or proximal to it. A count, in instances where the radiant does not join the opposite triradius, is made between the traced radiant and the triradius, along a line passing from the triradius to the radiant; this line is approximately in the long axis of the digit in whorls with outer tracings, and at right angles to the digital axis in whorls with inner tracings. Neither the radiant nor the triradial point is included in the count. The same principle applies in counting ridges between two traced radiants or between two triradii.

COUNTS PER CENTIMETER. As an indirect measure of ridge breadth, the number of ridges transecting a line of fixed length may be counted. The best device is a glass disc for insertion into the base of the finger-print magnifier and having in its center an engraved line exactly one centimeter in length. With the disc in place, the magnifier is oriented over the print so that the line crosses ridges at right angles. One end of the line is centered in the ridge with which the count is to begin. Every ridge which meets or transects the line is counted, following the rules before stated. The ridge touched or crossed by the opposite extremity of the line is the last ridge included in the count.

PATTERN SIZE (QUANTITATIVE VALUE)

The *quantitative value* of Bonnevie (44) is determined by ridge count from triradial point to point of core. This value is an expression of pattern size, and though an imperfect one, it has proved useful especially in studies of inheritance. The quantitative value is recorded as follows: two integers represent the ridge counts, one for that of the radial side of the pattern and one for the ulnar side. In an ulnar loop the only possible count is the standard loop count, but the value would be written so as to indicate the absence of a count on the ulnar side of the pattern, e.g., 18-0. In a radial loop the reversed notation, e.g., 0-18, shows that the count is on the opposite side. The two counts in true whorls and composites are recorded in the same way, e.g., 14-18. In arches, which have no counts, the value is 0-0. To minimize the effects of arbitrary elements in the rules governing ridge counting, Bonnevie groups the counts in classes. Beginning with class *0*, for plain arches, the classes ascend through *10*. Class *1* includes patterns which have one or two triradii but no ridge count. The succeeding classes, with their ridge counts, are: class *2*, 1-2 ridges; *3*, 3-4; *4*, 5-6; *5*, 7-8; *6*, 9-10; *7*, 11-13; *8*, 14-16; *9*, 17-20; *10*, 21 and higher.

The quantitative value of a pattern (in Bonnevie's original method, since superseded) is half the sum of its two class values. The class values of an ulnar loop having the count 18-0 are *9-0*, and the quantitative value is accordingly 4.5; in the whorl having the count 14-18, the classes are *8-9* and the quantitative value is 8.5. Either the original ridge counts or the class values provide for collective treatment of the characteristics of individuals, of single digits, and of right and left sides.

The adequacy of the class values, as just described, is questioned by Grüneberg (202) and Newman (225); in a later paper Bonnevie (154) acknowledges the deficiency. One weakness concerns the treatment of whorls. The larger count in a whorl, rather than the average of its two counts, should be compared with the count of a loop. Mueller (221), apparently without recognizing that his procedure serves at least partly to offset the inadequacies of the original Bonnevie method, adjusts the values of all typical loops having counts of three or more ridges by adding 25% to the actual count. The second chief weakness of Bonnevie's original class values is the assignment to one class of all counts greater than 20. In his modification of Bonnevie's class values, Newman assigns the value *1* to patterns having a zero ridge count and values from *2* through *17* to a succession of two-ridge classes. In whorls these values apply to the larger of the two counts. The assignment of a class value of *1* to patterns having no ridge count is a questionable beginning of a seriation which aims to measure pattern size in terms of numbers of ridges. The class values as

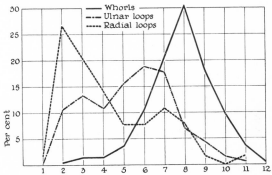

FIG. 54.—Frequencies of the quantitative values (Grüneberg's classes) in 113 individuals: ulnar loops, 735; radial loops, 64; whorls, 227. (*Data from Cummins and Steggerda.*)

revised by Grüneberg properly begin at *o*, for plain arches. Patterns having one or two triradii but no ridge count (tented arches and the arches which are transitional between true patterns and plain arches) have the value *1*. Beginning with class *2*, each is a three-ridge interval: class *2*, ridges 1-3; class *3*, ridges 4-6, and upward.

Whether pattern size is analyzed by absolute ridge counts or by class values, its variability is like that of other bodily characteristics expressible in measurements. In Roscher's counts of 3000 ulnar loops patterns of 12 to 16 ridges form the peak of the curve of distribution; over one third of the patterns lie within this range. The descent to a maximum of 30 ridges is an even slope, while the more frequent smaller loops elevate the opposite limb of the curve. Figure 54 presents the distribution in another sample of Grüneberg's class values for ulnar loops, radial loops and whorls. The curve of distribution of class values for ulnar loops is more depressed than Roscher's curve, because it is constructed from class values instead of direct ridge counts, but the irregularity associated with the disproportionate number of smaller ulnar loops is similarly evidenced. Radial loops exhibit a distinct shift to increased frequencies in the lower class values, while whorls conform to a binomial curve.

There are two chief deficiencies in ridge counts as measures of pattern size. (a) The rules for ridge counting introduce aberrations of this measure. The placing of the line of count is governed arbitrarily by end points that may shift without influencing the expanse of the pattern area. Two loops may be of the same actual size, as measured by the area included within the type line, though in one the ridge count is greater because the core is located farther from the delta. A count across the whole pattern area (Mairs' "full count") might provide a useful supplement to the usual count between the two termini. Arbitrary prescriptions for including or omitting ridges in the count seem to be necessary, and, in mass analyses, it is probable that discrepancies are equalized. (b) The ridge count as a measure of pattern size, without a correction factor for standardization of ridge breadth, yields an exaggerated value when ridges are narrow, and a minified value when they are broad.

PATTERN FORM

Patterns, even of the same type, are variable with respect to form of the pattern area. Some patterns are elongated in the axis of the digit, and others are broad. The variations in pattern form may be likened to variations in proportionate breadth and length of the cranium—long (dolichocephalic), broad (brachycephalic) and intermediate (mesocephalic) —or to variations in body build. In the same way that anthropometric indices express proportionate relations, such as that of cranial breadth and cranial length, the *index of pattern form* indicates the ratio of breadth to height of a pattern.

METHODS. Prints intended for measurements of pattern form should be made with care to minimize distortion of the pattern area in printing.

TABLE 3

VARIATION OF PATTERN-FORM INDICES IN PRINTS, OF THE SAME INDEX FINGER, MADE WITH DIFFERENT DEGREES OF PRESSURE

(*Mueller*)

	Rolled prints	Dab prints
Strong pressure	61	56
Moderate pressure	58	55
Weak pressure	57	53

The pressure should be even and gentle throughout the rolling process, to avoid foreshortening or narrowing of the pattern area. The indices listed in table 3 show that patterns are broader in rolled prints than in dab prints, and that in either process of printing, breadth increases with added pressure. In analyzing prints of young children it must be remembered that pattern form may undergo change with growth. Mueller (222) made repeated prints of four children, aged two to six years, through a period of 2½ years. He reports variations of pattern form in the same digit amounting to as much as 15 points of the index, and ranging downward to 1 index point.

Determinations of pattern form were first made by Bonnevie (44); only her later modified procedures (154) are here considered. Still different modifications are employed by Geipel (59, 197) and by Cummins and Steggerda (279). The differences among the methods lie mainly in orientation of the lines for measuring breadth and height.

The several methods have in common the use of one or another type of ruled transparent plate. This plate may be the commercially available glass disc for insertion in the base of a finger-print magnifier, or it may be made by photographing a coordinate ruling. The essential features of any plate intended for this use are two graduated lines intersecting at right angles. The intervals of graduation, providing they are constant and sufficiently fine, are immaterial since determinations involve proportion rather than absolute values. In the authors' plates the intervals are 0.35 mm. The two reference lines on the plate are named *base line* and *axis* when oriented for the reading of breadth and height respectively.

The following directions are selected from varying procedures adopted by different authors. The pattern area is first outlined, the tracing being carried far enough around the distal boundary of the pattern area to mark the height of the pattern (Fig. 55). Neither loops nor symmetrical meet whorls require special treatment in the height reading. Most whorls are distinguished by non-meeting of radiants, hence the more external of the two distal radiants and the more proximal of the two triradii are selected as landmarks for height measurement. In an asymmetrical whorl the tracing is begun from the triradius which is farther from the core; if the distal radiant passes inside that arising from the other triradius, a tracing is made also from the second triradius, so as to mark the true height of the pattern. Since there is no pattern area defined in arches, a peripheral boundary must be determined arbitrarily. To establish a peripheral boundary, Bonnevie and Geipel trace a ridge crossing fixed points (their 10 markings) on the base line of the plate. It is suggested that a ridge which is representative of the curvatures near the center of the "pattern area" might instead be chosen for tracing. Some personal variation in this selection is inevitable, though the method meets the difficulty at least as satisfactorily as the choice of fixed points on the base line.

Orientation of the measuring plate varies considerably in the practice of different investigators. There is agreement among all workers in reading breadth as half, or about half, of the total breadth of the pattern area (Fig. 55). Thus, a breadth/height reading of 8/10 would mean that the real proportion is $16 \pm /10$. The justification for so considering breadth is that loops have on only one side a fixed point for breadth measurement, the triradius. There is agreement also in reading breadth of true whorls and other patterns with two triradii on the side which yields the larger measurement. Finally, all workers orient the base line through a triradius (except in plain arches).

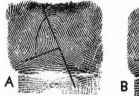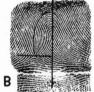

FIG. 55.—Two prints of the same pattern for illustration of the unlike methods of orienting the lines of measurement of breadth and height: *A*, according to both Bonnevie and Geipel; *B*, according to Cummins and Steggerda. The indices obtained by the two methods are: *A*, 70; *B*, 50.

For measuring height all workers align the axis of the measuring plate through the core. Both Bonnevie and Geipel place the axis so as to conform to the direction of the core and surrounding central features (Fig. 55,A). The cores of many patterns slant, and there is accordingly no fixed relationship between the long axis of the digit and the directions along which breadth and height are measured. A constant reference to the digital axis is provided by the method of Cummins and Steggerda. For the reading of pattern height the axis of the plate is placed through the core and parallel with the digital axis, and the base line is thus at right angles to the digit (Fig. 55,B). The distal interphalangeal flexion furrows aid in orientation of the base line, and prints prepared for studies of pattern form should include these furrows.

The pattern-form index of an individual finger—or the average of indices in a series of digits, the ten digits of an individual, or series of corresponding digits—may be assigned its place in a group classification. Bonnevie defines these classes of form indices:

—— 59	Elliptical
60–80	Intermediate
81 ——	Circular.

Geipel also considers three groups:

—— 91	Narrow
92–111	Intermediate
112 ——	Broad.

In genetic comparisons of the ten-digit averages Geipel allows an over-lapping, as follows:

—— 93	Narrow
90–113	Intermediate
110 ——	Broad.

Bonnevie favors exclusion of the thumbs in computing the average form index of the individual, holding that the extraordinary breadth of thumb patterns distorts the individual average. Geipel considers that the ten-digit average is not rendered inadequate by inclusion of the thumbs, which with his method of measurement elevates the form index of the individual by 5.2 points on the average. In the Cummins-Steggerda series of Dutch, where pattern form was measured by a different method, there is an equal difference between the ten-digit average and eight-digit average (the actual value of the difference, 4.6, being the same as in two of the series from which Geipel compiled his results).

Certain characteristics of pattern form, notably the conformation of the interior of the pattern, escape recognition in the index. Bonnevie's original method of registering pattern form is concerned with the breadth and height of the central area alone. Within patterns, especially whorls, variations in form of the central area may occur independently of the form of the pattern as a whole. The internal ridges of a whorl may spiral or they may form concentric figures. The spiral and concentric figures may be circular or elliptical, and the ellipses may be broad or narrow, sometimes much attenuated in the axis of the digit. Again, the central configuration may exhibit double-looped arrangements or other localized peculiarities. The recording of all such details necessitates the use of special descriptive methods.

Another feature deserving attention is the slant of the internal ridges with reference to the axis of the digit. In loops the cores may be in line with the digital axis, transverse to it or on an intermediate slant. The angle may be readily measured with the interphalangeal flexion furrows

TABLE 4
PATTERN-FORM INDICES, IN THREE SERIES, DETERMINED BY DIFFERENT METHODS

Digits	Germans, 2200+	Norwegians, 373	Dutch, 113
	Geipel	Bonnevie	Cummins and Steggerda
I	123.0	109.0	85.8
II	101.6	84.9	73.4
III	87.5	80.2	61.3
IV	94.7	75.9	58.1
V	100.4	84.7	59.0

as a line of reference. The angular relation may prove to have useful applications in biological studies.

STATISTICS. The distribution of the indices (ten-digit average) in one sample is shown in figure 56. The average form indices for single digits, in this series and in two other collections, are included in table 4. The

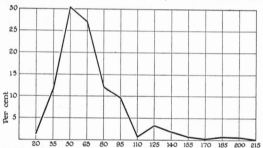

FIG. 56.—Frequencies of the pattern-form indices in 113 individuals. (*Data from Cummins and Steggerda.*)

data represent three national populations (Germans, Norwegians and Dutch). Possibly the unlikenesses among the three series are in part racial distinctions, but it is probable that the observed differences in pattern form are attributable at least mainly to differences of method. Nonetheless, the three sets of determinations indicate certain consistent differential trends among the digits, especially the increased pattern breadth of the thumb.

The mean pattern-form indices of different pattern types present no significant differences among whorls, ulnar loops and radial loops, but the distributions of individual indices indicate a trend in which the types diminish in breadth in this order: whorls, ulnar loops, radial loops. Arches are of course the broadest of all patterns, this being apparent without measurement. According to observations (197) on 315 males and 287 females, there are no sexual distinctions in pattern form.

Configurations of Middle and Proximal Phalanges

The few available studies of configurations on middle and proximal phalanges indicate that further investigation will be profitable. MacArthur (215) mentions a study in progress in which it is found that for the discrimination of monozygotic and dizygotic twins these regions present "features of high diagnostic value."

Whipple (147) was among the first to direct notice to the inclination of ridges on these segments, pointing out that their configurations form two systems of slanting ridges with opposed directions, an arrangement regarded by her as a provision against slipping in prehension. Ploetz-Radmann was the first to make precise studies of these configurations; her scheme of description is adopted by subsequent workers interested in these regions (63, 129).

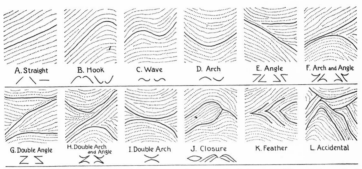

Fig. 57.—Types of configurations of middle and proximal phalanges. (*Traced from the prints illustrated by Ploetz-Radmann.*)

Ploetz-Radmann differentiates four basic types of configurations (Fig. 57,A-D: *straight, hook, wave, arch*), seven combination types (Fig. 57,E-K) and another class comprising rare configurations which do not conform to any one of the defined types. In figure 57 supplementary sketches distinguish the sub-types recognized by Ploetz-Radmann on the basis of directional characteristics.

Middle and proximal phalanges, imprinted by rolling, are investigated in 200 persons by Ploetz-Radmann. The two phalanges are separately formulated and the results brought together for various comparisons. The majority (80%) of all phalanges, whether proximal or middle, bear one or another of the four basic types. Enclosures and feathered configurations are confined to proximal phalanges. On digits I, II and III the characteristic slants are proximo-radial, while digits IV and V typically slant in the proximo-ulnar direction. Arches are most frequent on digit III, next on digit IV.

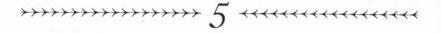

5

PALMS

TOPOGRAPHY

ANATOMICAL LANDMARKS. In describing palmar dermatoglyphics and in presenting methods of interpreting them it is necessary to make use of designations referring to the anatomy of the hand (Fig. 58).

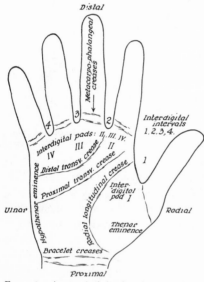

FIG. 58.—Anatomical landmarks in palmar dermatoglyphics.

Terms of anatomical direction (proximal, distal, radial and ulnar) are frequently employed in describing the locations of features and in indicating directions toward the respective palmar margins.

Interdigital intervals, the clefts between digits, are numbered in sequence beginning with the interval between the thumb and index finger.

Around the central *hollow* of the palm there is a series of six elevations, of varying prominence and expanse. Four of these are *interdigital pads*, each lying in proximity to an interdigital interval. Interdigital pads are distinguished by numbers, each having the number of the neighboring interval. Inter-

digital pad I is the least prominent member of this series, being usually hardly evident as an elevation. The *thenar eminence* occupies a large share of the proximo-radial quadrant of the palm; its elevation is due mainly to the location in this region of muscles which control the thumb. The *hypothenar eminence*, a more elongated elevation lying in the ulnar portion of the palm, is associated with muscles of the little finger, though in its proximal region there is commonly a localized bulge representing a true pad which has the same morphological significance as pads of the interdigital series (Chap. 9).

The major *flexion creases* are fairly constant in their arrangement in different palms, and those illustrated are useful as landmarks in descriptive dermatoglyphics. The most distal *bracelet crease* typically coincides with the proximal limit of ridged skin. Located at the bases of digits, the *metacarpo-phalangeal creases* form dividing lines between the free digits and palm. The *radial longitudinal crease* (the palmist's "line of life") curves to embrace the thenar eminence and the region occupied by interdigital pad I. The *distal transverse crease* (the "line of heart") and the -radial portion of the *proximal transverse crease* (the "line of head") form an incomplete proximal boundary of the region occupied by interdigital pads II, III and IV. The levels of termina-tion at the ulnar border of the

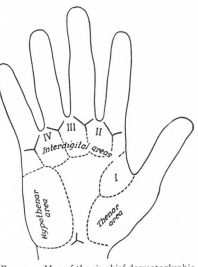

FIG. 59.—Map of the six chief dermatoglyphic areas of the palm.

distal and proximal transverse creases aid in defining zones for formulating palmar main lines.

DERMATOGLYPHIC AREAS. Corresponding to the described reliefs, the palmar surface is divisible into dermatoglyphic areas or configurational fields. Of these areas, six (Fig. 59) are included in the customary descrip-tive formulation: hypothenar, thenar and the four interdigitals. Each of the areas is a topographic unit, its individuality being expressed both by the existence in some palms of a discrete pattern and by the characteristic presence of partial boundaries formed by triradii and their radiants. A palmar area is comparable to the ball of a finger with respect to its nature as a unit, notwithstanding that the several areas are modified by their conjunctions and that their individuality as units is sometimes obliterated completely. The configuration of a palmar area is classifiable according to the general principles which govern the classification of finger prints.

TRIRADII. Characteristically, there are four *digital triradii*, located in proximal relation to the bases of digits II, III, IV and V (Fig. 60). In radio-ulnar sequence they are named *a*, *b*, *c* and *d*. The two distal, or digital, radiants of each triradius embrace the *digital area*, the zone

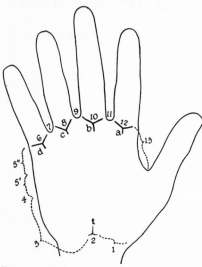

bounded by these radiants and the most proximal metacarpo-phalangeal flexion crease. The distal radiants thus embrace the base of the digit as they course to the interdigital intervals (in the instance of triradius *d*, in passing to the fourth interdigital interval and to the ulnar margin). The proximal radiant is directed toward the interior of the palm, and when fully traced this radiant is known as a palmar *main line*. The four main lines (Fig. 63) originating from digital triradii are named in radio-ulnar sequence *A*, *B*, *C* and *D*—each letter corresponding to the designation of the respective triradius but distinguished by capitalization.

FIG. 60.—The scheme of numbers for formulating palmar main lines.

Axial triradii (Fig. 60,*t*) are located most commonly at or very near the proximal margin of the palm, in the interval between the thenar and hypothenar eminences. They may occur, however, as far distal as the center of the palm. A palm may have one, two or three axial triradii, or rarely none. A composite of X-ray records of digital and axial triradii (Fig. 61) shows that the distribution of axial triradii is confined rather closely to the axis of the fourth metacarpal bone. This confirms the general observation in prints that these triradii, whatever their levels, are confined to a zone aligned with the axis of the fourth digit. The distal radiant of the axial triradius may be traced through the palm and considered as a main line (Fig. 63,*T*—named from the symbol of the axial triradius, *t*).

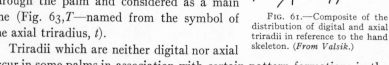

FIG. 61.—Composite of the distribution of digital and axial triradii in reference to the hand skeleton. (*From Valsik.*)

Triradii which are neither digital nor axial occur in some palms in association with certain pattern formations in the palmar areas. Under some circumstances accessory triradii related to interdigital areas are recognized as origins of supplementary main lines.

TRACING AND FORMULATION OF MAIN LINES

Basic Methods

TRACING. As they are traced on the palm print, the main lines are marked with a fine-pointed pencil, ordinary or colored. Lines *A, B, C*

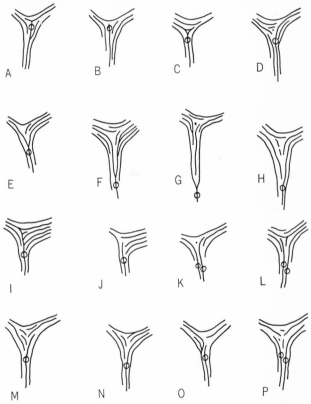

FIG. 62.—A series of representative digital triradii, illustrating selection of the ridge traced as a main line. The proximal radiant is marked by a circle; in cases (K,L,P) having two circles the ridge on the radial side is selected as the proximal radiant.

and *D* originate from the respective digital triradii as their proximal radiants, and line *T* is the distal radiant of the axial triradius. In cases presenting two or three axial triradii, line *T* is traced from the proximal one.

A main line is traced according to the same rules which apply to the tracing of type lines in finger prints, with the following supplements adapted to conditions in the palm.

(a) Selection of the ridge to be traced as the main line usually presents no difficulty (Fig. 62), but occasionally the triradial construction is such that either of two ridges appears equally entitled to recognition as the proximal radiant (Fig. 62,K,L,P). In such a case the ridge on the radial side is arbitrarily chosen as the beginning of the main line.

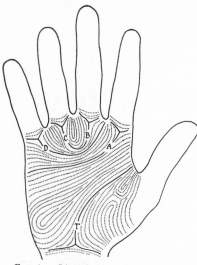

(b) Interruptions of ridges are frequent and the tracing of a main line beyond an interruption is definitely prescribed. Often another ridge is in a direct line, and if so the tracing is continued on that ridge. Otherwise, the tracing is transferred to an adjoining ridge in accord with the following rules. If one of the two neighboring ridges has a closer spatial or linear relationship with the ending the tracing is continued on it. If such discrimination can not be made the general course of the main line is projected visually, to determine which of these alternatives applies: when the sweep of the ridges is curved, the ridge toward the concavity is selected; when the course is relatively straight, the ridge is chosen which carries the line toward the ulnar side, rather than the radial, or toward the distal margin rather than proximally.

FIG. 63.—Identification of the main lines (A, B, C, D, T), in a palm having the formula: 11.10.8.5'.13-t-L^r.L/L.O.L.V.

(c) The tracing is made without anticipating the terminal relations of the line, to avoid bias in favor of tracing lines either to the palmar margin or to fusions with other main lines.

(d) Particular caution is exercised in meeting a flexion crease. Imperfect ridge formation and altered ridge courses within flexion creases (Fig. 37), as well as lapses of printing within creases, may require that the tracing be continued empirically. The main line is traced across the crease onto the ridge which is in most direct linear continuation.

FORMULATION. Completely traced, the main lines of a palm constitute a skeleton (Figs. 64–69) comparable to the type lines of a finger print. The general aspects of the palmar configuration may be largely reconstructed from inspection of the main lines alone (Fig. 70), or even from the descriptive formulation, since there is so intimate a relationship between the main lines and the other elements of configuration.

The formulation (classification) of main lines is based upon a numbered sequence of positions around the periphery of the palm, each traced line being described by the position in which it terminates. Numbers are applied to a series of 14 intervals and points (Fig. 60). The number sequence begins with the proximal part of the thenar eminence and continues around the proximal, ulnar, distal and radial borders of the palm.

Digital triradii and the axial triradius are points (axial triradius, *2*; digital triradii, *d*, *c*, *b* and *a* being numbered in order *6*, *8*, *10* and *12*). Mutual fusion of two main lines results when a tracing continues from one digital triradius to another digital triradius (Fig. 63, lines *B* and *C*); each of the two main lines is then formulated with the number assigned to the triradius from which the other line arises. When a line is traced to an interdigital interval it is formulated by the number of that interval (for example, a line *D* reaching the second interdigital interval, as it does in figure 63, is formulated *11*). A line terminating along the proximal margin of the thenar eminence anywhere on the radial side of the axial triradius, is formulated *1*. The four remaining intervals, embracing the proximal margin of the hypothenar eminence and the ulnar border of the palm, are not limited by definite anatomical landmarks (Fig. 60). The approximate midpoint of the ulnar border is determined as position·*4*; often the proximal transverse flexion crease reaches this point, and the termination of the crease in any case is a helpful guide in estimating the extent of distal and proximal halves of this border. The interval between positions *4* and *2*, including the proximal half of the ulnar border and the proximal margin of the hypothenar eminence, is position *3*. The distal half of the ulnar border is position *5*, which is itself divided into halves for more specific formulation of main lines, the proximal half being numbered *5′* and the distal half *5″*. Usually the distal transverse flexion crease ends at a level corresponding to the point separating *5′* and *5″*.

Having traced the four main lines, the symbols for their terminations are composed in a *main-line formula*. It is recorded in the order *D*, *C*, *B*, *A*, with periods separating the symbols. In figure 63, as an example, the formula is 11.10.8.5′. If it is desired to include line *T*, its symbol (in this case, *13*) is added as a fifth element in the formula.

Special Formulations

The foregoing methods of formulation are basic, but several special procedures remain to be described.

DOUBLE FORMULATIONS. Two circumstances demand double formulation. In *dual formulation* two determinations are actually realized on the palm, while *alternative formulation* is used when the interpretation is on the borderline or doubtful. Their symbols are distinguished typographically. The two elements in a dual formulation are separated by a slant line with the larger number first, while in alternative formulation the preferred interpretation is given precedence and the alternative element of the

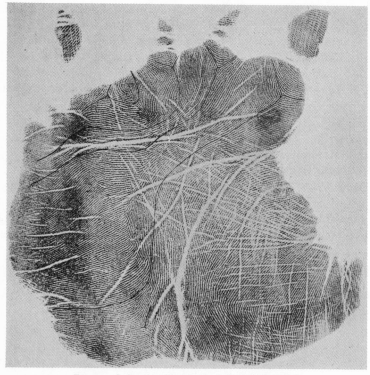

FIG. 64.—Left palm, formula: $7.5''.5'.3$-t-$A^u.O.M.O.L.$

symbol follows in parentheses. Examples of these usages are shown in figures 65–69.

ABSENCE OF A DIGITAL TRIRADIUS. In the absence of a digital triradius, a condition almost confined to triradius c, the digital area is not discretely bounded. The ridges in its territory are extended proximally as a progressively widening system of arciform ridges encroaching into the interdigital areas (Fig. 66). Lack of the triradius, and necessarily of the corresponding main line, is formulated by the symbol O, standing in the formula in the place assigned to the main line involved.

ABORTIVE MAIN LINES. Closely allied to the absence of a digital triradius is abbreviation of a main line. Line C is selected for illustration since it is the one principally involved. In the degree of least development there is, practically speaking, no main line at all, though the triradius is present. This condition is formulated x, regardless of the line involved. A more frequent abortive state, formulated X, is that in which the proxi-

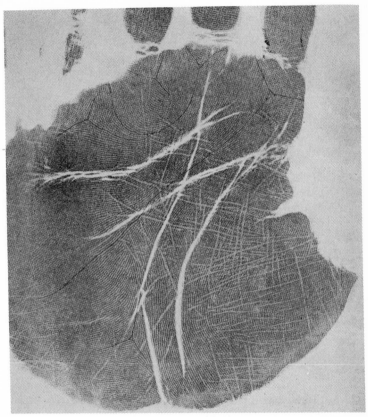

FIG. 65.—Left palm, formula: $10.X.7/6.3\text{-}t'\text{-}A^u/A^c.O.O.V.M.$

mal radiant can be traced for a short distance. It commonly forms the axis of a configuration resembling the tented arch of the finger-print series (Fig. 67), but with the convexity facing proximally rather than distally. A third type of abortive main line is formulated by the number of the triradius of origin, 8 in the case of line C. The line recurves to fuse with itself or with one of the digital radiants of its own triradius (Fig. 68). The distinction between a distal termination (position 7 or 9) and the abortive form (position *8*) is the independent course of the line reaching an inter-digital interval, as contrasted with definite fusion of the line with itself or with a distal radiant of its triradius of origin. The most reduced state of the line reaching *7* or *9* (Fig. 69) is closely allied to the abortive form, and the pattern which it encloses may be wholly dependent for its character as a pattern upon the line itself, the interior lacking recurved ridges.

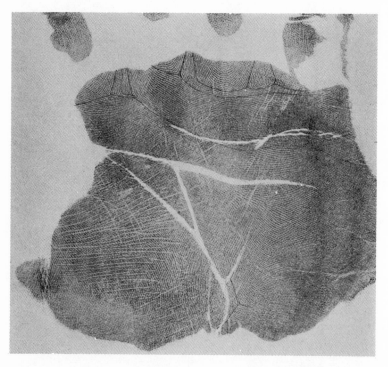

MUTUAL FUSION OF MAIN LINES. A main line may continue into the proximal radiant of another digital triradius. Such a tracing resolves the terminations of two main lines, each termination being complementary to the other. In figure 63, for example, line *C* is traced to triradius *b*, and two symbols of the formula are derived, namely,—.10.8.—.

Two main lines may have a limited extent of fusion, one or both being traceable beyond the zone of fusion to an independent termination (Fig. 71). Diverted courses of this sort are produced by centers of ridge multiplication, divergences of many ridges from a common point. Dual formulations are recorded for all cases of regionally limited fusion.

When two traced lines are separated even for a part of their course by no more than two ridges (Fig. 72), their intimate relationship is indicated in the formula by alternative formulation. The first symbol records the actual tracing, and the second symbol signifies the nearness of another line with consequent possibility of a variant tracing, e.g., $7(8).5''(6).5''.3$.

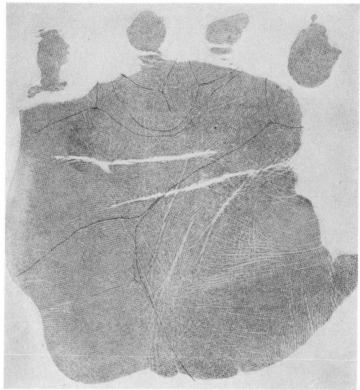

FIG. 67.—Left palm, formula: $11(10).X.7(6).4/1\text{-}1'\text{-}V/A^c.O.O.V.V.$

FUSIONS OF MAIN LINES WITH DISTAL RADIANTS OF FOREIGN DIGITAL TRIRADII. A main line may fuse with a distal radiant of a triradius other than the one giving origin to the line in question, a condition not to be confounded with fusion of two main lines. In these rare cases the main line is formulated as attaining the position entered by the radiant with which the line fuses. Thus, for example, if the terminal course of line A merges with the ulnar distal radiant of triradius d, the line is formulated $5''$, the zone entered by both radiant and main line.

TRACING MAIN LINES FROM ACCESSORY TRIRADII AS SUBSTITUTES FOR DIGITAL TRIRADII. The standards for formulating main lines require supplements in some cases. The main-line formula is a descriptive record, and the value derived from it in studies of mass samples exists largely in the fact that the formulation of lines D and A pictures the degree of transversality of ridges in the distal area of the palm. The courses of lines B and C add nothing of significance to the record of general ridge direction.

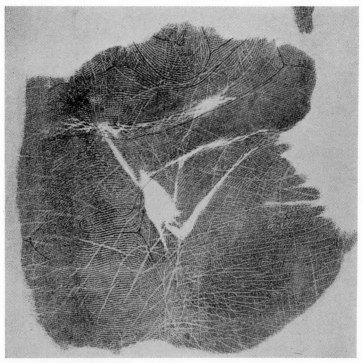

FIG. 68.—Left palm, formula: $11/7.8.7.5 - t'-L^r/A^c.O.O.V.d.$

Their courses are confined by lines D and A, and formulation serves only to describe local courses in the middle of the distal palm, these being often circuits around interdigital patterns. For example (Fig. 70,B), the formula $11.9.7.5''$ remains adequately descriptive of generalized ridge courses if lines B and C are omitted: $11.—.—.5''$.

There are fairly frequent accessory lines D and A, which, unless included, would render the main-line formula inadequate for description of generalized ridge courses. In figure 70,A, line D fuses with an accessory triradius associated with the fourth interdigital pattern; line D in this palm has two terminations (*11* and *7*), both of which are formulated. In figures 70,C and 70,D the aspect of the distal palmar configurations is the same as in figure 70,A, though in neither does line *D* fuse with a radiant of the neighboring pattern triradius. To make the formula complete, the course of the radiant of the accessory triradius must be recorded. This radiant simulates line *D* both in course and in the position of its triradius of origin. In formulating the accessory radiant a special symbol is applied,

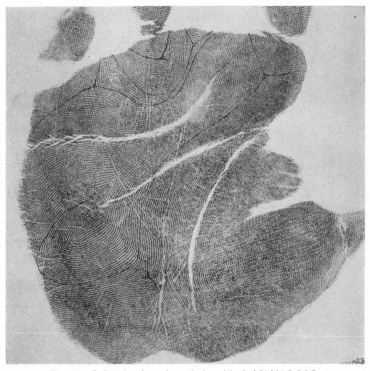

Fig. 69.—Left palm, formula: 11(10).9.7(6).3*h-t'-L^r*/*A^e*.0.0.1.0.

the two elements being separated by a dash (e.g., *11-7*) to denote the presence of an accessory radiant which assumes the character of line *D*, though not fused with it. It will be recalled that a true dual formulation (e.g., *11/7*) always signifies fusion of line *D* with an accessory triradius. An accessory radiant is not formulated unless it courses farther radially than does line *D*, hence the more radial of the two positions indicated in the symbol invariably stands for the accessory feature rather than the main line.

Line *A* presents an exact parallel to the situation described for line *D*. A radiant traced from an accessory triradius may fuse with line *A* or,

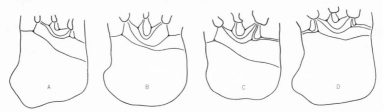

Fig. 70.—Tracings from four right palms, illustrating a typical set of palmar main lines (*B*) and three palms in which accessory lines have more descriptive significance than the main lines proper.

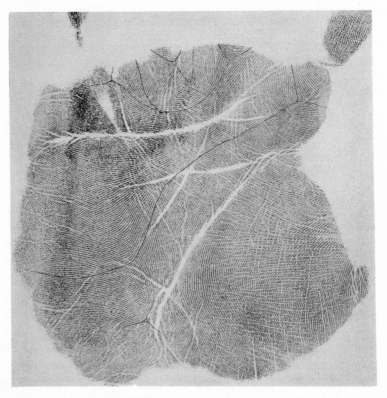

Fig. 71.—Left palm, formula: 10.9.7/6.3-*t*-*A*ᵘ.*O.M.L.M.*

without fusion, simulate a typical course of line *A*. If there is a fusion with the accessory triradius, the ordinary dual formulation (e.g., *11/5″*) is used. When the courses of line *A* and of the related accessory radiant are independent, the symbol for formulation has its elements separated by a dash (e.g., *11-5″*, as in figure 70,D). An accessory radiant is not formulated unless it terminates farther proximo-ulnarward than does line *A* proper.

These special conditions involving lines *D* and *A* require that each print be examined after routine tracing of the main lines. If accessory triradii occur in relationship to second and fourth interdigital patterns,

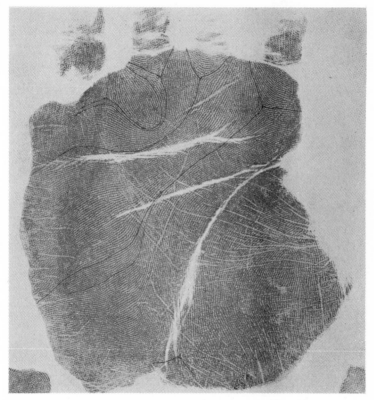

FIG. 72.—Left palm, formula: 7(8).5″(6).5″.3-*t*-*A*ᵘ.*V*.*O*.*O*.*L*.

their radiants are traced to determine whether they should be included in the formula. In writing the double symbol for either main line the larger number is written first.

INTERDIGITAL TRIRADII. In defining digital triradii emphasis is placed upon their characteristic location, one at the base of each digit except the thumb. Fluctuations from typical position introduce some modifications in formulating main lines. Displacement may be so extreme that in some cases there is an apparent supplanting of digital triradii by triradii occupying interdigital positions.

Triradius d may be shifted radially to be in line with the fourth interdigital interval, and there may be also a distal displacement. Similarly, triradius a is sometimes shifted in the ulnar and distal directions. Notwithstanding such departures in the positions of triradii a and d, their

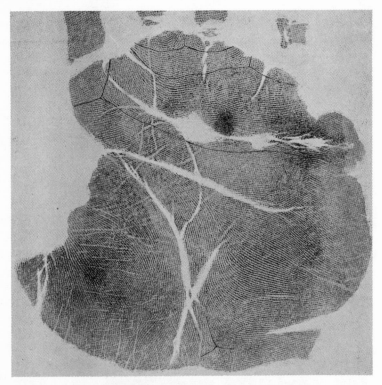

FIG. 73.—Right palm, formula: 11.OidO.5'-t-A^u.O.O.O.O.

proximal radiants retain the ordinary characteristics of main lines. Triradii b and c frequently approach each other, but there is commonly no difficulty in identifying their proximal radiants as main lines. In an occasional palm, however, triradii b and c appear to be wanting, being supplanted by a single triradius located in direct line with the third interdigital interval.

Figure 73 demonstrates both applications of the rule for formulating these interdigital triradii. The rule is: Apply the usual means of formulating main lines when the proximal radiant of an interdigital triradius assumes the character of a main line. When the usual means of formulation fail, consider the digital triradius as absent, and include the symbol *id* in the main-line formula, placing it, without punctuation, in the space corresponding to its position. Thus, line *D* in figure 73 presents no difficulty in formulation; notwithstanding displacement of triradius *d*, its proximal radiant follows a course characteristic of line *D*, reaching position *11*. In the same palm, the triradius related to the third interdigital interval is so unlike a digital triradius in position and direction of the radiants that the ordinary formulation does not apply. The special formulation indicates that digital triradii *b* and *c* are absent and that an interdigital triradius occurs in relation to the third interval: 11.oido.5′.

FORMULATION OF AXIAL TRIRADII

Commonly there occurs a single axial triradius at or very near the proximal palmar margin, in the depression between the thenar and hypothenar eminences. Some palms have two or even three axial triradii, lying at different levels in the longitudinal axis. Rarely there is no axial triradius. Axial triradii are distributed within a narrow field aligned with the axis of the fourth digit (Fig. 61). Formulation records the number and levels of axial triradii. In the palmar formula, the symbol or symbols for axial triradii follow the main-line formula, separated from it and from the succeeding pattern formula by dashes (see legends of figures 64–69).

An axial triradius at or very near the proximal margin is formulated *t*. The most distally situated position of an axial triradius, near the center of the palm, is *t″*, and one which lies at an intermediate level is *t′*. In the absence of an axial triradius the symbol *O* is used, and should there be question as to presence of a *t*, due to incomplete printing, the symbol *?* indicates that the determination can not be made. In some palms where there is no *t*, the ridges of the thenar and hypothenar areas diverge in its expected position to form a parting, *p*. When two or three axial triradii occur they are formulated in proximo-distal order (e.g., *tt′t″*), the symbols not being separated from each other by punctuation marks.

The distinction between *t* and *t′* and between *t′* and *t″* is not always clear. Lacking precise means of discrimination, this formulation has proved the least satisfactory of all elements of the palmar formula. It is possible that more refined methods might be developed to evaluate the levels. Norma Ford[1] suggests that the level of *t′* be more specifically indicated, her practice being to append to the symbol *t′* the letter *l*, *m* or *h*, the respective initial letters of low, middle and high. It will be apparent that

---

[1] Personal communication, February 14, 1942.

"low" and "high" should be considered as indicators of possible alternative formulations. At least many cases of $t'(l)$ are instances which might be interpreted as t, and in the same way some examples of $t'(h)$ might otherwise be interpreted as t''; thus, the formulae of these border-line instances might be written $t'(t)$ and $t'(t'')$ in accord with the usual notation of alternative formulations.

FORMULATION OF CONFIGURATIONAL AREAS

The six configurational areas of the palm are formulated individually. The configuration of each area is recorded by a descriptive symbol, and the series of symbols is set down as the *pattern formula* in this order: hypothenar, thenar/interdigital I, interdigital II, interdigital III, interdigital IV. When there is a question regarding classification of the configuration type an alternative formulation is made, giving precedence to the preferred interpretation, e.g., $V(M)$. When a configurational area bears two discrete configurations it is formulated with a dual symbol; a hypothenar area might have two patterns, for example L^u/L^u, or a pattern and an arch, L^r/A^c.

Hypothenar

The prevailing directions of ridges of the hypothenar configuration are slants which approach the transverse, in contrast with the generally longitudinal direction of the thenar system. Typically there is a marked multiplication of ridges from a point near the center of the palm; from this point ridges fan out over the hypothenar area.

The configuration of the entire hypothenar eminence constitutes the *hypothenar system*, but the only configurations which are formulated are those of its proximal portion (82). This area bears the proximal hypothenar pad. The area is approximately bounded on its radial side by a line drawn from the base of the ring finger to position *2* of the palmar border. It will be recalled that axial triradii are distributed in close relation to this line. Axial triradii are intimately associated with the hypothenar configuration, their radiants forming boundaries or penetrating the configuration. When t' is present, its ulnar radiant commonly divides the hypothenar configuration into distal and proximal elements (see duplex configurations, below).

PRIMARY TYPES OF CONFIGURATIONS. There are three primary types of true patterns in the hypothenar area: whorls, loops and tented arches. The other primary configurational types are not true patterns: plain arches, open fields, multiplications and vestiges.

True *whorls*, as in finger prints, are distinguished by concentric ridges. Typically, however, there are three triradii instead of two. The triradius on the ulnar margin may be extralimital, potentially present at a point lying outside the area of ridged skin. The symbol for the whorl is *W*. Whorls presenting spiral or double-looped centers, enclosed by a concentric periphery, are qualified in formulation by adding *s* as a superscript

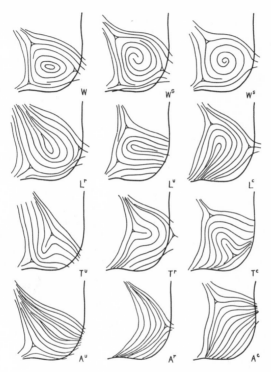

FIG. 74.—The four primary types of hypothenar configurations with their varieties and symbols, illustrated as in prints from right palms.

(Fig. 74). Whorls having no more than eight ridges from the core to the nearest triradial point, may be formulated as small by using the symbol *w* instead of *W*.

Hypothenar *loops* are morphologically like loops of finger prints, but in the hypothenar area there are three instead of two directions of opening: the radial margin, the ulnar margin, the proximal (carpal) margin. The symbol for all loops is *L*, and superscript letters are added as abbreviations of the directions of opening: L^r, L^u, L^c (Fig. 74). Loops having no more than eight ridges may be distinctively formulated, *l*.

Tented arches in the hypothenar area are morphologically like tented arches of the fingers, though here it is the general aspect of the configuration rather than a rigorous distinction between tented arches and loops which governs the formulation. Tented arches are oriented in three different directions; the concavity of the arch may face ulnarwards, radially or proximally (toward the wrist, carpus). The symbol for all tented arches

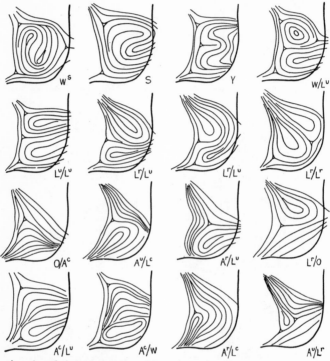

Fig. 75.—A series of derived varieties of hypothenar configurations, with their symbols, illustrated as in prints from right palms.

is T, with a superscript abbreviation of the direction of the base: T^u, T^r and T^c (Fig. 74).

Plain arches, a special form of open field, have an arched form as in finger prints. A is the symbol for a plain arch, and the same superscript letters are used as in tented arches to indicate the facing of the concavity: A^u, A^r and A^c (Fig. 74).

Open fields (symbol: O) are configurations in which the ridges are essentially straight instead of arched. Such configurations are exceedingly rare.

Vestiges lack the sharp recurvatures of ridges which distinguish true patterns, though well developed vestiges may show resemblance to definable types of patterns. Ordinarily a vestige is merely a local dis-arrangement of ridges which converge abruptly or a system of straight and parallel ridges which differ in direction from those surrounding the vestige area. The symbol for vestige is V, and when a vestige presents a recognizable affinity to a particular pattern type the symbol of that pattern type is prefixed, e.g., L^rV.

SOME SPECIAL VARIANTS OF PATTERNS. The hypothenar area may dis-play a duplex configuration: two true patterns, a pattern and an arch or open field, two arches, or two open fields. Often the two configurations are separated by the ulnar radiant of an intermediate axial triradius, t', but they may be discrete even without this separation—discrete in the sense that from neither configuration do ridges enter the pattern area of the other. In either case, each of the two configurations is independent and it conforms structurally to one of the primary types. The usual dual formulation is applied to signify the presence of two discrete configurations. The symbols of the two features are separated by a slant, the distal configuration being recorded first. Figure 75 shows a series of duplex configurations and their symbols. Qualify-ing symbols to indicate patterns of small size and pattern affinities of well developed vestiges follow the rules outlined for typical single configurations.

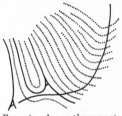

FIG. 76.—A parathenar pattern.

S-patterns (symbol: S) are double-looped designs, in which the two elements are interlocked by a flow of ridges from one into the other (Fig. 75).

Complex configurations not assignable to any of the types above characterized are formulated as Y.

PATTERNS WITHIN PATTERNS. Whorls, loops and sometimes other patterns may contain central configurations unlike the arrangement which gives character to the pattern as a whole; even an arch may enlodge a pattern within its concavity. Thus, an L^r may enclose a whorl, like the central pocket in finger prints. Since its general aspect is that of a loop, it is formulated as L^r with the addition of the symbol w (small letter, written on the same line rather than as a superscript, e.g., L^rw). Enclosed patterns are entitled to distinctive formulation only when they are of small size. When an enclosed whorl or loop exceeds a ridge count of eight it alone is formulated as the hypothenar pattern.

Parathenar patterns are assigned to the hypothenar area in routine formulation but are of doubtful morphological relationship to it (Chap. 9). When the area is patterned it appears as a narrow distally opening loop on the radial side of the hypothenar area proper (Fig. 76).

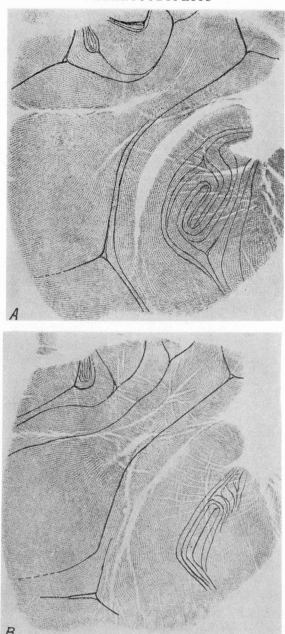

FIG. 77.—Two left palms with illustrative thenar/first interdigital configurations: Palm A, W^s/V; Palm B, L/V. (*From Wilder.*)

Thenar and First Interdigital Areas

The configurations of the thenar and first interdigital areas are closely related anatomically. In these two areas the varieties of configurational combinations are: (a) No indications of patterns or vestiges, the thenar eminence and the adjoining territory bearing a continuous open field. (b) A single pattern or vestige centered in an intermediate position with reference to the thenar and first interdigital areas (Fig. 72). (c) A pattern or vestige in the first interdigital area, the thenar configuration being an open field. (d) A pattern or vestige in the thenar area, the first interdigital area being an open field. (e) A pattern or vestige in each of the two areas (Fig. 77).

The patterns are whorls and loops. The vestiges are localized disarrangements of ridge course, frequently of the type shown in figure 78. The ridges composing open fields either course in a gentle curve or are sharply angulated over the thenar eminence (Fig. 71). The symbols are as described for configurations elsewhere, the initial letters of the names of the configurations: *W, L, V, O*. The directions of opening of loops might be indicated, but since the directions are nearly constant such formulation is hardly profitable. A single symbol is used for those configurations which lack a recognizable distinction of thenar and first interdigital areas. Dual formulation is made when the thenar and first interdigital elements can be differentiated, the symbol for the thenar being recorded first (Fig. 77). Bettmann presents detailed descriptions of these configurations.

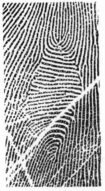

FIG. 78.—A common type of thenar/first interdigital vestige, occurring either as an isolated configuration or in company with separate indications of thenar and first interdigital. (*From Bettmann.*)

Second, Third and Fourth Interdigital Areas

The configurational area lying between digital triradii *a* and *b* is interdigital II, that between triradii *b* and *c* is interdigital III, and the configurational area between triradii *c* and *d* is interdigital IV. When a digital triradius fails or is much displaced the midpoint of the base of the corresponding digit affords a landmark separating the interdigital areas on either side. The configuration of an interdigital area may be a true pattern (whorl or loop), a vestige or an open field (including the special form of open field known as a multiplication). In one interdigital area there may be two configurations, each entitled to formulation. The usual type of dual symbol is used in formulating an interdigital area presenting two patterns, two vestiges or a pattern and a vestige—the feature on the radial side being written first, e.g., L/D.

Whorls (W) of the interdigital areas are invariably of small size and are accompanied by accessory triradii.

Loops characteristically open into the nearest interdigital interval. Other directions of opening are rare, hence formulation of these patterns does not record the direction of opening. A loop unaccompanied by an accessory triradius is formulated L, or l if the pattern is small. A loop of an interdigital area is formulated as small when the ridge count across its greatest width is no more than six ridges; the count is made at right angles to the long axis of the loop, the termini being the main line bounding the pattern. A loop accompanied by an accessory triradius is distinctively formulated, D (or d, if the count is no more than six ridges).

Vestiges (V) are conspicuous local disarrangements of ridges, not conforming to the definition of a true pattern but suggesting an approach toward the construction of a pattern. A vestige may be a group of sharply converging ridges, ellipsoidal in shape if convergences occur in both extremities, or a group of straight parallel ridges forming a distinctive field within a zone of ridges of different course.

Open fields (O) are patternless configurations. The increased width of an interdigital area at and near the level of the digital triradii (as in interdigital areas II and III of figure 72) is associated with curvatures of ridge course and with *multiplication* of ridges; multiplication signifies a greater number of ridges at the level of increased width of the area. Multiplications of this type are formulated merely as open fields because the multiplication is more or less evenly distributed across the interdigital area, contrasting with a localized region of multiplication wherein there is a concentrated spraying of ridges. Such a relationship is accentuated by tracing the ridges which border the multiplying system. Some degree of concentration of ridge multiplication commonly occurs in open fields of the interdigital areas II and IV, toward line A in the second area and toward line D in the fourth (e.g., Fig. 71). In formulation, multiplications of this type may be differentiated from simple open fields by using the symbol M instead of O. In many biological studies no distinction is made between a multiplication and an ordinary open field.

For the occurrence within a single interdigital area of two vestiges, two patterns, or a pattern and a vestige dual formulations are standard. An interdigital area having only a single pattern or vestige may justify dual formulation when that pattern or vestige is neither centered within the area nor expanded to fill its whole width. The symbols in such cases are O/L, L/O, etc., the radial element being entered first in the dual symbol. This principle of formulation applies to any interdigital area, but only in interdigital IV is there noteworthy frequency of such conditions.

OTHER METHODS OF FORMULATION

The foregoing exposition of methods of formulating palmar main lines, axial triradii and configurational areas is largely extracted from an account of revised methods (85) published in 1929. As a preliminary to the revision, a study (84) was made of the error incident to determinations, carried out by the methods then current, and the revision was designed to minimize inconstancy in formulation. The revised methods have not been subjected to such a test, but it will be evident that there remain some points (especially the discrimination of vestiges and of the levels of axial triradii) which are open to personal variation in interpretation. A test of the methods would be desirable, carried out perhaps in the same manner as before, with several workers independently formulating a large series of prints, made in manifold so that all workers would have identical sets.

Some suggestions toward revision of current methods already have been made, especially concerning more refined subdivision of the terminations of main lines. Valsik (99) and Meyer-Heydenhagen (219) subdivide position 3, in the belief that the portion of the palmar border ordinarily formulated under this one symbol is too extensive. The latter author distinguishes three levels of position 5, instead of the current two.

Valsik is critical of the landmarks generally employed in formulating main-line terminations, insisting that they should be confined to dermatoglyphic features; presumably he would resort to ridge counting to define zones of the ulnar border. Ride (92) uses ridge counting for this purpose. He designates the triradii by number: axial triradius, *1*; digital triradii *d*, *c*, *b* and *a* are *2*, *3*, *4* and *5* respectively. The zone on the radial margin of the axial triradius has the value from 0 to 1, the extensive interval from the axial triradius to triradius *d* has the value from 1 to 2, and so on through the first interdigital interval, which has the value from 5 to 6. Ridges are counted between the consecutively numbered triradii, and the termination of a line is expressed as a percent fraction of the distance from the triradius of the lower number to the triradius of the next higher number. Thus a main line terminating at the midpoint of the ulnar border would be formulated as 1.50. In determining the distance between consecutive digital triradii, Ride finds that direct measurement is usually satisfactory, but he prefers ridge counting especially for the ulnar border, where a curved line of count is drawn roughly parallel to that border; this line crosses ridges approximately transversely. Special provision is made for the two intervals which lack one end-point triradius, positions *1* and *13* of the standard formulation. In our opinion, such refinement of method gives a false appearance of precision.

Other classifications are proposed by Beletti, Ferrer, Lecha-Marzo, Pond, Sharp and Stockis. The methods need not be detailed here, since they are adapted especially for personal identification. Schlaginhaufen's method of descriptive classification (144), concerned with number and placement of triradii, is applicable both in palms and in soles.

METRIC ANALYSES

The procedures of ridge counting for determining quantitative values of finger patterns and for obtaining an indirect measure of ridge breadth (Chap. 4) are adaptable to the palm (and sole). Ridge counting also may be used as a measure of other dimensional relations, for example the distances between successive digital triradii or, as mentioned above in connection with Ride's proposal, the distance between a main-line termination and a designated triradius. In some studies calling for determination of certain dimensions, absolute measurements are no less satisfactory than the tedious and time-consuming method of counting ridges, which is itself faulty as a metric procedure because of variability in ridge breadth. Direct measurement is suitable when differences in total hand size are too small to be of any consequence, as in comparisons of all four hands in twins. For comparisons in which individuals of unlike hand size are concerned, the method is obviously unsuitable (98) unless there is an appropriate correction factor for the varying hand sizes.

Direct measurements have been made in several studies. In an analysis of bimanual differences (86) and in an attempt to determine whether such differences vary with handedness (351), the following procedure was adopted, supplementing qualitative comparisons of the palmar dermatoglyphics. In preparing prints for these studies, particular care was taken to minimize the error which is associated with variability in pressure and in spreading of the hand.

The measurements involve distances between triradii and between triradii and certain lines (Fig. 79). The instrument employed is a caliper having sharp points for fixation within triradii and on lines, and long jaws which serve as verticals for some of the measurements. The following intervals are measured, the results being discussed elsewhere (Chap. 11): (a) Intertriradial interval *a-b*. (b) Intertriradial interval *b-c*. (c) Intertriradial interval *c-d*. (d) Intertriradial interval *a-d*. (e) The distance from triradius *d* to the level of the marginal termination of line *D*, measured from *d* along the line *a-d* to the point of intersection of *a-d* and a vertical dropped to it from point *D*; this measurement and *a-d* give the *line-D index*. (f) The vertical distance from *a-d* to the axial triradius, or to the one most proximal if there are two or three axial triradii. (g) The distance from the axial triradius to a vertical dropped proximally from triradius *a*, the interval being measured along a line parallel to *a-d*. (h) The distance

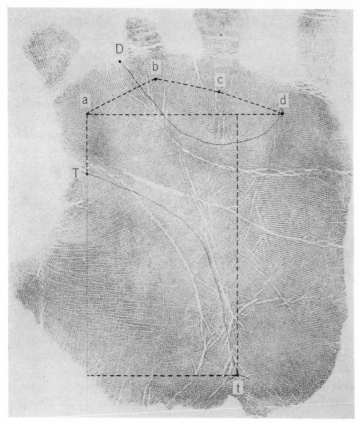

FIG. 79.—A right palm, illustrating reference points for several measurements, including those for determination of the line-D index.

from the terminal portion of line *T* to triradius *a*, measured along a vertical intersecting line *a-d*.

In her study of twins Meyer-Heydenhagen (219) introduces three other measures, none of them having reference to fixed base lines: (a) The distance from triradius *a* to the nearest major flexion crease, variably the proximal transverse crease or the radial longitudinal crease. (b) The distance from triradius *d* to the distal transverse flexion crease. (c) The distance from triradius *b* to axial triradius.

Determinations of pattern form may be made in at least some of the configurational areas by the same methods as those used for finger prints. Meyer-Heydenhagen measures the breadth and height of loops in interdigital areas II, III and IV. She places the axis of the measuring disc through the middle of the loop, and the base line through the nearest triradius. Width is read along the base line from the axis to the triradius; height is read along the axis from the base line to the intersection of the axis with a line traced around the pattern from the triradius (usually a main line, but sometimes the radiant of an accessory triradius). It will be evident from the topography of the palmar interdigital patterns, that the morphological "base" of the pattern faces distally, rather than proximally as in finger prints.

STATISTICAL TRENDS

The workings of the methods of formulation may be appreciated through examination of a sample of mass data, a collection of 1281 German males chosen from available unpublished materials.[2] Terminations of main lines, occurrences of axial triradii and configuration types of palmar areas are presented in tables 5–10. It should be understood that differing trends associated with race, sex and constitution would be disclosed in other samples. However, as in the presentation of finger-print characteristics, the fundamental directions of variation are here exhibited.

Main Lines

The list of main-line formulae for a series of palms is tallied in two different ways. One tally is devoted to individual main lines, the terminations in each of the several positions being counted. Another tally is concerned with the main lines in combination, that is, a count of the numbers of different main-line formulae, or combinations of main lines of individual palms. In the compilation, the second symbol of an alternative formulation is disregarded. Dual formulations of line D have one symbol representing a radiant which extends farther radially than the other; it is this symbol which is tallied. Dual formulations of line A have one symbol representing a radiant extending to a position farther ulnarward or farther proximally than the other; this symbol is entered in the tally. The stated choice of one symbol in dual formulations of lines D and A is governed

---

[2] The Poll Papers (15) include a collection of palm prints and finger prints. The finger prints had been analyzed and reported by Poll. He had not worked at all with the palm prints, which have been since traced and formulated in accord with the "Revised methods." The data here recorded in tables 5–10 are from this collection.

by the fact that the general courses of ridges over the palm are best registered by this means.

Line T usually is not included in the tabulations, though it may be noted that its terminations are most frequently in position *13* and next in *12* and *11*. The line runs nearer the thumb in right hands (86, 93, 293).

TABLE 5

PERCENT FREQUENCIES OF TERMINATIONS OF PALMAR MAIN LINES IN 1281 GERMAN MALES
(Bold-faced type emphasizes the preponderant terminations)

Posi-tions	Line D		Line C		Line B		Line A	
	R	L	R	L	R	L	R	L
1	....	....	....	....	....	....	1.3	11.3
2	....	....	....	....	....	....	1.8	5.2
3	....	....	....	....	0.1	0.5	**20.0**	**38.6**
4	....	....	....	....	0.2	1.0	**17.6**	**14.9**
5′	....	....	....	0.2	**3.4**	**10.9**	**46.8**	**25.1**
5″	0.1	0.1	**7.7**	**15.6**	**31.8**	**47.5**	11.6	4.8
6	....	....	2.7	1.8	**6.5**	**8.6**	0.4	
7	**7.4**	**15.5**	**20.6**	**33.2**	**52.3**	**31.1**	0.5	
8	2.7	2.0	....	0.2	3.5	0.1		
9	**25.1**	**42.2**	**54.0**	**31.9**	2.0	0.2		
10	6.6	8.9	3.5	0.1				
11	**57.1**	**31.2**	2.0	0.2				
12	0.2							
13	0.5							
X	....	0.2	4.5	10.1	0.1			
x	....	....	0.2	0.6				
o	0.2	....	4.8	6.3	0.2	0.2		

ANALYSIS OF INDIVIDUAL MAIN LINES. Table 5 lists the percent frequencies of the several positions of termination. The distribution of figures in the table indicates that the four main lines have differential trends. Terminations of line D are almost limited to the distal border, mainly in positions *11*, *9* and *7*. Line C terminates usually in the more ulnar regions of the distal border and the distal portions of the ulnar border, the largest frequencies being in positions *9*, *7* and *5″*. Line B carries this shift still farther. Terminations in the distal border are almost limited to positions *7* and *6*, and there is a much larger share of terminations in the distal part of the ulnar border than is the case for line C. Line A continues the ulnar-proximal progression, since it nearly always reaches the ulnar and proximal borders of the palm.

Line C is noteworthy for its relatively frequent absence and for its tendency to be abortive. Closely allied to the abortive state is the condition in which the line recurves distally to fuse with itself or with a digital radiant. In the present series no other main line of this character occurs, and though the condition is rare in line *C*, its confinement to this line is a significant correlate of the relative abundance of abortive states. Even a line *C* which reaches position *7* or *9* may not be far removed from the condition formulated as *8*, since the smallness of many loops enclosed by it (Tables 9 and 10) indicates a trend of suppression of line *C*. All the varieties of suppression of line *C* are more frequent in left hands.

Morphological limitations exclude the possibility of main-line terminations in certain positions and may reduce potentially higher frequencies in others. There are varying degrees of association of the main lines in individual palms (83). In the rare instance of termination of line *D* in position *13*, line *A* necessarily courses to the distal border of the palm. This is an obligative relationship, determined by morphological boundaries. When line *D* terminates in position *11* or in a position farther ulnarward, line *A* is topographically freed for a course to the proximal or ulnar border. Notwithstanding such topographic independence, line *A* tends to reach positions more and more proximally in correlation with the more ulnarward terminations of line *D*. Similar associations exist between line *D* and other lines, and between line *B* and others.

The distribution of frequencies of terminations of a main line does not conform to a regular curve of variation, as may be illustrated by reference to line *D*. Its terminations in positions *8* and *10* are limited in number because these positions are points (digital triradii), while the expanse of the interdigital areas allows for more frequent entrances of main lines. Depressions, separating peaks of sharply increased frequency, are not due entirely to this fact nor to a default of the method of formulation. They appear also when the level of termination of line *D* is determined by ridge counting (93) or by measurement (86). The method of measurement and its results are as follows:

With line *D* completely traced, its radialward extent is expressed in reference to the length of a line connecting digital triradii *a* and *d* (Fig. 79). A vertical to line *a-d* is dropped from the terminal point of line *D*. The distance between the intersection and triradius *d* is stated as a proportion of line *a-d*, the percent fraction being multiplied by 100 to convert the result to a whole number, the line-*D* index. In one series of European-Americans, the average index in right hands is 64.7 and in lefts 55.8 (86). The line-*D* index is more variable in left hands.

Figure 80 demonstrates both the conspicuous bimanual difference of the line-*D* index and the trimodal frequency distribution which is a correlate of the. topographic relationships of the positions in which line

D terminates (interdigital intervals and digital triradii). The peaks in this graph correspond to terminations in interdigital intervals, while the two sharp depressions of frequencies are associated with the more restricted terminations in triradial points.

ANALYSIS OF THE COLLECTIVE MAIN-LINE FORMULA. In an analysis of mass statistics it is not sufficient to consider the main lines singly, dismembered from their combinations in individual palms. At the same time, a mere tally of different main-line formulae is pointless, since the four main lines are so variously combined in different palms; there occur, for example, over 170 different formula in one series of about 4000 palms (276). Some elements of the formula are irrelevant to its import as a descriptive device in the common statistical applications, while others are subject to grouping in morphologically related classes.

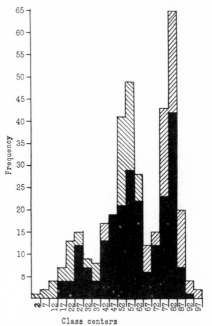

Several schemes of summating single main lines and collective formulae have been proposed. One procedure consists in bringing together, for individual main lines, the terminations which are closely related. The advantage in such grouping is the reduction of the effects of artificialities attending initial formulations—for example, in the discrimination between terminations of line D in positions 7 and 8 or in positions 9 and 10. For line D it has been suggested (276) that the ter-

FIG. 80.—Frequency distribution of the line-D index in 300 right palms and 300 lefts. Common distribution of right and left, solid black; right alone, ////; left alone, \\\\.

minations be grouped in three modal types. These types are designated 7, 9 and 11. *Type 7* includes positions 7, 8, X and 5; *type 9* embraces positions 9 and 10; *type 11* includes positions 11, 12 and 13. In the same manner the endings of line A may be brought together under three modal types (95): *type 5*, including positions 7, 6, $5''$ and $5'$; *type 3* includes positions 4 and 3; *type 1* includes positions 1 and 2. Lines B and C might be treated in a similar manner; but from the practical standpoint the gain would be insignificant. In racial comparisons (Chap. 15) the available data are chiefly in the form of frequencies of types 7, 9 and 11 of line D. These data are perforce used, though the method is obviously inferior to the main-line index now to be described.

The main-line formula serves to describe generalized direction of ridges, but of the four main lines, D and A are adequate to depict the general ridge direction in all palms. A record of the terminations of lines D and A, as combined in individual palms, is the *main-line index*, a useful and simple device (83) for recording the most significant features of the total main-line formula. This index is in a sense an expression of the direction of a neutral line, its inclination being determined by the courses of lines D and A. The index is not a proportion but a summation of values describing the courses of these two main lines. Values are assigned to the

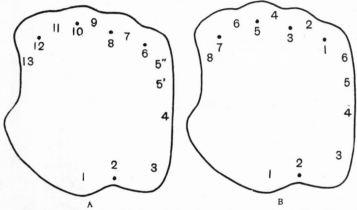

Fig. 81.—The symbols employed in formulating the terminations of main lines (A) and their equivalents as values (B) in the main-line index.

positions used in the scheme of formulating main lines (Fig. 81). For line A the original numerical symbols of the ulnar and proximal borders are adopted as values, with the single exception that value 6 is assigned to position $5''$. It will be apparent, therefore, that the series 1 through 6 stands for a progressive shift from longitudinal to transverse alignment of line A. Line-D terminations are evaluated so that slants in the distal palm receive values which are essentially equal to those given corresponding slants of line A. Thus, values 1 through 8 are substituted respectively for positions 6 through 13 in the scheme of formulation. The index is the sum of the values of lines A and D. Reference to several examples will elucidate its descriptive service. In a palm having the formula 11.—.—.5″ the courses of both lines indicate transversality, and the sum of the respective values (6 + 6) for these positions is an index very near the maximum. Another palm, with the formula 9.—.—.4 (for which the values are $4 + 4$) is an intermediate slant between the transverse and longitudinal. The association of the courses of lines A and D is not rigidly fixed, and their courses, unlike the two examples cited, may not be of the same rank of transversality. The formula 9.—.—.2 (values $4 + 2$) is an instance of this relationship, and it will be noted that in all such cases the index is as adequately expressive of the totality of ridge direction as in the cases where both lines possess the same value.

The main-line index may be computed from independent tallies of terminations of lines A and D, but for statistical purposes each palm is rated separately. In the German series (Table 5) the average index of the 2562 palms is 8.66. Right palms alone average 9.50 and lefts 7.82. As measured by the index, therefore, transversality is 21% more pronounced in right palms.

Axial Triradii

The frequencies of axial triradii at the different levels and in various combinations, in the German series, are listed in table 6. In a large majority of palms there is but one axial triradius, most commonly situated at or

TABLE 6

FREQUENCIES OF TYPES AND COMBINATIONS OF AXIAL TRIRADII IN 1281 GERMAN MALES

Types	Right	Left	Types	Right	Left
t	61.0%	64.8%	tt''	6.5%	4.1%
t'	20.7	21.7	$t't''$	0.8	0.3
t''	2.3	1.9	ttt''	. . . . .	0.1
tt	0.2	0.2	$tt't''$	0.2	0.5
tt'	6.5	6.2	$t't't''$	0.1	
$t't'$	0.4	0.3	?	1.5	0.1
			(O or t)		

very near the proximal border (t). Among the combinations of two triradii in single palms, tt' and tt'' are the most common. Combinations of three triradii are rare. The lack of precision in the method of formulating axial triradii is to be kept in mind if these features are compared in racial or other samples. The exceedingly rare combinations of two triradii lying at the same level (tt; $t't'$) denote the presence of parathenar patterns (Fig. 76) or vestiges.

Configurational Areas

HYPOTHENAR. Hypothenar configurations of the 2562 palms composing the German series are of 44 differently formulated types (Table 7). The level of variability compares closely to that of another series (82) in which there are 48 formulae for 2827 palms. Each of the primary types with its variants (Fig. 74) is represented, and a number of the derived forms (Fig. 75) occur.

TABLE 7

FREQUENCIES OF THE TYPES OF HYPOTHENAR CONFIGURATIONS IN 1281 GERMAN MALES

Types	Right	Left	Types	Right	Left
A^u	44.1%	50.0%	L^u/A^c	0.4%	0.2%
A^c	1.6	1.4	L^r/A^r	0.1	
A^r	1.5	0.2	$A^u/L^u/A^{c\cdot}$	0.3	0.2
A^u/A^c	16.0	16.7			
			W	0.7	0.5
V	0.9	0.9	W^s	1.4	0.6
$A^u/V/A^c$	......	0.1	A^u/W	0.5	0.2
A^u/V	0.1	0.3	A^u/W^s	....	0.1
V/A^c	0.3	0.1	A^r/W	0.1	
SV	0.1		W/A^c	0.3	
			W^s/A^c		0.1
T^r	0.5	0.1			
T^u	0.1				
T^c	......	0.1	L^r/V	0.2	
			$A^u/L^u/V$	....	0.1
L^r	15.7	13.6	V/L^u	0.1	0.1
L^u	3.0	2.4	T^r/L^u	0.1	
L^c	0.8	0.5	L^r/L^u	0.5	1.2
A^u/L^r	0.2	0.1	L^r/L^r	0.4	
A^u/L^u	4.5	4.6	L^u/L^u	0.1	0.2
A^u/L^c	0.5		S	1.6	0.9
A^r/L^r	0.1		A^u/S	0.1	
A^r/L^u	0.1		S/A^c	0.1	0.2
A^c/L^u	......	0.1	W/L^u	....	0.2
L^r/A^c	3.3	4.4	$W/L^u/A^c$	0.1	

The majority (65.7%) of these hypothenar configurations are plain arches, chiefly A^u and A^u/A^c; vestiges occur in 1.4% of the cases, and the remainder (32.9%) are patterns of various types. The frequencies of pattern types are: tented arches, 0.4%; one loop, either alone or in company with a plain arch, 27.4%; one whorl, either alone or in company with a plain arch, 2.2%; two loops, S-patterns and varied combinations, 2.9%. Counting plain arches, vestiges and true patterns together, 71.4% are single configurations and 28.6% are duplex (or triplex in a few instances). True patterns are slightly more abundant in right palms than in lefts, the respective frequencies being 35.4% and 30.4%. (The values listed in this paragraph are obtained from absolute frequencies in the original data, thus avoiding the error incident to summation of percent frequencies for the numerous types, as listed in table 7.)

THENAR AND FIRST INTERDIGITAL. Table 8 lists the configuration types of these two areas in the German series. Eighteen different formulations are required. Both areas, in 85.1% of the palms, lack vestiges or

TABLE 8

FREQUENCIES OF THE TYPES OF CONFIGURATIONS OF THE THENAR/FIRST INTERDIGITAL AREA
IN 1281 GERMAN MALES

Types	Right	Left	Types	Right	Left
O	90.5%	79.8%	V/V	0.7%	1.4%
V	2.7	6.1	V/L	0.3	0.4
L	0.3	1.2	L/O	1.2	0.6
W	0.2		L/V	1.5	3.9
W*	0.1		L/L	0.2	2.3
O/V	0.6	1.3	W/O	0.2	0.5
O/L	0.1	0.2	W/V	0.2	0.6
O/W	......	0.1	W/L	.....	0.2
V/O	1.2	1.5	W/W	0.1	

patterns. A vestige or pattern is present in one or both of the areas in the remainder, 14.9%. The coexistence of separate vestiges or patterns in both the thenar and first interdigital areas is the most frequent relationship, amounting to 5.9% of the whole series of palms; in 2.6% the thenar

TABLE 9

FREQUENCIES OF THE TYPES OF CONFIGURATIONS OF THE SECOND AND THIRD INTERDIGITAL
AREAS IN 1281 GERMAN MALES

Type	Interdigital II		Interdigital III	
	R	L	R	L
O	83.8%	92.7%	36.1%	56.7%
V	7.4	2.8	3.2	10.2
l	.....	.....	4.4	6.6
L	.....	.....	54.9	25.6
d	1.4	0.7		0.1
D	7.4	3.7	1.4	0.6
W	.....	.....	0.1	0.2

alone bears a vestige or a pattern, and in 1.2% the first interdigital is thus distinguished. There are 5.2% of palms displaying a single vestige or pattern placed in an intermediate position and not expressly assignable to the thenar or the first interdigital area. There is a distinct bimanual difference in the frequency of vestiges and patterns, the left palm having the greater number.

SECOND, THIRD AND FOURTH INTERDIGITAL AREAS. Since there are no duplex configurations in the second and third interdigital areas of the German series, the number of possible configurational variants is limited to the seven types listed in table 9.

Of the three interdigital areas in the distal palm, the second area presents the lowest frequency of vestiges and patterns. In the German series the patterns are invariably loops having an accessory triradius. Of all

TABLE 10

FREQUENCIES OF THE TYPES OF CONFIGURATIONS OF THE FOURTH INTERDIGITAL AREA IN 1281 GERMAN MALES

Types	Right	Left	Types	Right	Left
O	51.4%	27.7%	l/V	0.1%	1.2%
V	7.3	10.0	L/V	0.5	2.7
l	2.2	6.4	L/d	0.1	0.1
L	27.6	35.6	V/D	0.1	
d	0.8	0.6	l/D	0.1	1.6
D	8.0	9.5	L/D	0.5	2.3
W	1.4	2.1	l/W	. . . . .	0.1
V/V	. . . . .	0.1	L/W	. . . . .	0.1
All single patterns and vestiges.				47.3	64.2
All duplex combinations of patterns and vestiges.				1.3	8.0

palms in the collection, 6.6% bear this type of configuration. Vestiges occur in 5.1% of the palms. Vestiges and patterns of the second interdigital area are more abundant in right hands than in lefts.

The third interdigital area is marked by a vestige or pattern in 53.6% of the palms. The most common pattern is a loop (without accessory triradius), occurring with a frequency of 45.8%. A loop with an accessory triradius is infrequent (1.0%) and whorls are extremely rare (0.15%). Vestiges amount to 6.7% in the whole series. Well developed patterning of this area is a distinctive trend of right hands, but small loops and vestiges occur more commonly in left hands.

The fourth interdigital area (Table 10) shows a relatively frequent occurrence of duplex combinations of patterns or vestiges, 4.7%. Single patterns or vestiges occur in 55.8% of all hands. The most common pattern type, whether single or in combination, is the loop without an accessory triradius. Loops with the accessory triradius as well as whorls are more common than in the second or third interdigital area. There is marked bimanual asymmetry of patterns and vestiges, 72.3% of the left hands bearing single and duplex combinations, as against 48.6% in right hands.

Summary

Each palmar main line, notwithstanding individual variability, courses within a prescribed field. Line D is extended radialward in the distal region of the palm, terminating along the distal border with only rare exceptions. Line C extends in a field characteristically occupying only the ulnar portion of the distal border and the distal part of the ulnar border; this line is distinctive in the frequency of complete and partial suppression. Line B involves a still more ulnarward restricted portion of the distal border of the palm, and in compensation there is an increased entry into the distal half of the ulnar border. Terminations of line A are virtually confined to the ulnar and proximal borders of the palm. The distinctive bimanual trends exhibited in main lines indicate a greater tendency in right hands toward transverse coursing of ridges. The suppressed states of line C are more frequent in left hands.

The frequencies of patterns and vestiges vary widely among the several configurational areas. Combining true patterns and vestiges (in the German series, here used as a sample), the fourth interdigital has the highest frequency (60.5%), the third interdigital next (53.6%), and there is a rapidly diminishing frequency from hypothenar (34.3%) to the thenar/first interdigital combined (14.9%) and second interdigital (11.8%). The following areas display larger frequencies of patterns in right hands: hypothenar, second interdigital and third interdigital. The thenar, first interdigital and fourth interdigital areas have higher frequencies of patterns and vestiges in left hands.

SOLES

TOPOGRAPHY

STANDARD anatomical terms are applied for designating directions and describing the locations of plantar features. *Distal* and *proximal* have the same meanings in hand and foot, but in the foot the equivalent of radial is *tibial* and the equivalent of ulnar is *fibular*. The terms tibial and fibular are derived from the names of the two bones of the lower leg, tibia and fibula, which respectively are on the sides of the big toe and little toe.

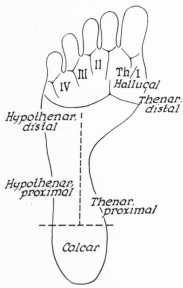

FIG. 82.—Topography of plantar configurational areas. Broken lines indicate approximate boundaries.

CONFIGURATIONAL AREAS. There are eight plantar configurational areas (Fig. 82), which should be compared to the previously described palmar areas. The region of the foot corresponding topographically to the hypothenar eminence of the palm is much more elongated, occupying the fibular region of the sole and the entire heel. The heel region is the *calcar* area of dermatoglyphic topography. The remainder of the fibular region of the sole constitutes the *hypothenar* area proper; this area is divisible into *distal* and *proximal* sections. The homologue of the region of the thenar eminence in the palm is likewise elongated, and is separated into *distal* and *proximal* thenar areas. The distal thenar area is a component of the tibial portion of the ball of the foot. In the ball region there are four dermatoglyphic areas, which in tibio-fibular sequence are: *hallucal* (representing the *distal thenar* and *first interdigital* combined), the *second, third,* and *fourth interdigitals*. These four areas usually may be individually distinguished not only through the presence of triradii and radiants which limit them but also by the fact that each often bears a discrete pattern covering its entire expanse. In the fetus and infant the individuality of the areas of the ball region is evidenced further by their slight elevation as pads. The configurations of all plantar areas are classifiable, and as in fingers and palms they may be treated by the method of "pattern intensity."

As in the palm, the distal radiants of each digital triradius typically embrace a *digital area*. In the sole there are five digital areas instead of four, since in relation to the big toe there is commonly a digital triradius that has no counterpart in the palm.

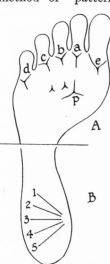

TRIRADII. The characteristic topography of the triradii of the distal sole is shown in figure 83,A. It is appropriate to name the digital triradii in accord with the system applied in the palm, so that *a*, *b*, *c*, and *d* are homologous in palm and sole, though the triradius at the base of the big toe requires a new literal designation, *e*.

In the proximal region of the ball there commonly occurs a triradius, or more than one; such triradii mark the conjunctions of configurational areas when the designs of the opposed configurations are of unlike directions. Called "lower deltas" (i.e., lower triradii) by Wilder, and not otherwise named here except for the one (*p*—for proximal) associated with the conjunction of the hallucal and second interdigital areas, they correspond to the accessory

FIG. 83.—*A*. The plan of triradii in the distal sole. *B*. Diagram of ridge directions, with numerical symbols applicable in description of the alignment of ridges in the mid-region and calcar area.

TABLE II
SYMBOLS FOR PLANTAR TRIRADII

Literal Symbols		Numerical Symbols of Schlaginhaufen
d		17
c	Digital triradii	3
b	(in fibulo-tibial	2
a	order)	19
e		13
p		9
—	Proximal triradii	15
—	(in tibio-fibular	11
—	order)	16

triradii of certain types of palmar interdigital configurations (D, d and W). Harkness-Miller suggests that these lower triradii, perhaps especially p, might be homologous to axial triradii of the palm.

Except for the work of Wilder (101, 114) and of Schlaginhaufen (144) little attention has been given to the systematization of the plan of plantar triradii. Table 11 identifies the foregoing designations of triradii with Schlaginhaufen's numerical symbols, which have been adopted by a few workers (for example, Bychowska, 127).

FORMULATION OF MAIN LINES

The proximal radiants of the five digital triradii may be considered as main lines and traced on sole prints in accord with the rules outlined for the palm. Occasionally "pseudo-digital triradii" (105) occur; they may be compared descriptively to displaced digital triradii (Fig. 90: the triradii proximal to the second and third toes). The radiants of triradius p, or indeed of any lower triradius, likewise may be traced to their terminations. These traced lines, whether issuing from digital, pseudo-digital or lower triradii, may be formulated like palmar main lines.

Certain technical difficulties arise in application of the method. (a) One or more digital triradii may not be included in the print and the lines originating from them accordingly are not traceable. (b) Triradius p, the radiants of which might be useful as an indicator of general ridge direction, is frequently absent. (c) A main line may enter an interdigital area, and become involved in its pattern, so that its course is of no significance for describing generalities of ridge direction. The formulation of such lines is extremely intricate (166), and the detail has only limited usefulness in biological analyses. (d) Main lines frequently extend to positions on the tibial and fibular borders, where there are no definite anatomical landmarks for the establishment of intervals and points.

Despite these difficulties, it is desirable at times to describe plantar main lines in terms of the positions of their endings along the plantar borders. The distal border lends itself to the same system followed in the formulation of palmar lines, with interdigital intervals and digital triradii numbered to indicate positions of termination. The lines, including radiants from triradius p, may course to the distal portions of the tibial and fibular borders, and, if they are to be formulated at all, it is fitting that the procedure take into account the morphological affinities of palm and sole. These relationships are here presented from the viewpoint of comparative dermatoglyphics (141).

Figure 84 is designed to emphasize the parallelisms between palm and sole by applying to the sole the symbols used for homologous intervals

and points in the palm. The numbers for positions along the distal border
are those originally proposed by Wilder (114) in an exposition of methods
which few workers have since adopted owing to the technical difficulties
mentioned. Reference already has been made to the elongation in the sole
of the regions corresponding to the palmar hypothenar and thenar areas.
Methods of formulating terminations of main lines along the plantar
borders have not been standardized. The present suggestion of zones for
formulation goes little farther than to draw at-
tention to homologies, with a view to securing
uniformity in the treatment of palm and sole.
Along the fibular border the most distal segment
is here designated 5, and, though there is no
landmark to separate its distal and proximal
regions, zones 5″ and 5′ might be distinguished
as in the palm. There is likewise no proximal
boundary, and the only criterion of the individuality of this zone is the frequent presence of
a distal hypothenar pattern (Fig. 92) and the
appearance in the fetus of a localized pad in this
region. It is the maximum expanse of the distal
hypothenar pattern and of the corresponding
fetal pad which sets the proximal boundary of
zone 5 (Fig. 84). Point 4 of the fibular border is
located somewhat distal to the mid-level of the
margin. The proximal hypothenar territory
(position 3) is markedly elongated. Position 3
includes about two-thirds of the fibular border
and the entire heel margin. The inclusion under
one symbol for formulation of so prolonged a
share of the foot margin is not a disadvantage
inasmuch as plantar main lines do not extend

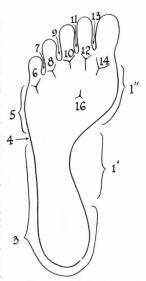

Fig. 84.—Border positions
of the sole, with their symbols.
Homologies with the palm
are indicated by the use of
the same numerical symbols,
with the addition of 14 and 16
for two triradii which have
no counterparts in the palmar
scheme.

far proximally. The tibial margin distal to the heel corresponds to position 1 in the palm, but it may be subdivided into distal (1″) and proximal
(1′) halves for descriptive formulation.

Since the main lines do not extend farther proximally than the middle
of the sole, their formulation affords no indication of the general alignment
of ridges in a large share of the plantar surface. Some workers accordingly
have adopted Schlaginhaufen's practice of describing the variable alignments. In figure 83,B five grades of alignment are indicated. The slants
may be characterized by describing them in terms of coursing from the
fibular to the tibial margin:

1—Pronounced slant proximally

2—Slight slant proximally

3—Transverse

4—Slight slant distally

5—Pronounced slant distally.

It will be apparent that distinctions between consecutive grades can not be sharply drawn without resort to angular measurements, a procedure which has not been adopted by investigators employing this descriptive method.

FORMULATION OF CONFIGURATIONAL AREAS

Many workers limit their analyses of the plantar dermatoglyphics to the frequencies of configuration types in the several areas, often only the four areas of the ball region. For identification purposes the suggested classifications are naturally so limited (79, 109). Even in the ball region faulty technique in printing may make it necessary to exclude some prints of a series. If the extreme distal border is incompletely registered, lapses involving some pattern types might lead to erroneous classification (e.g., a loop having its head in the unprinted zone would appear as an open field, or a whorl would appear as a loop having its opening in an interdigital interval).

The following account of configuration types and symbols for their formulation is based mainly upon the methods of Wilder, of Schlaginhaufen and of Montgomery. There is only partial agreement of scope and method among these three writers. In instances of their discrepant treatment of the same configurational areas our choice of methods aims to secure maximum descriptive usefulness and the greatest possible conformity to methods applied in the fingers and palm. Modifications of description and formulation are introduced at some points (especially in connection with the hypothenar), which in the light of new information call for a more extended or a different analysis.

The ten sole tracings illustrated in figures 85–94 depict most of the varieties of configuration occurring in each of the eight areas, and their legends supply the formulations of the configuration types.

HALLUCAL AREA. The hallucal area, occupying the tibial part of the ball region, presents four primary types of configuration: whorls (in the sense of Galton), loops, tented arches, open fields. Each of the primary types, as described below, exhibits different varieties. In addition to these, there may occur in any area a vestige (symbol, V), characterized as in the palmar configurational areas.

Whorls, as in finger prints, may be considered either as a comprehensive group, or the group may be subdivided. If subdivided, the types may be formulated by using *W* as the primary symbol, adding abbreviations of the names of sub-types for all except the typical concentric or spiral whorl. Otherwise primary status may be given to each of the types,

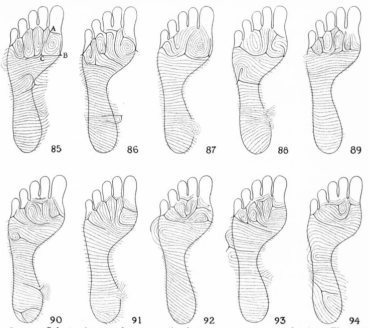

FIGS. 85–94.—Sole tracings, each a composite from two or more actual prints. The pattern formulae are:

85.—$W.L^d.L^d.L^d.L^t/L^f.O.V.$
86.—$W.L^p.W.W.V.O.L^f.$
87.—$Sm.O.L^d.L^p.V.O.L^f.$
88.—$LP.O.L^d_+ IV.L^t/L^t.O.V/V.$
89.—$CP^d.W.W.L^d.V/O.O.O.$
90.—$L^d.V.L^p.O.W/V.L^t.L^t.$
91.—$L^t.O.O.O.O.V.V.$
92.—$L^f.V.W.O.L^t/O.O.O.$
93.—$T^d.L^p.W.W.L^t/L^t.O.V.$
94.—$O.L^d.O.O.L^t.L^t.O.$

thus: *W* for the true whorl, *CP* for central pocket, etc. The main types, with symbols, are:

(a) A typical concentric or spiral whorl (*W*: Figs. 85, 86).

(b) A whorl presenting an S-shaped central design (*WS*).

(c) Seam, a whorl showing abrupt interruption of the concentric circuit, with a number of ridges ending in a right-angled relation to a part of the system (W^{sm}: Fig. 87).

(d) Lateral pocket, or two interlocked loops; tracings from the two cores reach the same plantar margin (*LP*: Fig. 88).

(e) Twin loop (*TL*), or two interlocked loops, differing from the above in that core tracings reach different plantar margins (e.g., tibial and distal). Lateral pockets and twin loops may not justify distinction in many biological analyses.

(f) Central pocket, a loop having one or more recurved ridges in its center, corresponding morphologically to the central pocket occurring in finger prints. Since there are three types of loops distinguished by the directions of their openings (L^d, L^t, L^f—see below), superscripts are added to indicate these types—CP^d (Fig. 89); CP^t; CP^f.

Loops of the hallucal area have their open extremities pointed in three directions: distally (L^d, Fig. 90); to the tibial margin (L^t, Fig. 91); to the fibular margin (L^f, Fig. 92). (L^d, L^t and L^f correspond respectively to Wilder's types *A*, *B* and *C*.)

Tented arches (*T*, Fig. 93) usually are not subdivided, though the system adopted for the palmar hypothenar might be applied here. A tented arch may be described in terms of the facing of its base, using the initial letter of that direction as a superscript in the symbol.

Open fields (*O*, Fig. 94), which actually are plain arches, ordinarily are not designated by their directions, but the method of formulating plain arches of the palmar hypothenar may be applied. Wilder (101) recognizes three classes of open fields on the basis of non-appearance of specific triradii. The rationale of Wilder's classification of open fields is a series of morphological affinities traceable from the relationships of triradii in a whorl. In a typical whorl of the hallucal area (Fig. 85) there are three triradii: *A*, lying distal to the pattern; *B*, on the tibial side; *C*, on the fibular side. His designations of hallucal loops (*A*, *B* and *C*) indicate the directions of their openings, each type being interpreted as if it were converted from a whorl to a loop by suppression of the triradius on the side of its opening. In turn, types of open fields (*AB*, *AC* and *BC*) are individually distinguished by reference to the location of the two triradii which are assumed to have disappeared in each. In accord with this interpretation the open field in figure 94 is *BC*.

SECOND, THIRD AND FOURTH INTERDIGITAL AREAS. These are the "plantar areas" of Wilder, as distinguished from the hallucal area, and they are respectively the first, second and third interdigitals of many writers. The hallucal area is morphologically a fusion of the distal thenar and first interdigital (Chap. 9), hence it seems desirable to adhere to a scheme of numbering the three "plantar areas" which agrees with their true identities as second, third and fourth interdigitals.

All the areas exhibit the same general types of configurations:

Whorls (*W*: Galton's inclusive sense, the occasional deviations from the construction of true whorls not being recognized in formulation). See figure 86, areas III and IV; figure 89, areas II and III.

Loops may open distally (*U*, or *L^d*: Fig. 85, II, III and IV) or proximally (*Ω*, or *L^p*: Fig. 86, II; 87, IV).

Vestiges (*V*), localized disarrangements of ridge direction, especially in the form of abrupt convergences, lacking the recurvatures which characterize true patterns.

Open fields (*O*), as previously defined for palmar interdigital areas (Fig. 87, II; Fig. 91, II, III and IV).

Departures from the typical relationships of interdigital areas sometimes occur. A pattern or vestige may not be centered in exact alignment with an interdigital interval; interdigital II in figure 90 is displaced in this manner, being as closely related to the third interdigital interval as to the second. In such cases, however, the sequence of configurations in the ball region may offer a clue to their individualities. It is not uncommon that two adjoining configurational areas are united as a single pattern (Fig. 88, III and IV). Here, too, the identities of the configurational areas involved are clear; in formulating, any convenient symbol (e.g., note legend of figure 88) might be chosen to indicate the fusion of two configurational areas.

The typical relationship of interdigital configurations which open into interdigital intervals (*O*, *L^d*, and some vestiges) is that ridges flowing from an interdigital area enter the interval of corresponding number. Not infrequently, however, the opening ridges may be deviated to another interval (Fig. 87, where ridges from area II reach the first interdigital interval; Fig. 94, where the configuration of III enters the fourth interval). Such a deviation, which is associated with suppressions of digital triradii and fusions of the related digital areas, might be recognized in formulation by adding to the symbol of the configuration type, as a superscript, the number of the interdigital interval receiving the aberrant opening of the configuration.

HYPOTHENAR. The hypothenar area demands a special formulation adapted to the variable relationships of configurations in its distal and proximal territories. Sometimes the distal and proximal regions are separately recognizable (Fig. 93), but the two may be blended either into one pattern (Fig. 94) or vestige (Fig. 87), centered at an intermediate level, or into a continuous open field (Fig. 91). Dual formulation is applied in all cases in which the identities of distal and proximal elements are recognizable, even if one of them is an open field (e.g., Fig. 92, *L^t/O*). In the duplex symbol the distal element is recorded first. Single formulation is reserved for the instances of blended configurations, where there is a continuous open field or a pattern centered at an intermediate level. Configuration types of the hypothenar area are of the same fundamental classes as those occurring in other areas. They are formulated with the initial letters of their names, with superscripts indicating the directions of the open extremities of loops as exemplified in the legends of figures 85–94.

When it is desired to indicate the general alignment of ridge courses the numerical scheme illustrated in figure 83,B is useful. These numerals might be attached as superscripts to the initial letters which stand for configuration types, or the ridge alignments might be formulated independently of the configuration types. If they are combined in one scheme of formulation it would appear to be superfluous to write the symbol for an open field (O) in addition to the number; use of the number alone will simplify the cataloguing of a series of prints.

CALCAR AREA. The configuration of the calcar area is very rarely other than an open field (O). The occurrence of a whorl (W), a loop $(L^t$, Figs. 90 and 94; $L^f)$ or a vestige $(V$, Fig. 91) may be formulated by the usual symbols. Ridge directions may be designated by the numerical scheme of figure 83,B.

PROXIMAL THENAR AREA. So little study has been accorded the territory of the proximal thenar configuration that all the possible variants probably have not been observed. The usual symbols should meet any likely need in formulation, as exemplified in figures 85–94.

DIGITAL AREAS. Absence of plantar digital triradii, mentioned earlier, has its parallel in the palm, where the chief localization is in triradius c instead of in a and b as in the sole. In the absence of a digital triradius there are no radiants to confine the digital area, which accordingly blends into the main configuration of the distal sole (Figs. 87, 94). Digital triradii also may be shifted (Figs. 86, 90, 92, 93), and replaced or supplemented by interdigital triradii or by pseudo-digital triradii (Fig. 90). With the disappearance or proximal shifting of digital triradii the digital areas adjoining two or more digits are thus fused (Figs. 86, 87, 90, 92, 93, 94). Such fusions have morphological importance, and any device which indicates the digital areas involved may be improvised for the tallying of a series of soles.

COMPLETE PLANTAR FORMULA. The writing of a complete descriptive formulation of the sole has not been a general practice. In formulating configurations of the distal sole the order adopted for listing the several symbols is: hallucal, interdigital II, interdigital III, interdigital IV, distal hypothenar. Restriction to these areas is an adaptation to the frequently incomplete recording of other regions in prints. When the prints are adequate, and when there is reason to extend an analysis to other areas, the following are appended in this sequence to the preceding formula: proximal hypothenar, calcar, proximal thenar. The complete formula would then include eight symbols. The advantage of catalogues of complete formulae is that they admit ready analysis of the associations of configuration types in individual soles. In special studies, the plantar formula might be enlarged to include features additional to the configuration types of the eight areas: absence and displacements of digital triradii, fusions of digital areas, courses of at least some main lines, inclination of ridge courses in different regions.

STATISTICAL TRENDS

Extracts of data (Tables 12–16) from a study of plantar dermatoglyphics by Takeya will illustrate the directions, and to some degree the extent, of individual variation, though the trends displayed in the statistical results are modified by the racial composition of the series.[1] The material comprises the prints of 1000 Chinese at Fushun, near Mukden. The prints were exhaustively analyzed by Takeya, and the results are here presented only in part.

TABLE 12

FREQUENCIES OF THE POSITIONS OF TERMINATION OF THE FIBULAR AND DISTAL RADIANTS OF TRIRADIUS p, FORMULATED BY THE NUMERICAL SYMBOLS SHOWN IN FIGURE 84
(*Data on Chinese, from Takeya*)

	Fibular radiant					Distal radiant			
	9	8	7	6	5	$1''$	13	12	11
Right (533 soles)	25.7%	2.2%	58.5%	0.7%	12.8%	0.7%	68.7%	4.5%	26.1%
Left (458 soles)	9.8	1.1	56.8	1.6	30.6	0.2	32.3	11.1	56.3

TRIRADIUS p. This triradius is present in 53.3% of the right soles and 45.8% of the lefts, or 49.5% of the entire series.

---

[1] A similar, though not so extensive a study, is that of Montgomery (108). It deals only with the four configurational areas of the ball region and the distal hypothenar, in a series of 2000 persons. The frequencies of configuration types in each area are presented, but without separate listings of right and left sides. Harkness-Miller presents complete formulations of plantar configuration types and main lines in the soles of 100 persons.

The fibular radiant (Table 12) is directed into the fourth interdigital interval in 57.9% of the soles, and the next most common terminations are in the distal portion of the fibular border (20.9%) and the third interdigital interval (18.3%). Rarely does this radiant fuse with digital triradius d (1.1%) or c (1.8%). There is a definite bilateral distinction in the frequencies of positions of termination of the fibular radiant. In right soles the tendency is for the radiant to extend farther tibialward than in

TABLE 13

RIDGE COURSES OF OPEN FIELDS OF THE MIDDLE OF THE SOLE AND OF THE CALCAR AREA, FORMULATED BY THE NUMERICAL SYMBOLS SHOWN IN FIGURE 83,B

(Data on Chinese, from Takeya, based on 1000 right and 1000 left soles, each less 7 soles for the calcar area, which bear patterns instead of open fields)

	Middle of sole				Calcar area			
	1	2	3	4	2	3	4	5
Right...........	0.7%	21.2%	68.5%	9.6%	3.1%	52.3%	41.7%	2.2%
Left.............	0.3	10.1	64.0	25.7	0.9	18.4	69.9	10.8

lefts, where the inverse tendency is reflected in a sharp rise in the number of endings on the fibular borders and decrease of endings tibialward. The distal radiant, which most commonly terminates in the first or second interdigital interval (Table 12), displays the same trend, suggesting an interdependence of the two radiants as if they were both pivoting on the triradius of origin. Corresponding distinctions between right and left soles are exhibited in the courses of main lines originating from digital triradii (105). All these statistical differences between right and left soles are the plantar counterpart of the bilateral distinction manifested in the courses of palmar main lines.

RIDGE DIRECTIONS PROXIMAL TO THE BALL. The alignments of ridges in the middle and proximal (calcar) sections of the sole are recorded in table 13. Two-thirds of the soles exhibit transversely coursing ridges in the mid-region, and the remainder are nearly equally divided between fibulo-distal and fibulo-proximal slants (of slight obliquity, grades 2 and 4). There is a tendency of right soles to favor the fibulo-proximal slant, and of lefts, the fibulo-distal slant.

In the calcar region 55.8% of the soles present a slight fibulo-distal slant, and the next most common direction is transverse (35.3%). Right soles tend more to the transverse alignment, while lefts display a greater frequency of inclinations in the fibulo-distal direction, as is true of the mid-sole.

TABLE 14

FREQUENCIES OF TYPES OF CONFIGURATIONS IN THE HALLUCAL AREA

(*Data on Chinese, from Takeya, based on* 1000 *right and* 1000 *left soles*)

	W	L^d	L^t	O	X (?)
Right	30.2%	50.7%	6.3%	11.9%	0.9%
Left	31.1	46.2	8.2	12.5	2.0

CONFIGURATIONAL AREAS. The most common configuration in the hallucal area is a loop opening into the first interdigital interval. It occurs in 48.5% of soles (Table 14, L^d). Whorls are next in frequency, 30.7%, and open fields follow with 12.2%, then loops opening to the tibial border, 7.3%.

TABLE 15

FREQUENCIES OF TYPES OF CONFIGURATIONS IN THE SECOND, THIRD AND FOURTH INTERDIGITAL AREAS

(*Data on Chinese, from Takeya, based on* 1000 *right and* 1000 *left soles*)

	Interdigital II				Interdigital III				Interdigital IV		
	O	L^d	L^p	W	O	L^d	L^p	W	O	L^d	L^p
Right	89.6%	8.1%	2.1%	0.2%	40.8%	58.4%	0.2%	0.6%	90.7%	9.2%	0.1%
Left	92.8	5.1	2.0	0.1	42.3	57.0	.....	0.7	93.1	6.9	

The most common configurational type in the second and fourth interdigital areas is the open field (Table 15). The third interdigital area differs in presenting an excess of patterns over open fields. Throughout the three areas a loop opening distally (L^d) is the most frequent pattern type.

TABLE 16

FREQUENCIES OF TYPES OF CONFIGURATIONS IN THE DISTAL AND PROXIMAL HYPOTHENAR AREAS

(*Data on Chinese, from Takeya, based on* 1000 *right and* 1000 *left soles. The original formulations by Takeya are in terms of Schlaginhaufen's types, which are here combined as follows: Open fields = types* 1, 6, 7 *and* 8; *Vestiges = types* 2, 3 *and* 4; *Loops = type* 5)

	Distal hypothenar			Proximal hypothenar		
	O	V	L	O	V	L
Right	31.4%	34.9%	33.7%	79.4%	16.5%	4.1%
Left	22.6	39.3	38.1	83.9	14.0	2.1

The configurations of the distal and proximal hypothenar areas are listed in table 16. Vestiges and patterns occur more frequently in the distal area than in the proximal area.

The calcar area is patterned in only 14 soles of the entire series of 2000, thus giving a frequency of 0.7%.[2] The remaining configurations are open fields, their ridge alignments being discussed above.

Except for the distal hypothenar area, where the relationship is reversed, right soles bear a greater proportion of patterns in each of the six configurational areas considered. The bipedal differences are greatest in the instance of the distal hypothenar area and least in the hallucal. The statistical reliability of some of the smaller differences is questionable. Bipedal differences of pattern frequencies in the calcar and proximal thenar areas cannot be analyzed in the available material.

---

[2] The calcar pattern is rare in all races, though it is possible that some populations may double or triple the frequency here indicated for Chinese. For example, de Pina (Sobre figuras papilares da região plantar em portugueses e negros de Africa. J. med. Gal.-Port., Sept. 1935) finds in a series of 296 Portuguese two individuals having the calcar area patterned unilaterally and three who bear bilateral patterns—making an incidence of 1.7% of the individuals who are patterned on one or both soles. The same author reports a frequency of 2.2% in a series of 268 West African Negroes, three cases of unilateral and three cases of bilateral calcar patterns. It is possible, of course, that families characterized by frequent calcar patterns are included in the material reported.

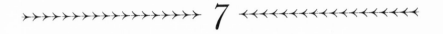

7

TOES

SCANT material relating to toe prints is available in the literature, but it is sufficient for comparison with the data on fingers. The most extensive analysis of toe prints is that of Takeya. His material consists of 1000 Chinese, the same subjects dealt with in Chapter 6. Another important contribution is the study by Newman. It is based upon a much smaller number of subjects, 100 European-American males, but its value is enhanced by the conjoint analyses of toes and fingers of the same individuals. Steffens investigates toe prints and finger prints in 100 pairs of twins (German), 50 pairs each of monozygotics and same-sexed dizygotics, the sexes being in equal numbers in either group. She presents data not only embracing the total material but also for a series composed of one member from each pair, selected to eliminate possible vitiation of the statistics by the inclusion of twin partners. Hasebe (286) presents

TABLE 17
FREQUENCIES OF THE TYPES OF CONFIGURATIONS OF TOES

	Whorls			Fibular loops			Tibial loops			Arches		
	R	L	R + L	R	L	R + L	R	L	R+L	R	L	R + L
Chinese............	20.4 %	21.0 %	20.7 %	60.6 %	53.9 %	57.2 %	1.4 %	3.8 %	2.6 %	17.6 %	21.3 %	19.4 %
Japanese..........	17.2	17.2	17.2	62.8	55.6	59.2	0.6	3.0	1.8	19.4	24.2	21.8
European-Americans*...........	21.2	22.2	21.7	67.6	60.4	64.0	1.0	1.4	1.2	10.0	16.0	13.0
Germans (Steffens).			21.7				59.0					19.0

* Newman's original figures for whorls and fibular loops are here modified by transferring from his class of whorls the several examples of invaded fibular loops.

the frequencies of configuration types in toes of 100 Japanese males. Féré records pattern-type frequencies for the big toe alone in 182 subjects, and for all toes in 34.

The configurations of toes conform to the topography described for finger prints (Chap. 4); they present, moreover, the same basic types and the same manifestations of transition from one type to another and are subject to identical methods of analysis. Only passing comment has been made with regard to pattern form and pattern size (118, 119), and there is no information at all in reference to the middle and proximal phalanges. With regard to the occurrences of pattern types, the chapter is extended to include pertinent comparisons with fingers.

STATISTICAL TRENDS

TOTAL FREQUENCIES OF PATTERN TYPES. The frequencies of the basic types of patterns, in the four available collections, are listed in table 17. Whorls and tibial (radial) loops are less abundant than in fingers, while arches are more frequent. Comparisons of fingers and toes in the same racial populations demonstrate consistent direction of this intermembral difference. In Newman's collection of 100 European-Americans, whorls are 67% more frequent in fingers than in toes, and arches are nearly six times more abundant in toes than in fingers. Steffens' German series presents a whorl frequency in fingers which is 40% greater than that in toes; arches are 4½ times more frequent in toes. Hasebe's Japanese series displays an even more striking difference in the same direction, whorls being 2½ times more abundant in fingers, and arches nearly 8 times more abundant in toes. The fingers of Japanese have a much greater abundance of whorls than do the fingers of European-Americans or Germans, yet the toes of Japanese as compared with European peoples show a lesser number of whorls. Thus there appears to be an inverse relationship between the occurrences of whorls and arches in toes and fingers. As is generally true in mass statistics of fingers, the incidence of arches decreases with elevation of whorl frequency.

TABLE 18
FREQUENCIES OF SUBTYPES OF WHORLS, COMPARED IN TOES AND FINGERS

	Toes		Fingers
	Takeya	Newman	Scotland Yard (Table 1)
True whorls..................................	2.4%	5.6%	20.1%
Central pockets.............................	0.1	0.1	2.1
Lateral pockets and twin loops...................	14.1	15.3	3.1
Accidentals.................................	4.1	0.7	0.1

The subtypes of whorls represented in the total frequencies of 20.7% in the Chinese series and the 21.7% in the European-American series are distributed as indicated in table 18, which includes also corresponding data for fingers. The proportionate representation of each of these classes differs widely in toes and fingers. True whorls and central pockets are much less abundant in toes, the proportions of double-loop patterns and accidentals being several times greater than in fingers.

TABLE 19

FREQUENCIES OF BICENTRIC WHORLS (LATERAL POCKET LOOPS, TWIN LOOPS, ACCIDENTALS) COMPARED IN TOES AND FINGERS

Toes			Fingers	
Takeya	Newman	Steffens	Scotland Yard (Table 1)	Steffens
87.9%	73.7%	88.9%	12.6%	35.7%

Whorls may be classified also according to the presence of one core or two: monocentric (true whorls and central pockets); bicentric (lateral pocket loops, twin loops and accidentals). The frequencies of bicentric patterns, in percent of all whorls in the inclusive sense, are listed in table 19; the implied percent remainders are the frequencies of monocentric patterns. Toes differ from fingers in presenting a considerable increase in the proportion of bicentric patterns.

TABLE 20

FREQUENCIES OF THE TYPES OF CONFIGURATIONS ON TOES
(*Data on 1000 Chinese, from Takeya*)

Digit	Side	Whorls	Fibular loops	Tibial loops	Arches
I	R	6.3%	78.0%	4.8%	10.9%
	L	9.3	67.7	10.4	12.6
	R + L	7.8	72.9	7.6	11.8
II	R	17.9	74.6	0.5	7.0
	L	19.9	69.0	0.8	10.3
	R + L	18.9	71.8	0.7	8.7
III	R	60.2	36.6	0.3	2.9
	L	55.3	36.4	1.7	6.6
	R + L	57.8	36.5	1.0	4.8
IV	R	17.4	65.0	0.7	16.9
	L	19.8	50.9	4.4	24.9
	R + L	18.6	58.0	2.6	20.9
V	R	0.4	48.8	0.7	50.1
	L	0.7	45.4	1.9	52.0
	R + L	0.6	47.6	1.3	51.1

The noteworthy trends evidenced in the digital distribution of pattern types (Table 20 and Fig. 95) are emphasized in the occurrences of whorls, tibial loops and arches. The total of fibular loops may be regarded as a pool which enlarges or contracts with decrease or increase of these other types. The differential trends of pattern frequency among the five toes are best appreciated by stating the incidence on each digit in terms of the total of each pattern type rather than in reference to the total of all patterns.

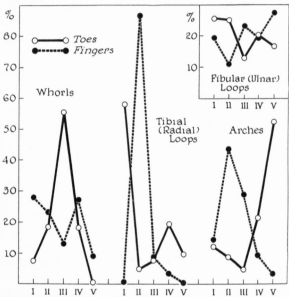

FIG. 95.—Frequency distributions of pattern types on individual digits, for comparisons of toes and fingers. Data from tables 1 and 15, converted to indicate the percent of the total of a particular pattern type borne by each digit.

Digit I bears a larger number of tibial loops (58%) than any other toe. It has next to the lowest frequency of whorls (7.5%).

Digit II is the site of minimum frequency of tibial loops (5.0) and next to the lowest frequency of arches (8.9%).

Digit III carries by far the highest frequency of whorls (55.7%) and the least frequency of arches (4.9%).

Digit IV bears next to the highest frequencies of tibial loops and arches, but its chief distinction lies in the fact that no other digit, toe or finger, reaches this degree of leveling of frequencies of the four pattern types (the closest approach to it being the index finger). Of the total frequency of each type, 18.0% of the whorls are on this toe, 20.2% of the fibular loops, 19.5% of the tibial loops, and 21.5% of the arches. This distribution is in sharp contrast with widely unequal distributions in all other toes and fingers. The corresponding values for the fifth toe may be cited in illustration: whorls, 0.5%; fibular loops, 16.5%; tibial loops, 9.9%; arches 52.6%.

Digit V has the highest frequency of arches and the lowest frequency of whorls.

These digital distributions of maximum and minimum pattern-type frequencies differ significantly at some points from the conditions existing in fingers: (a) The maximum frequencies of whorls in fingers occur in digits I and IV, while in toes these patterns are more concentrated on one digit, III. (b) The maximum frequencies of radial (tibial) loops are in finger II and in toe I. (c) Arches are concentrated in finger II and in toe V.

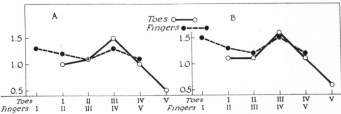

FIG. 96.—Average pattern intensities of individual toes and fingers, with the superimposed graphs shifted for demonstration of similarities. *A*. Data from tables 1 and 15. *B*. Data from Newman.

According to Newman, the pattern distributions on fingers and toes show greater similarities if toes I, II, III, and IV are compared respectively with fingers II, III, IV and V. Of the intermembral distinctions just listed, the localization of radial (tibial) loops is a clean-cut illustration of this principle. Further demonstration is afforded in comparisons of pattern intensity. Pattern-intensity values have been computed for individual digits, converted from the frequencies in tables 1 and 20 and from Newman's data on toes and fingers. A fairly close fit between the graphs (Fig. 96) for toes and fingers is obtained only between toes I-IV and fingers II-V. Toe V and finger I are thus left unpaired in the pattern-intensity comparison. It might be suspected that racial differences create a false showing in the comparison between fingers of the Scotland Yard series and toes of Chinese (Fig. 96,A). However, the same relationships are present in Newman's series (Fig. 96,B), which indicates that the difference here observed is independent of race.

Steffens shows that there is a relationship between fingers and toes with regard to the total frequencies of pattern types. When the toes present frequent arches, the fingers show arches and loops, with no whorls or at best a limited number. When there are many loops on toes the fingers also bear loop patterns. The coefficient of correlation of arch-frequencies on toes and fingers of the same individuals is 0.50, and for whorls it is 0.36 (see Chap. 11, Association of patterns).

BIPEDAL DIFFERENCES. In each of the toes, except III, whorls are more abundant on the left side than on the right (Table 21), the reverse of the bilateral distinction characterizing fingers (Table 1, where it will

TABLE 21

TOTAL FREQUENCIES, SEPARATELY FOR RIGHT AND LEFT SIDES, OF ARCHES, LOOPS AND WHORLS
ON TOES

	Arches		Loops		Whorls	
	R	L	R	L	R	L
European-Americans (Newman)...	10.0%	16.0%	67.8%	61.0%	22.2%	23.0%
Germans (Steffens).............	17.2	20.8	62.6	56.0	20.2	23.2
Japanese (Takeya).............	17.6	26.0	62.0	57.7	20.4	21.0
Japanese (Hasebe).............	19.4	24.2	63.4	58.6	17.2	17.2

be noted that the dextral excess in whorls is at its minimum in finger III). Tibial loops likewise are more frequent on left toes, indicating a reversal of the trend noted in radial loops of the fingers. Arches are more frequent on left toes, but in this instance the trend agrees with that observed in fingers, where only the index finger presents a higher frequency on the right side, but the excess is very slight. Bilaterally different trends of the main pattern types are expressed also in their total frequencies. Though only European stocks and Japanese are represented in the data of table 21, the likeness of results of bilateral comparison suggests that the trends are a common human characteristic.

PATTERN COMBINATIONS. Pattern combinations in individuals may be treated by the "manuar" method of Poll. The significant trends are evidenced both in the "unipedar" and "bipedar," the latter alone being illustrated (Fig. 97).

Two points of special interest appear in the bipedar. (a) Unlike the case in fingers, individuals presenting five arches and five whorls do occur. Two individuals in Takeya's series of 1000 present this combination. It will be recalled that the combination has not been recorded in fingers, though on mathematical grounds it might be predicted in two individuals of about 500,000 if the assortment were determined by chance alone. (b) The fields of the bipedar assigned to combinations of 9 whorls and of 10 whorls are vacant, and it is possible that they would remain unfilled even in a much larger series. Toe V has so low an incidence of whorls, and arches are generally so frequent in toes, that the combination involving ten whorls may be in the same category of rarity as the combination of five whorls and five arches in fingers.

PATTERN FORM. Even in the absence of quantitative determinations, certain general statements may be made about the shape and general character of toe patterns. In toes patterns tend to be broader, or less highly vaulted, and smaller than in fingers (118). Loops in toes tend to be perpendicular to the proximal ridges of the pattern area, contrasting with the more general slant of loops in fingers. The erect looped pattern

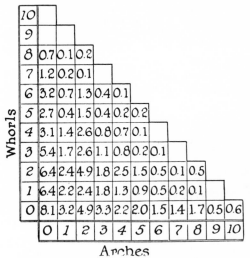

FIG. 97.—"Bipedar" showing the percent frequencies of pattern type combinations of toes in individuals. (*Data on 1000 Chinese, from Takeya.*)

area may be sharply marked off from the transversely coursing ridges at its base (119).

QUANTITATIVE VALUE. Inspection alone indicates that toe patterns tend to be smaller than finger patterns. This is borne out in the ridge counts reported by Steffens (Table 22). The data are obtained from 100 German children, one partner from each of 100 twin pairs (though Steffens shows that the results do not differ when both partners are included). The data are of particular importance because quantitative values of fingers and toes are determined in the same individuals.

The average ridge count for all fingers in Steffens' material is 14.3 ± 0.46, and for all toes, 10.6 ± 0.57. Inasmuch as arches are very frequent in toes, and the zero ridge counts of these configurations lower the average values, it is important to note that a difference persists when arches are excluded from the determinations. Excluding arches, the figures (based upon the whole series of 100 twin pairs) are: average count in fingers, 15.0 ± 0.22; average in toes, 12.9 ± 0.16.

TABLE 22

RIDGE COUNTS (QUANTITATIVE VALUES) COMPARED IN FINGERS AND TOES
(*Data on 100 Germans, from Steffens*)

	Fingers					Toes				
	I	II	III	IV	V	I	II	III	IV	V
All configurations.	17.4	11.7	12.8	16.8	14.0	11.9	10.6	17.3	10.4	3.1
Loops only........	15.7	9.8	12.1	14.8	13.6	11.8	9.0	9.8	11.2	7.1
Whorls only......	20.4	17.4	17.4	19.2	16.8	18.7	18.4	22.6	19.0	16.3
Average, all digits.	14.3 ± 0.46					10.6 ± 0.57				

The seriations of ridge counts, for all configurations including arches, are:

$$\text{Fingers} \quad \text{I} > \text{IV} > \text{V} > \text{III} > \text{II}$$
$$\text{Toes} \quad \text{III} > \text{I} > \text{II} > \text{IV} > \text{V}.$$

Slightly different orderings are obtained when loops and whorls are singled out, indicating that toe III owes its large ridge count to whorls; when loops alone are considered this digit shifts to third place in the list, and digit I takes first place as in the hand. Toe V retains last place in the list as the digit with minimum ridge count, whether all patterns are involved or loops or whorls alone are considered. Finger V also presents the least ridge count of all fingers in the case of whorls.

Part 3

BIOLOGY

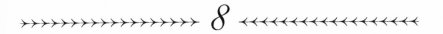

ELEMENTS OF FINGER-PRINT
IDENTIFICATION

A KNOWN individual is recognized ordinarily at a glance. His stocky build, ruddy face, stubby nose, blue eyes, light hair, mannerisms, habits of dress and other qualities are appraised without conscious effort. Sight recognition is effective because two individuals seldom present closely similar total combinations of such characteristics, notwithstanding their likeness in some traits. Sight recognition, however, is not infallible. Extraordinary resemblance makes for confusion of individuals, and intentional alterations and changes brought about by ageing or disease may lead to lack of recognition. Such lapses in identification usually are of little consequence in every-day life, but an absolutely reliable means of establishing identity is demanded in many situations.

Scientific methods of personal identification originated about sixty years ago, when Bertillon devised the system which bears his name. He revised the inexact descriptive methods previously employed in criminal identification and proposed the use of eleven body measurements. As a systematic method adapted to the needs of agencies of law enforcement, the Bertillon procedure is naturally more reliable than sight recognition. Measurements lend themselves to classification, classification being requisite for ready search of the filed records essential in systematic personal identification. The Bertillon system, cumbersome and often fallible, was gradually superseded by the immeasurably superior method of finger-print identification, which is now employed universally for the registration of criminals and increasingly for various civil and military purposes.

Finger prints are ideally suited to the needs of an identification system. Their characteristics are permanent, as well as classifiable for filing under headings which may be subdivided without limit. The classified finger prints of an individual afford means to determine quickly if that person has been previously entered in the identification file; the search in the file is directed by finger-print characteristics alone, without reference to name or other data that might be falsified. If present in the file, the finger-print card will reveal the identity as well as the recorded prior history. Finger prints have the additional advantage, in criminal investigation, of being impressed in the touching and handling of objects, so that a person makes unwittingly an identifiable record of himself.

The world's greatest file of finger prints is that of the Federal Bureau of Investigation, which functions as a central clearing house of identification records. From police agencies throughout the United States duplicate finger-print cards are sent to the Bureau. Additionally, there is an international exchange of cards which (in January, 1941) embraces 89 foreign countries, territories and possessions. The *Law Enforcement Bulletin*, published monthly by this organization, carries numerous reports of identifications established through its facilities. Identifications obviously can be made only if the finger prints are on file. At present the persons so identifiable are largely those with criminal records, but there is gratifying increase in the filing of cards of law-abiding citizens.

The Argentine Republic has made greater advance in promoting civilian finger-printing than any other nation. Starting with the printing of applicants for appointment to the police force, in 1891, compulsory registration has been gradually extended to include employees of banks and of the postal system, students on matriculation, electoral officials, government employees, immigrants, domestic servants, chauffeurs and taxi drivers, some classes of tradesmen, and members of all the regulated professions—including physicians and dentists. Finger-print cards representing about half of the national population are now on file at Buenos Aires.

Though special mention is made of finger prints, the principles which hold true for them apply also to palms, soles and toes. Dermatoglyphics of these areas are equally permanent and individually variable. They are classifiable in the same general manner, though descriptive classification calls for adjustments to the morphological peculiarities of these regions. In the case of palms (79, 80, 90, 91, 94, 96) and soles (79) several schemes have been devised, some of them being in routine use.

Chance prints of toes, palms and soles are presented occasionally in evidence of personal identity. The nature of this evidence is in all respects comparable to the finger print, and the qualified finger-print expert is competent to deal with it (124).

CLASSIFICATION AND FILING

Classification of finger prints provides for orderly placing of finger-print cards in a file. With systematic filing of an original card, any subsequent card of that individual falls in the same section of the file, and a search of the section quickly yields the earlier record. Classification may be extended as far as the size of the finger-print collection warrants. In a small file only the more comprehensive classes are separated; the larger the collection, the more subdivision is necessary. Each section in the file, whether devoted to a comprehensive class or to one of the subdivisions, will contain a number of cards. Thus the final step in searching for a prior record of an individual involves inspection of a group of cards having the same filing formula, for comparison of finger-print characteristics which are not differentiated by that formula.

In *primary* classification of ten-finger sets under the Henry system, the digits are considered in "pairs." The consecutively numbered squares of the standard finger-print card (Fig. 41) indicate the order in which the pairs are composed, beginning with the right thumb and the right index. The five pairs are numbered in order as indicated below. The pairs are written in the form of fractions, with the even-numbered member of the pair placed in the position of numerator:

Pair 1.	Pair 2.	Pair 3.	Pair 4.	Pair 5.
(2) $\overline{R. \text{ index}}$	(4) $\overline{R. \text{ ring}}$	(6) $\overline{L. \text{ thumb}}$	(8) $\overline{L. \text{ middle}}$	(10) $\overline{L. \text{ little}}$
(1) R. thumb	(3) R. middle	(5) R. little	(7) L. index	(9) L. ring

This fractional notation is important in constructing the primary classification formula, which is derived from numerical values assigned only to whorls (inclusive sense—thus including all patterns with two or more triradii). Arches and loops (i.e., patterns with no triradius or but one) have zero values. The presence of a whorl determines a numerical value for each digit of the ten-finger set. The numerical value assigned to a whorl depends on the pair to which the digit bearing it belongs, but is the same whether the digit occupies the position of numerator or denominator:

Pair 1.	Pair 2.	Pair 3.	Pair 4.	Pair 5.
16	8	4	2	1

Entering these values in the fractional notation, a finger-print set in which all patterns are whorls would appear:

Pair 1.	Pair 2.	Pair 3.	Pair 4.	Pair 5.
$^{16}\!/_{16}$	$^{8}\!/_{8}$	$^{4}\!/_{4}$	$^{2}\!/_{2}$	$^{1}\!/_{1}$

Another set, with whorls in both thumbs and both ring fingers, but in these digits only:

Pair 1.	Pair 2.	Pair 3.	Pair 4.	Pair 5.
$^{0}\!/_{16}$	$^{8}\!/_{0}$	$^{4}\!/_{0}$	$^{0}\!/_{0}$	$^{0}\!/_{1}$

To obtain the classification formula, the numerators of the five pairs and the five denominators are added separately. These sums, in the first example, are $\frac{31}{31}$, and in the second, $\frac{12}{17}$. Early in the history of finger-print identification an expedient in the filing system was adopted to compensate for sets in which all patterns have o values, the addition of 1 to the numerator and 1 to the denominator. Accordingly, a finger-print set in which there are no whorls will have the primary classification number $\frac{1}{1}$, rather than $\frac{0}{0}$, and the two examples become $\frac{32}{32}$ and $\frac{13}{18}$ respectively.

The series of numbers selected for the values of whorls in the different pairs form a progression in which the value for any one pair is twice the value of the succeeding pair. One advantage of this geometric progression is that the classification number may be decoded. Practical finger-print workers, familiar as they are with classification numbers, recognize the distributions of finger-print patterns without decoding. The decoding may be illustrated by the second example, where the classification number is $\frac{13}{18}$. The fraction first is reduced to its original value, $\frac{12}{17}$ (by subtracting $\frac{1}{1}$). There is no pair in which the value for one whorl is 12. Since the only possible combination which yields 12 is 8 and 4 (assigned respectively to pairs 2 and 3), it is clear that the right ring finger and left thumb bear whorls, and that other digits in numerator positions have no whorls. The denominator, 17, breaks down into 16 and 1, with no other possibilities. The value 16 in denominator position stands for a whorl in the right thumb, and the remainder, 1, indicates a whorl in the left ring finger.

The 1024 combinations of numerator and denominator, each ranging from 1 through 32, serve as primary divisions in the file. In the filing cabinet the finger-print cards are arranged in the sequences of this numerical classification. Thirty-two divisions are first separated by the sequence of denominators; then each of these is divided into 32 parts by the sequence of numerators. All cards classified as $\frac{1}{1}$ are filed in the first section. This section is followed by the group of cards classified as $\frac{2}{1}$, and this group by $\frac{3}{1}$, $\frac{4}{1}$ and onward in the sequence of the numerators through $\frac{32}{1}$. The next primary division, beginning with $\frac{1}{2}$, continues through $\frac{32}{32}$, and the next following division would carry the cards indexed from $\frac{1}{3}$ through $\frac{32}{3}$—and so on through $\frac{32}{32}$.

It will be evident that the group location of a finger-print card in the primary division of the file is as precisely determined as the location of a word in the dictionary. The search for a finger-print card in a primary division of a file, if it were not subdivided, might be compared to hunting for a word in a jumbled dictionary where the only grouping is by initial letters. The searcher in a finger-print file finds in a primary division a large number of cards which must be examined individually to determine whether there is a finger-print set identical with that of a person whose prints have been made. Such searching is minimized by secondary classification.

The *secondary* classification breaks the primary divisions into subclasses. Unless a file is very small this subdivision is necessary, since the number of cards falling in some primary divisions becomes so large that it is impracticable to inspect them all at each search through the file. The primary division $\frac{1}{1}$, for example, would contain about 25% of the total number of cards in a collection. One kind of secondary classification is based upon the pattern types of the index fingers: arches, tented arches, ulnar loops, radial loops. The occurrence of a plain arch, a tented arch or a radial loop on any digit other than the index also is recorded. These pattern types, symbolized by initial letters of their names, are entered in the classification formula in numerator-denominator form, right hand in the numerator and left hand in the denominator. Using capital initials for the index finger, small letters for the other digits, and adhering to a standard sequence of notation, the divisions of the primary classifications are thus arranged for systematic filing.

More subordinate divisions are made, using the ridge counts of loops and the ridge tracings of whorls. The technology of classification involves much detail, pertinent only in works designed as manuals for the identification worker.

Single finger-print classifications have been devised for dealing with chance prints found at the scene of crime. Only in exceptional circumstances does the standard ten-finger filing system aid in the identification of a chance print, as when there are grounds for suspecting a particular person, whose filed finger prints may be then compared with the chance print. Single finger prints, like complete finger-print sets, are classifiable. The classification is necessarily carried beyond that required for ten-digit sets, taking into account the more minute features of the print. Manuals designed for the identification worker may be consulted for details of method (43, 49, 66).

INDIVIDUALITY OF THE FINGER PRINT

Routine finger-print identification is practicable because finger prints lend themselves to classification. The validity of identifications established by finger prints rests on two cardinal facts. (a) The patterns and the characteristics of single ridges are permanently fixed. Except for enlargement in the course of bodily growth, there is no change in the ridge characteristics of a finger pattern throughout the lifetime of the individual, and they persist after death until the skin is decomposed. Once legible prints of a person are registered, that record is a means of positive identification, regardless of the lapse of time intervening between the original and the later finger-printings. (b) The complex of ridge details in a single finger print, or even part of one, is not duplicated in any other finger.

From the practical standpoint, the crucial test of the individuality of the finger print is an identification determined from a chance print of a single finger. The chance print is developed, if necessary, and photo-

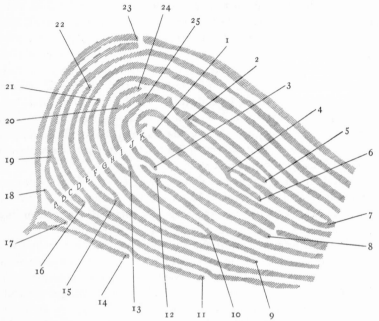

FIG. 98.—A tracing of the pattern area of the finger print shown in figure 53, with minutiae indexed for description and comparison.

graphed for examination. This *evidence print* is compared with the *identifying print*, obtained from the file or made from a suspected person.

Let it be imagined, as an example, that the loop illustrated in figure 53 is an identifying print and that another impression of unknown origin is at hand for comparison. Figure 98 is a tracing of the pattern area of this print, and for the purpose of discussion it is considered an evidence print. The first comparison concerns major features of the patterns. These two prints are loops having the same ridge count, 11, and the same general appearance of ridge details. Since the minutiae are apparently identical, each detail will now be singled out for comparison in the two prints. Figure 98 is designed for illustrating the procedure of comparison.

The ridges transected by the line of count are here identified by letters, and 25 ridge details within the pattern area are labeled with numbers. Beginning with ridge *A*, it will be noted that it ends abruptly at the point marked *18*, just distal to the triradius; the opposite extremity, at *11*, is either an ending or an imperfectly printed union with ridge *B*. Ridges *B* and *C* arise from a bifurcation at *19*. Ridge *B* continues ulnarward without a break, while ridge *C* terminates after a short course, at *16*. Ridge *D* sweeps through the entire pattern area without presenting any feature of note. Ridges *E* and *F* spring from a bifurcation at *15;* the ridge from which they arise has an ending short of the opening of the pattern area, at *9*. Ridge *E* comes to an end at *22*, while *F* continues without interruption to the opening of the pattern. In this manner each detail is matched in the two prints.

Having considered that one print is an evidence print of unknown personal origin, and that the other is an identifying print, the question is: Are both prints from the same finger? This question is answered in practice by making point for point comparisons of the minutiae of the evidence print and the identifying print. Every detail in the pattern area of the print shown in figure 98 is duplicated in figure 53, and these details are found to lie in the same topographic positions and in the same sequence in reference to individual ridges. That the two prints are identical is obvious. It should be noted that the tracing in figure 98 is an incomplete record of the details which are available in figure 53, both outside the pattern area and, within it, in the form of numerous incipient ridge details which are not included in the tracing. If sweat pores were imprinted, the number of points of comparison would be tremendously increased. The 25 labeled minutiae are, however, more than enough to illustrate the discussion which follows.

The reasoning leading to the conclusion that two identical prints must originate from the same finger is now to be examined. Complete observational proof that prints from two fingers are never identical is unattainable. Even if it were possible to compare every finger pattern with every other one now available, the investigator could only arrive at a conclusion based upon experience with a fraction of the fingers that have existed and that are to come into being. It would be unnecessary, as a matter of fact, to consider such a task, since a significant experience is already accumulated. There are millions of finger-print cards on file, and thousands of experts working with them. Constantly it is necessary to compare the details of patterns, yet never has there been discovered an instance of duplication of different fingers. To make the case stronger, the prints of "identical" twins (Chaps. 12, 13) have been studied exhaustively, without encountering a single case of duplication. The possibility of duplication is put to severe test in these twins, for the two members of the pair have the same inheritance. In spite of the control by the same genetic factors, their finger-print characteristics are never identical, and at best there is merely a close resemblance (Fig. 144).

It is a familiar observation that the structures of plants and animals are widely variable. Corresponding parts of the same species may seem to present little or no difference if the inspection is merely casual. But many unlikenesses become apparent if the objects are examined closely, and the number of differences increases as attention is directed to more and more minute characters. The philosopher Leibniz contended, as have many others before and after him, that "there are never in nature two beings which are exactly alike, and in which it is not possible to find a difference." Thomas de Quincey relates that Leibniz was once explaining the matter to a royal personage; to give point he turned to a gentleman in attendance with a challenge to produce from any tree or shrub two leaves duplicating each other in venation. The challenge was accepted—but the duplicate leaves could not be found. As with leaves, so it is with finger prints. The London newspaper, *News of the World*, was quite safe when in 1939 it offered a prize of £1000 to the person having a finger print identical with any one of a series of prints published for the contest.

The unique character of every biological aggregate—a single leaf, a finger print, an ear of corn, the striped pattern of a zebra—has been recognized in the axiom, "Nature never repeats." Without questioning the intended meaning of this axiom, the suggestion might be offered that it read "Nature never repeats exactly." If nature did not repeat at all, there would be no multiples of the same class—trees and men, whorls and loops, and indeed no universe of fingers to bear whorls and loops. Such repetition, however, is confined to the general molds of things, and in the last analysis of detail "Nature does not repeat."

In spite of diligent search, an instance of duplication of two finger prints never has been found. This is not unexpected in view of the operation of the law of simple probability, or chance. The occurrence of minutiae at specific points is governed at least in large part by developmental processes which yield random results. Accordingly, the presence and locations of forks, ends and other ridge details may be considered from the same mathematical approach which applies, for example, to the chance of throwing a particular face of a die, or the head of a coin. To some degree finger-print minutiae are subject to control through inheritance (Chaps. 12-14), but even the maximum possible "loading" by inheritance is insufficient to counteract the random production of these details.

Pearl[1] refers to the tossing of a coin as "a classical event" because this act has been so frequently used in the discussion of probability. Following tradition, the same example may be chosen here. Imagine first the random tossing of a penny. Because the coin is a thin disc, it is bound not to stand on edge after an ordinary toss. This much is certainty, but no one can be certain of throwing a head, or a tail. The face which lies upward after the throw may be either head or tail, and that each has an equal chance in the result can be determined by trial. If the coin is tossed many times, it will be found that equal numbers of heads and tails have appeared and that no toss can influence the result of any other. The chance of a head, or a tail, may be expressed as the fraction $\frac{1}{2}$. "Head" has one in two chances and "tail" has one in two.

Having dealt with this problem in its simplest terms, with the toss of one penny, the chance involved with the use of two pennies is next to be considered. At the toss each coin has an equal chance of falling head up. What is the chance of heads for both pennies? Of the three possibilities—two heads, one head and one tail, and two tails—there is one chance in four that two heads will appear. The mathematical formula for determining this result is simple. Knowing the chance involved in each of the two events, the probability of their occurring together is the product of these two chances: $\frac{1}{2} \times \frac{1}{2} = \frac{1}{4}$. On this same principle, the chance of all heads in the toss of any number of pennies may be calculated. If there were 25 pennies the chance of falling all heads is $\frac{1}{2}$ raised to the 25th power, or $1/35,554,432$.

The chance of all heads in a toss of 25 pennies is small, but an enormous reduction of the chance of obtaining a prescribed result would be introduced by imposing specific restrictions. Assume that the coins are marked for identification, each of them with a different letter, and that the floor on which they are tossed is laid off in 25 squares correspondingly lettered. Postulating that mechanical provisions for the toss insure that one coin will lie in each of the squares, what is the chance that each coin will fall head up within the square corresponding to its identifying mark? The judgment of common sense is that the chance must be exceedingly small; it may be calculated by the formula previously used. The chance of one coin lying head up within its proper square is the product of the chances of these two independent events, namely $\frac{1}{2} \times \frac{1}{25} = \frac{1}{50}$. The chance that all 25 coins satisfy this requirement is $\frac{1}{50}$ raised to the 25th power, or

$$\frac{1}{2,980,232,238,769,531,250,000,000,000,000,000,000,000,000}.$$

[1] *Introduction to Medical Biometry and Statistics*, 3rd edition. Philadelphia, W. B. Saunders Co., 1940.

The chance of the occurrence is therefore so infinitesimally small that from a practical view it may be completely disregarded.

Probability, or chance, is subject to experimental proof in applications such as coin tossing. Though this experimental proof is feasible only in the higher brackets of chance, the correspondence of computed expectation and actual result is a comforting sign that the same law holds when the chance is lowered through increase in the number of items that must be satisfied.

The accelerated diminution of chance, with progressive increase of the number of coins fulfilling the double requirement of "head" and "lying in proper square," is hardly appreciated unless one actually sets down the numbers. There are good odds that one of the coins will conform to requirement, the chance being $\frac{1}{50}$. The chance that two will conform sinks to $1/2,500$; for each additional conforming coin the chance is only $\frac{1}{50}$ of the preceding, thus: 3 coins, $1/125,000$; 4 coins, $1/6,250,000$; 5 coins, $1/312,500,000$; 6 coins, $1/15,625,000,000$, etc.

How does this apply to the individuality of a finger print? In brief, the concatenation of 25 specific ridge details existing in the finger-print example chosen may be likened to a successful result in the tossing of the 25 coins. In the finger print the result is already in existence, having been brought about during the period of differentiation of the skin ridges, several months before the person was born. The cogent question is whether an identical result ever might be realized in some other finger. The practical answer to this question is *no*.

The occurrence of a particular ridge detail in a particular place is not a strictly random event, but that the element of randomness plays the chief rôle in producing it is evidenced by the differences which occur in "identical" twins. Inheritance is the factor which may influence randomness, but even in two individuals having the same inheritance the combinations of details are widely different. For treatment of chance in reference to finger-print details it seems safe to apply the usual computation for the concurrence of random events, only remembering that in closely related individuals the chance is increased. The increase, however, can not be mathematically corrected. The only correction which is available is to set the chance of duplication of the single items at a figure which is undoubtedly much higher than actuality.

Only to a limited extent would it be possible to determine the actual frequencies of the finger-print characteristics. The pattern used in this discussion is an ulnar loop. Ulnar loops are common, as instanced by their 64% occurrence in the Scotland Yard series (Table 1). Disregarding the varying frequencies of ulnar loops on different digits, there is thus a mathematical chance of $1/1.6 \pm$ that two prints from different digits might both be ulnar loops. The pattern in question is an ulnar loop having a count of 11 ridges, and if this feature be also taken into account the chance of duplication of the two characters (pattern type and ridge count) is much smaller. Roscher's data (75) on ridge counts of 3000 ulnar loops show only 154 having counts of 11 ridges. Still ignoring unlikenesses among different digits, there is a chance of $1/19.5$ that two randomly chosen ulnar loops would have counts of 11 ridges. Employing the usual mathematical formula, the chance of concurrence of this particular pattern type and ridge count in two fingers is

$$\frac{1}{1.6} \times \frac{1}{19.5} = \frac{1}{31}.$$

There are no data on the frequencies of specific minutiae occupying specific positions in patterns. Balthazard and others discuss the chance of duplication of two prints on the basis of a $\frac{1}{4}$ probability of repetition of a single detail. This figure exaggerates the chance of coincidence. Wentworth and Wilder (79) point out that the real probability would be closer to $\frac{1}{50}$, or even $\frac{1}{100}$. Avoiding both undue exaggeration of chance and the possibility of minimizing it through the use of too low a value, we may choose $\frac{1}{50}$ as a working figure. If each of the 25 details indicated in figure 98 might be duplicated by chance in a pattern of another finger, the mathematical setup for the chance of duplicating the entire series of details is exactly that which applies to the problem of tossing the 25 coins onto 25 squares, the requirement being that each coin fall head up within the square having its own letter. That chance as shown above is expressed in a fraction in which the numerator is one and the denominator is a number having 43 places!

It must be realized that numerous details are available in a finger-print comparison. Twenty-five are selected in the example discussed, but the number present in one print often reaches a much higher figure, 60, 80 or 100. Another circumstance deserving emphasis is that negative characteristics are not included in the enumeration; the lack of an interruption or fork in an extent of a ridge (e.g., the whole length of ridge D in figure 98) is a feature which is just as important in the mathematics of chance as the presence and positions of particular minutiae. The mathematical chance of duplication is therefore even smaller than the figure cited above. Even if only pattern type and ridge count are considered in addition to the 25 minutiae, the chance is reduced 31 times; each ridge detail added to the series would reduce the chance by 50 times. The chance of duplication of this finger print is therefore so extremely small that common sense rejects as fantastic the idea of an actual realization. The mathematical treatment is perforce used in evaluating the chance. It is unfortunate that this approach carries the implication that a complete correspondence of two patterns might occur, when as a matter of fact the mathematical reasoning merely supplements observations indicating that such duplication is beyond the range of possibility. Under the circumstances it is impossible to offer decisive *proof* that no two fingers bear identical patterns, but the facts in hand demonstrate the soundness of the working principle that *prints from two different fingers never are identical.*[2]

We are reminded in this connection of the distinguished scientist Carl Ernst von Baer, 1792–1876, who in his eightieth year declared his conviction that he might not die. The reasoning upon which he based that opinion was: "Thus far, all human beings eventually have died. The saying 'All men must die' goes too far; actually it should only claim 'All men so far have died.' Even so, the statement is based only upon an experience to which there might be exceptions."[3] The claimant for actuality of duplication of patterns on two different fingers would take a position about as defensible as that of von Baer on exceptions to the law of mortality. To be sure, a defendant before a court of law might argue the possibility of duplication of finger prints. It might be claimed that an incriminating chance print, shown in expert testimony to be identical with one from a finger of the defendant, is in truth that of another man. The advocate for the defense hails the coincidence as the realization of an occurrence predicted by mathematics! Such a claim, instead of demonstrating that prints from two different fingers are duplicates, proves the weakness of a defense which must resort to patent misrepresentation of the attitude of science.

Workers familiar with finger-print minutiae all affirm that there are no two duplicate prints of different fingers. They recognize many qualities other than the mere occurrences of details. The minutiae, like total patterns, have individuality. The interruption between two ridge ends may be short or long, the ridges may or may not deviate in direction as

---

[2] There is an extensive literature on the philosophy of proof, as it relates to questions such as that here concerned with individuality of a finger print. *The Problem of Proof*, by Albert S. Osborn (2nd ed., Newark, The Essex Press, 1926) presents an excellent discussion of the canons of proof in legal applications; though the problems are illustrated especially by disputed documents, the general arguments (see especially his Chap. 25) and references to the literature are equally pertinent to the issue of finger-print proof. The tenets and history of the theory of probability are succinctly outlined by Florian Cajori in his *A History of Mathematics* (2nd ed., New York, The Macmillan Co., 1931).

[3] From A. Ecker, *100 Jahre einer Freiburger Professorenfamilie*, 1886—Quoted by E. Stemplinger, *Von berühmten Ärzten*, R. Piper & Co., 1938.

they terminate; bifurcations exhibit varying spreads, and many similar individual distinctions of minutiae occur.

When all these finer qualities are appreciated, it is not surprising that identifications of individuals are possible when only partial prints are available. Some chance prints contain a limited number of ridge details, the impressions being fragmentary. Authorities agree that demonstration of 12 correspondences of minutiae (and of course no discordances) proves that two prints originate from the same finger. Others are willing to go further, holding that in some circumstances correspondence of six or eight points establishes a positive identification (79). In the routine of identification, there is naturally no question of the possibility of duplication, since prints of all ten fingers are available for comparison with a new finger-print set. The individual distinctiveness of the complete finger-print set is expressed in the combination of the various pattern types, ridge counts, pattern form and other conspicuous features as well as in the complex of details in each print.

>>>>>>>>>>>>>>>>>> *9* <<<<<<<<<<<<<<<<<<

COMPARATIVE
DERMATOGLYPHICS

Ridged Skin

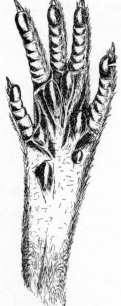

THE ridged skin of palmar and plantar surfaces is often termed "friction skin." Its structural specialization is adapted to locomotion, grasping and the reception of tactile stimuli. This specialization characterizes all primates (prosimians, monkeys, apes and man) and it occurs sporadically in some other groups of mammals. The present

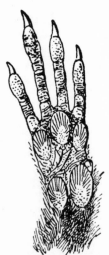

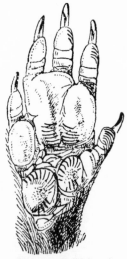

FIG. 99.—Left hind foot of the field mouse, Microtus. (*From Whipple.*)

FIG. 100.—Right fore foot of the squirrel, Sciurus vulgaris. (*From Kidd.*)

FIG. 101.—Right fore foot of the hedgehog, Erinaceus europaeus. (*From Kidd.*)

chapter surveys the occurrence of ridged skin and its configurations in the whole class of mammals.

DISTRIBUTION AMONG MAMMALS. Quadrupedal animals characteristically have no dermatoglyphics. Part of the under surface of the paw

156

of the cat or dog, for example, is hairy; though the foot pads are bare, ridges do not occur. The pads serve as cushions in walking, and the absence of hair on them is an adaptation to the walking function. When dermatoglyphic specialization does occur in quadrupedal mammals, it is apparently associated with prehensile use of the members. At any rate, the specialization is linked with function rather than with the place of the animal in the systematic classification.

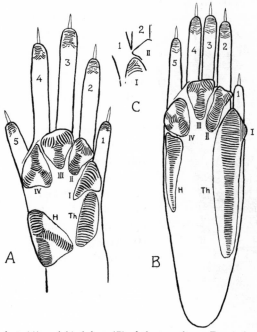

FIG. 102.—Fore foot (A) and hind foot (B) of the tree-shrew, Tupaia lacernata lacernata.

The field mouse (Fig. 99), typical of generalized rodents, possesses prominent walking pads which do not bear dermatoglyphics. Another rodent, the common squirrel (Fig. 100), has ridges partially covering some of the pads. Insectivores also are diverse with respect to the presence of dermatoglyphics, which in this group are at best only incompletely developed. Both the hedgehog (Fig. 101) and tree-shrew (Fig. 102) possess patches of ridged skin, but the arrangements of ridges are quite different in these two insectivores. Most carnivores lack dermatoglyphics, though in some forms the development of ridged skin is fairly advanced, as in the arboreal kinkajou of South America (Fig. 103). The marsupials are widely variable. Some marsupials have no dermatoglyphics and others, like Tarsipes, display ridges over the pads; Marmosa (Fig. 104) has more extensive ridged skin, and in Phalanger (Fig. 105) the sole is completely covered with ridges. No primate lacks at least some ridge-bearing areas, but the members of the group vary widely in the extent of the specialization.

ORIGIN OF RIDGES. Epidermal ridges are modified scales, primitively imbricated in arrangement. Each scale is associated with one hair, or a hair group, and a sweat gland. In the evolution of friction skin the hairs disappear, and scales aggregate into ridges. The story of this evolution is traced by Whipple, from whose work the following digest is extracted.

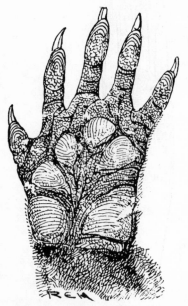

FIG. 103.—Left fore foot of the kinkajou, Cercoleptes caudivolvulus. (*From Kidd.*)

Among mammals other than primates there is considerable variation in the intimate structure of epidermal ridges, both as evidenced on the skin surface and in histological organization. Only the conditions in primates are to be mentioned. Prosimians, the lowest primate group, afford a good illustration of progressive stages of ridge formation. The prosimians, unlike man, apes and the majority of monkeys, exhibit large areas in which ridge formation is incomplete. The pads bear fully developed ridges, other regions displaying structures designated by Whipple as epidermal "warts" and epidermal "rings."

The probable evolutionary steps in ridge formation, as seen in the lemur, are illustrated in figure 106. The incomplete ridges are represented by minute elevations, warts (islands), each bearing in its center the orifice of a sweat-gland duct. Epidermal rings are annular conglomerates of such warts. The larger rings are elongated in the same directions as the neighboring ridges. Continuous long ridges would result from fission of the extremities of elongated rings, followed by end-to-end junctions with similarly disjoined elements of rings. Some primates lack rings, but the warts gather in lines which are "prospective" ridges. The transition from warts to rings or from either to long ridges is not to be pictured as a sequence in the developmental history of the individual. Instead, it is an expression of an evolutionary process which has been halted in successive phases, since ridges develop in the individual without passing through these steps. The successive pore-bearing segments of a ridge, like single islands, are morphologically equivalent to warts. Even in those primates where ridges are continuously developed over the whole palmar and plantar surfaces the zones of junction between ridged skin and the unspecialized skin of the dorsum show transitions from ridges to islands.

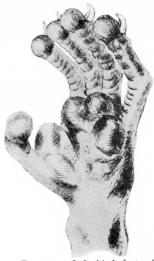

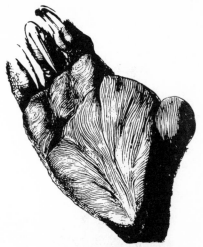

FIG. 104.—Left hind foot of Marmosa murina, a marsupial of the opposum group. (*From Dankmeijer.*)

FIG. 105.—Right hind foot of Phalanger maculatus, a phalangerine opossum. (*From Dankmeijer.*)

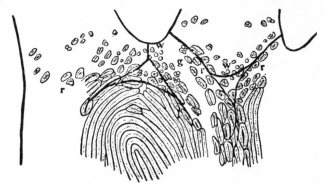

FIG. 106.—A portion of the distal palm of a prosimian, Lemur. (*From Whipple.*)

The minutiae of epidermal ridges in non-human primates are comparable to those in the human hand and foot. These details, together with variations in pattern construction, are applicable in individual identification as in man. Indeed they are put to this use in the chimpanzee colony maintained by the Yerkes Laboratories of Primate Biology, Yale University.

THE MORPHOLOGIC PLAN OF VOLAR PADS AND OF CONFIGURATIONAL AREAS

The feet of certain groups of mammals bear cushion-like elevations, the *walking pads* or *volar pads*. Epidermal ridges in some forms are limited to these pads. Volar pads are the background of a systematic topography of configurational areas. The pads are subject to considerable variation, evidenced in lowering, expansion and mutual fusion. In spite of such departures some degree of conformity to the basic morphologic plan of volar pads is apparent in all primates. That plan is well exemplified in the

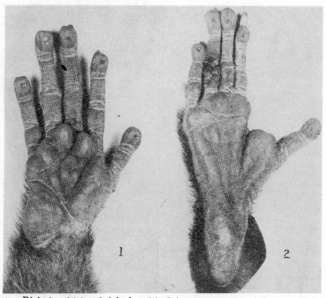

FIG. 107.—Right hand (1) and right foot (2) of the night monkey, Aotus zonalis, tor illustration of volar pads. The legends of figure 108, applying to configurational areas, are equally descriptive of the pads.

night monkey, Aotus, which has pads presenting a nearly primitive arrangement (Fig. 107). The plan of pads is correlated with the topography of configurational areas (Fig. 108).

The terminal segment of each digit bears an *apical* pad, and on palm and sole there are pads composing a marginal and a central series. Seven of the palmar or plantar pads are included in the marginal series. Of these, four are the distally placed *interdigital* pads (pads I, II, III, IV—the series being numbered in accord with the interdigital intervals with which they are related). The proximal elements of the marginal series are: a *distal hypothenar* pad (H^d) and a *proximal hypothenar* (H^p), in the respective regions of the ulnar or fibular border; a *thenar* pad (*Th*), in the radial or tibial region, which in the sole may be divided into two elements, *distal thenar* (*Th^d*) and *proximal thenar* (*Th^p*). In addition to the seven pads above enumerated there are two smaller and less constant components of the marginal series. They are *accessory* pads, adjuncts to interdigitals II and IV (designated II^r and IV^u in the palm, II^t and IV^f in the sole—the Roman numerals identifying their relation to the respective

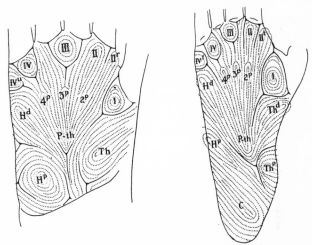

FIG. 108.—Morphologic plan of the dermatoglyphics in palm (left figure) and sole. *I, II, III* and *IV* are interdigital areas, designated by the respective numbers; *II^r* is a field occasionally found on the radial side of *II*, and *IV^u* represents a similar accessory feature in close relation to *IV*. The elements of the central area are termed 2^p, 3^p and 4^p, emphasizing their proximal relation to the corresponding interdigital patterns. The hypothenar area is represented with separate distal and proximal components, *H^d* and *H^p*. The thenar (*Th*), occupying the thenar eminence, usually is separated from the hypothenar configuration by a definite parathenar configuration (*P-th*).—With the exception of the necessarily different notations of accessory patterns *II^t* and *IV^f*, the distal, central and hypothenar portions of the sole correspond to the plan of the palmar dermatoglyphics. The thenar territory occasionally presents a separation of distal and proximal elements (*Th^d* and *Th^p*), and on the heel a calcar pattern (*C*) occurs occasionally.

interdigital pads, and the superscripts giving the initial letters of anatomical directions). Finally, there are three *central* pads located in the central area of the palm or sole in proximal relation to interdigital pads II, III and IV (these central pads being accordingly named 2^p, 3^p and 4^p).

Proximal to the central pads the palmar or plantar surface is depressed, representing the *parathenar* area (*P-th*). The heel region, which is interpreted as a prolongation of the hypothenar zone, is the *calcar* area (*C*).

Almost never is the full complement of volar pads expressed. The accessory pads related to interdigitals II and IV have been observed only in the slow loris, the night monkey and fetal man, though their occurrence as reflected in the dermatoglyphics is known to be more widespread. Central pads likewise are only infrequently present in primates. The major pads of the marginal series may be variously modified.

The consistent disposition of pads and of such surface irregularities as the parathenar area is manifested in the morphological plan of dermatoglyphics (Fig. 108). The plan of configurational fields is in the main a counterpart of the volar reliefs which have been described. However, a species which in the adult has vaguely marked pads may present conspicuous pads in the fetal period (Chap. 10). The epidermal ridges over the surface of a pad may form a pattern, though, as in the human palm and sole, the pad area often bears an open field. Sometimes, as in the parathenar area, a discrete pattern or open field is associated with a depression. The close correlation between dermatoglyphics and modeling of the volar surface reflects the fact that in fetal development the surface irregularities and ridge alignments are conditioned by the same factors of differential growth (Chap. 10).

Variation in Primates

Extent of Formed Ridges. The prosimians, comprising the lowest primates such as lemur, tarsier, bush baby, loris and potto, are variable with regard to the extent of ridge formation. In the bush baby definitely formed ridges occur only on the pads. The slow loris, in contrast, has the palmar and plantar surfaces continuously ridged except in flexion furrows and occasionally in the central portion of the palm. Other members of the group show different degrees of spread of the ridged area.

In monkeys of the New World, including marmosets, the howler, night monkey, spider monkey and capuchin monkey, there is also considerable diversity. The night monkey shows the least extensive ridge formation, areas other than pad surfaces presenting only islands and very short ridges. Occasional individuals among marmosets and capuchins exhibit incomplete ridge formation in the central portion of the palm or sole and in the proximal extremity of the sole. Continuously ridged skin is characteristic in other New World monkeys, in monkeys of the Old World, in apes and in man.

Incomplete ridge formation is less extensive and less frequent in the foot than in the hand. Inasmuch as ridge formation represents an advance in structural specialization, it is evident that in this respect the foot is more advanced than the hand.

Ridge Breadth in Primates. Measurement of ridge breadth is stated indirectly through the count of the number of ridges crossed by a 1-cm. line. For the human hand (young adult males), the average count, including the five finger patterns and five areas of the palm, is 20.7. It has not been possible to make exhaustive determinations in other primates, but the available observations are of interest when compared with findings in man.

TABLE 23

Counts of Ridges per Centimeter in the Palmar Hypothenar Area in Adult Primates, Arranged in the Order of Increasing Hand Lengths

(*Only one specimen of each form except where a number is indicated, the figures in these instances being averages of the individual determinations*)

	Hand length cm.	Ridge count	Hand length × 100 / Ridge count
Saimiri (squirrel monkey)	5.2	31	17
Aotus (night monkey)	5.4	25	22
Cebus—2 (capuchin monkey)	7.1	21	34
Erythrocebus (patas monkey)	8.2	24	34
Lemur	8.3	36	23
Cercocebus (mangabey)	9.5	22	43
Lagothrix (woolly monkey)	10.5	30	35
Macaca—2 (macaque)	10.7	20.5	52
Magus (Celebes macaque)	10.9	21	42
Pygathrix (langur)	12.0	20	60
Homo—200	19.2	18.5	104
Alouatta (howler monkey)	20.0	27	74
Pan—3 (chimpanzee)	20.8	21.3	98
Pongo—4 (orang)	23.9	20.6	117

Comparative observations must take hand size into account, since ridge breadth in man is loosely correlated with hand size. Table 23 lists the determinations in a series of genera, entered in the order of increasing hand lengths, from about 5 cm. in the squirrel monkey and night monkey to as much as 24 cm. in one of the large apes. Comparison of the hand lengths and ridge counts suggests a trend, even if an irregular one, toward an inverse relationship between them. Three forms (squirrel monkey, woolly monkey, howler monkey), having hand lengths which compare as 1:2:4, present ridge counts that are about equal. Then again, forms having equal hand lengths may exhibit quite different ridge counts, as in the howler monkey and man. These departures from inverse correlation between hand size and ridge breadth indicate a partial independence of the factors which condition ridge breadth.

The foregoing comments concern adults alone. For man and chimpanzee there are observations on both adults and juveniles, so that it is possible to state the relationship between hand length and ridge count in association with age differences. Variability is here less than that among adults of different genera presenting corresponding unlikenesses of hand size. In the chimpanzee series the coefficient of variation of the hand length/ridge count index is 12.0, and in the series of human individuals

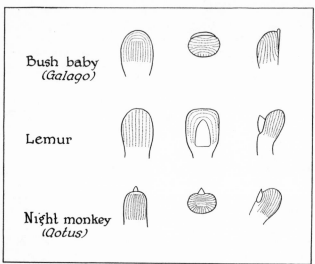

Bush baby
(Galago)

Lemur

Night monkey
(Aotus)

FIG. 109.—Finger patterns of three lower primates. (*Lemur and Galago after Schlaginhaufen.*)

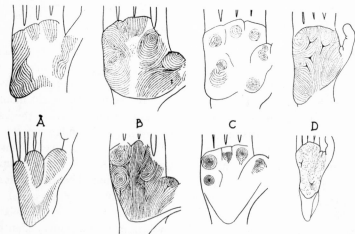

A   B   C   D

FIG. 110.—Palms and soles of four prosimian genera. *A*. Tarsius. *B*. Nycticebus. *C*. Galago. *D*. Lemur.

having hand lengths equal to those of the chimpanzees the coefficient of variation is 12.8. In a comparison of thirteen different primate genera the variation is more than four times as great, with a coefficient of 55.7.

This fact strengthens the conclusion that the characterization of a genus by distinctively fine or coarse ridges is in a measure divorced from the factor of hand size.

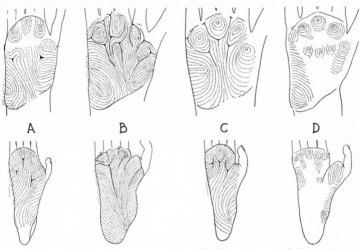

FIG. 111.—Palms and soles of four genera of New World monkeys. *A.* Oedipomidas. *B.* Alouatta. *C.* Saimiri. *D.* Aotus.

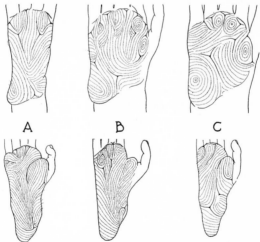

FIG. 112.—Palms and soles of three genera of New World monkeys. *A.* Ateles. *B.* Lagothrix. *C.* Cebus.

Intergeneric variation in ridge breadth is confined to a relatively narrow range, which suggests that proper functional performance of epidermal ridges depends in some way upon restricted variation in ridge breadth.

The "Primitive" Pattern. Varieties of patterns, as emphasized in the description of human finger prints, may be arranged in a series of

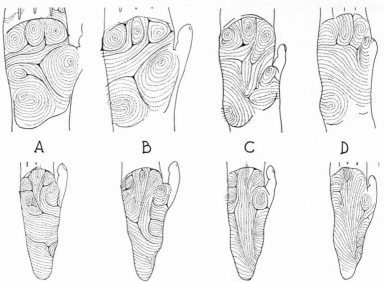

Fig. 113.—Palms and soles of four genera of Old World monkeys. *A*. Papio. *B*. Pithecus. *C*. Pygathrix. *D*. Colobus.

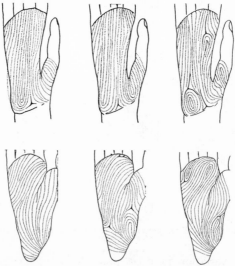

Fig. 114.—Palms and soles of the gibbon, Hylobates.

transitions between dissimilar types. Thus as shown in figure 48, one may trace various lines of descent from the typical whorl to the simple arch:

progressive reduction in the size of a whorl and final conversion of the pattern area into an arch; or degradation of a whorl into a loop and regression of that loop into an arch. These steps compose a pictorial

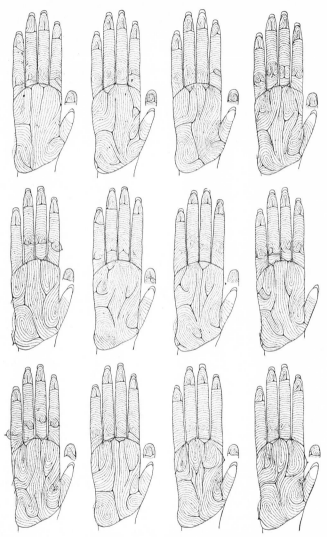

FIG. 115.—Palms of the orang, Pongo.

sequence which may be read in either direction. The whorl may be considered as degenerating, or, reading in the opposite direction, it may be regarded as evolving from the simple arch. There is, of course, no real conversion from one configuration type to another, since in the fetal period a pattern is formed in its fixed character. Nevertheless, the seriation aids in orienting a problem which presents itself in any comparative treatment of configuration types, namely, the tracing of pattern types from an assumed primitive status. This problem can not be finally resolved, but as a working hypothesis the whorl is considered primitive.

It is generally granted that volar pads primitively serve as cushions in walking, and that their lowering and loss of outlines are adaptations

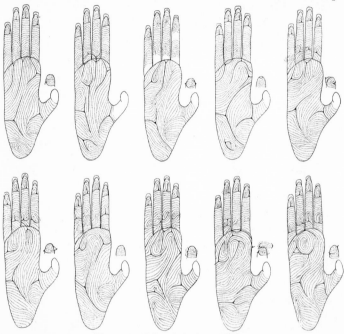

Fig. 116.—Soles of the orang, Pongo.

to prehensile use of the hand and foot. Since the shape of a pad is so intimately associated with the character of its pattern, the pads afford an indirect approach to the question of the primitiveness of patterns. In primates the apparently primitive volar pad is an elevation with a circumscribed base and a more or less pointed summit. This conformation of a pad is developmentally correlated with the presence of a whorl (Chap. 11). It may be assumed therefore that the whorl is the primitive pattern type and that other pattern types are advanced, being correlated with regressive changes of pads.

APICAL CONFIGURATIONS. Most New World monkeys, all Old World monkeys and apes (Figs. 115–116) present apical patterns which are morphologically comparable to those already described in human fingers and toes. These general morphological similarities are evident even if the observations are limited to a single specimen or only a few specimens representing a genus, but owing to limitation of material statistical comparisons are possible only in a few genera. The frequencies of pattern types

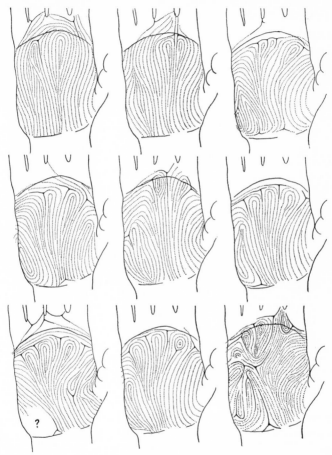

FIG. 117.—Palms of gorilla.

on fingers of chimpanzee (129) may be cited in illustration of the statistical comparison that eventually may be made in other primates. In chimpanzee the frequencies are, in round numbers: whorls, 50%; ulnar loops, 40%; radial loops, 9%; arches, 2%. The ridge counts of loops in chimpanzee average 11.4 ridges, hence pattern size is comparable in chimpanzee and man. These frequencies approximate the distribution of pattern types in man, yet there are several noteworthy peculiarities of the chimpanzee patterns: (a) Whorls are more evenly distributed among the digits. (b) The whorls are chiefly twin loops, lateral pocket loops and accidentals. Monocentric whorls form little more than one-third of the total, as compared with the proportion of about four-fifths in human fingers. The

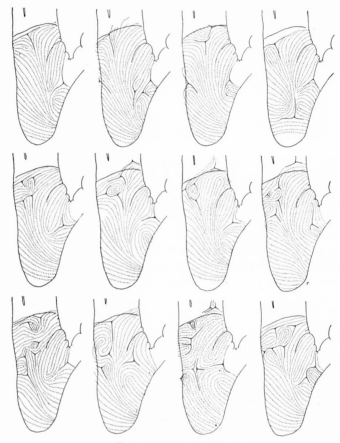

FIG. 118.—Soles of gorilla.

frequencies of monocentric and bicentric whorls in chimpanzee fingers compare closely, however, with the frequencies of these types in human toes. The toe patterns of chimpanzee (144) show 63% whorls, of which nearly half are monocentric, and the remaining patterns are chiefly fibular loops. (c) Radial loops in chimpanzee fingers are almost confined to digit I, contrasting with the characteristic concentration of these patterns on digit II in man. (d) Probably because of their location on the more expanded ball of the thumb, radial loops in chimpanzee have counts (15.9) larger than ulnar loops. (e) Arches occur chiefly on finger V instead of on fingers II and III as in man.

The morphology of apical configurations in prosimians and some New World monkeys is dissimilar to that of human patterns. Apical configurations of two prosimians and of one New World monkey are illustrated in

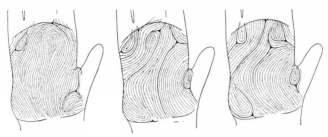

FIG. 119.—Palms of chimpanzee.

figure 109 as representatives of such non-conforming patterns. In the bush baby the central portion of the apical pattern is a series of longitudinally aligned ridges enveloped distally and on the sides by ridges forming a looped frame of the pattern area. The system of looped ridges extends also to the dorsal aspect. In lemur the looped frame is shifted dorsally and is not evident from the volar aspect. Thus in the bush baby and lemur the pattern area is so expanded as to encroach onto the digital

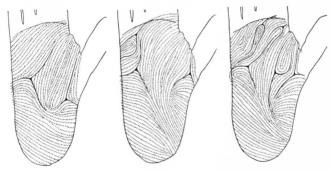

FIG. 120.—Soles of chimpanzee.

margins. The night monkey also shows an expanded pattern area but the convergences of ridges, distally and proximally, indicate more definitely the limits of the main pattern area. Some authors consider such a sequence of patterns as steps in the evolution of the specific pattern types appearing in higher primates. More probably they are merely associates of highly specialized pads, pads which are flattened and expanded.

PALMS AND SOLES. In characterizing palms and soles each genus or group is to be described in terms of general trends. All primates display individual variations in configurational arrangements, the magnitude of these variations being greatest in the apes and man. The illustrations (Figs. 110–122) are limited in many cases to one representative palm and sole of each genus. Numerous illustrations would be required to indicate the scope of individual variation.

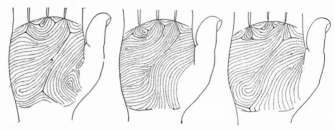

FIG. 121.—Human palms.

Adherence to the basic plan of dermatoglyphics (Fig. 108) indicates lack of specialization. Since no primate conforms fully, and since only the seven (or in the sole, eight) marginally placed configurational areas approach any degree of consistency throughout the primates, major emphasis is placed upon these marginal areas. In most genera the sole presents greater divergence from the morphologic plan than does the palm.

The genera of lowest primates (prosimians) are diverse (Fig. 110). Of the four genera illustrated, the tarsier deviates conspicuously from the

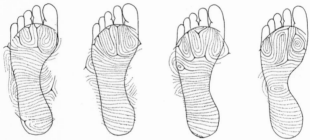

FIG. 122.—Human soles.

morphologic plan. It is the most specialized prosimian, as indicated by absence of whorls and infrequency of other true patterns. The group of New World monkeys (Figs. 111–112) has both primitive and advanced representatives. Some are so primitive that they lack complete ridge formation over the palm and sole, a feature otherwise limited to some prosimians. The most highly advanced form in this group is the spider monkey.

Departures from the basic plan occurring in Old World monkeys (Fig. 113) are almost confined to fusions of the thenar and first interdigital areas. The characteristic patterns on all areas are whorls.

In higher primates the order of increasing modification of the basic plan is: man (Figs. 121–122), orang (Figs. 115–116), gorilla (Figs. 117–118), chimpanzee (Figs. 119–120), gibbon (Fig. 114). Possibly the positions of gorilla and chimpanzee in this list should be transposed.

PROXIMAL AND MIDDLE PHALANGES. In some adult primates the proximal phalanges bear pads, their positions conforming to a consistent plan like the main pads of the palm and sole. Inclusion of phalangeal pads

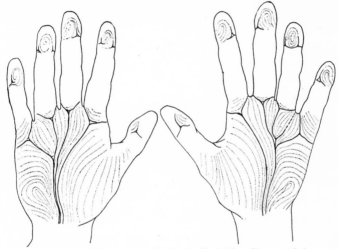

FIG. 123.—The palms of a White woman, the longitudinal ridge alignment being an exception to the characteristic of human palms. (*From Wilder.*)

in a basic morphologic plan would be justified. In the human fetus such pads have been noted, and since they subside in the course of development, it is quite likely that other primates which lack pads in the adult state may possess them transiently in the fetal period. The fairly common occurrence of sharply localized configurations on these phalanges furnishes further proof that such pads had existed in the fetus (Chap. 10). The dermatoglyphics of middle phalanges indicate that fetal pads might occur there also.

Localized patterns are exemplified in the orang (Figs. 115–116), where there is wide variability in the frequency and varieties of configurations on these segments. The occasional paired patterns on the proximal phalanges in the orang is of interest in connection with their frequent appearance in some other forms, the capuchin monkey for example. In man such patterns rarely occur, and their restriction to the proximal phalanx is in keeping with a higher frequency in other primates of patterns on proximal phalanges than on middle phalanges. In most primates the configurations of the phalanges collectively form slanting systems of ridges (Chap. 4).

The proximal and middle phalanges of prosimians usually are devoid of ridges, and in a few New World monkeys the skin of these regions is incompletely ridged.

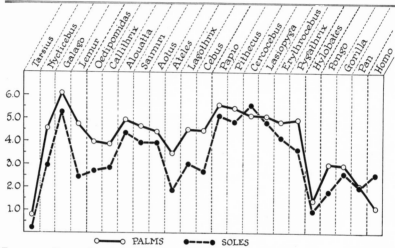

Fig. 124.—Pattern intensities of palms and soles of primates. Increasing values indicate greater number and complexity of patterns.

RIDGE DIRECTION. The directions of ridges, in areas of palm and sole which are undisturbed by local patterns, vary from longitudinal to transverse. The trends exhibit no orderly distribution with regard to the systematic classification of primates. In gibbon and the great apes the direction ranges from longitudinal to oblique. In chimpanzee it has been shown (129) that in spite of the generally longitudinal alignment of palmar ridges there is a bimanual distinction equivalent to that of the human palm, the tendency being for ridge courses to incline more to the transverse direction in right hands. In man the palm presents a combination of longitudinal and diagonal alignments; on the sole ridges course transversely or on a slight slant.

Wilder (101) records a pair of human palms (Fig. 123) presenting remarkable similarity to the longitudinal configuration observed in apes. Only one other instance of this singular relationship is known (291). The authors reporting this second case term the condition "orangoid," and they regard the longitudinal alignment as an atavism. In contrast to

Wilder's subject, where the peculiarity distinguishes both hands, in the second instance only the left palm presents the distinctive longitudinal direction; the main-line formula is 1.1.1.1.

PATTERN INTENSITY. The method of pattern intensity described in Chapter 4 is applicable in analyzing the configurations of palms and soles, though in practice it has been modified with regard to the numerical evaluations of configuration types (141). Without entering into the detail

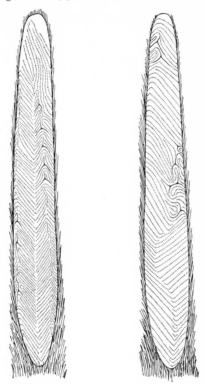

FIG. 125.—Dermatoglyphics of the tail, woolly monkey.

of the evaluations, but keeping in mind that higher values indicate greater number and complexity of patterns, two general results are to be mentioned. (a) The intensity values of palm and sole may be combined as a measure of the status of pattern development in a genus. The general trends are evident in figure 124, though the values for palm and sole are separated. It will be noted that the prosimian genera (Tarsius, Nycticebus, Galago, Lemur) are widely variable among themselves, and that as a group the Old World monkeys (Papio, Pithecus, Cercocebus, Lasiopyga, Erythrocebus, Pygathrix) present the highest values. New World monkeys

(Oedipomidas, Callithrix, Alouatta, Saimiri, Aotus, Ateles, Lagothrix, Cebus) have lower values. Gibbon (Hylobates), the great apes (Pongo, Gorilla, Pan) and man have still lower pattern intensity. Fluctuations of pattern intensity are not correlated with the group classification of primates, though the main trends within a group, as in Old World monkeys, may be consistent. (b) In all primates except man and Cercocebus (the latter being discounted in view of the limited number of hands and feet on which the values are based) pattern intensity is higher in the palm than in the sole. The distinctive position of man is therefore of peculiar interest. Lessened pattern intensity is regarded as indicating advance in specialization, hence in man the sole is in this respect less advanced than is the palm.

CAUDAL DERMATOGLYPHICS. The distal portion of the tail in three genera of New World monkeys (spider monkey, woolly monkey, howler) bears dermatoglyphics. The fundamental ridge arrangement is a herringbone configuration, which may or may not be disturbed by local vestiges or patterns (Fig. 125). Monkeys which possess caudal dermatoglyphics use the tail as if it were a hand—for suspension, prehension and exploration. It is therefore evident that the ridged skin on its ventral surface would have the same functional significance as palmar or plantar skin in preventing slipping and in enhancing tactile sensibility.

PRIMATE AFFINITIES

By combining all observations of descriptive morphology and pattern intensity, comparisons of primate groups may be made with a view to tracing affinities among them. The following condensed statement of the results of such comparison is extracted from the summary of a recent study by the present authors (141).

The consideration of affinities among primates is based upon the following premises.

(a) The conditioning of specific dermatoglyphic configurations is a by-product rather than an immediate vehicle of the evolutionary process. The features primarily concerned in the evolutionary process are the volar pads and other gross qualities of form and relief of the member. The dermatoglyphic configurations are reflections of particular forms and reliefs of the members in their fetal development.

(b) Prominently elevated and circumscribed volar pads are considered primitive; lowering of pads and obliteration of their boundaries indicate modification incident to prehensile use. Whorls and whorl-like patterns are associates of the primitive condition of the pads, while patterns of lesser complexity and open fields accompany states of regression of pads. In terms of pattern intensity, higher values thus indicate primitiveness.

(c) Adherence to the basic plan is a mark of primitiveness and degrees of specialization are indicated by departures from the plan, including such variants as suppression of individual configurational fields and fusions of neighboring fields.

(d) Approach to equally high pattern intensities of the several configurational fields, singly or grouped as described above, is an indication of primitiveness. Likewise an approach to equality in high total intensity values of the palm and sole is evidence of primitiveness.

(e) Minor degrees of bilateral asymmetry in pattern intensity are ranked as primitive, and increase in dextral and sinistral differences points to specialization.

Dermatoglyphics are subject to convergences in the evolutionary process. In marsupials and prosimians, for example, the dermatoglyphics cover a range of variation which may be compared closely to that of New World monkeys, and what is more to the point, the specific trends of variation comprised in any one of these groups are closely matched in the others.

The tracing of affinities is complicated by the apparent independence of the structural expressions which give measures of primitiveness and specialization. The different criteria lead to different orders of resemblance and unlikeness among the forms compared. The divergent results are summated, however, in arriving at judgments of relationship.

The prosimians are heterogeneous; it should be noted that the dermatoglyphics contraindicate simian origin from a tarsier-like stem. Old World monkeys, with the exception of langur, exhibit least specialization of dermatoglyphics; in respect to expanse and character of patterns, they have even exaggerated signs of primitiveness. The resemblance of langur to some New World monkeys is closer than to other Old World monkeys. The New World monkeys are diverse. The most primitive members are the night monkey and marmoset-like monkeys, the most specialized being the spider monkey. The squirrel monkey and capuchin are neither so primitive as the night monkey and marmoset-like forms nor so specialized as the woolly monkey and howler. Gibbon is the most specialized simian. The three great apes and man present specializations which follow different directions. While these divergent specializations render comparison difficult, the order of increasing specialization indicated by the pooled evidence is orang, gorilla or chimpanzee, man. Especially in adherence to the basic plan of configurations, man is even more primitive than orang; inasmuch as that plan is so fundamental a characteristic, it is concluded that man stemmed from an ancestral stock more primitive than any recent ape, having dermatoglyphic traits more closely allied to those of monkeys.

>>>>>>>>>>>>>>>> *10* <<<<<<<<<<<<<<<<

EMBRYOLOGY

B ROAD understanding of the dermatoglyphics in human beings can be gained only with knowledge of their phylogenetic and ontogenetic history. The phylogenetic history, traced through comparative anatomy, is outlined in Chapter 9. In presenting the ontogenetic history, or embryology, volar pads call for first attention. Volar pads are significant both in connection with the morphologic plan of dermatoglyphics and as a correlate of individual variation. The fetal development of these pads parallels their phylogenetic history. The differentiation of epidermal ridges will be traced from a period in which the epidermis is thin and smooth, and the factors responsible for production of patterns, vestiges and open fields also will receive attention. Except for several references to pads in other primates, the chapter is confined to human embryology.

VOLAR PADS

HAND. The volar pads (159) first to appear (second, third and fourth interdigitals) are evident at about the sixth week of development. At this time the hand is still paddle-like and, though the five digital rays are indicated, the free portions of digits are only broad scallops of the distal border. At the close of the second month, when the total length of the fetus is about 2.5 cm., the digits are elongated and separate. The pads of palm and fingers are evident as localized bulges, conforming in their placement to the morphologic plan which has been described. During the ensuing four weeks the pads become more rounded and individualized (Fig. 126). Beginning at about the thirteenth week, when the fetus measures about 7 cm. from crown to rump, regression of pads is apparent. Their elevations become relatively reduced and the boundaries indefinite. Some pads, notably the thenar and hypothenar, are precocious in their involution.

The central area of the palm is at first bulged, but the region soon becomes depressed. Scattered nodules of thickened epidermis appear within this sunken area. These nodules are transient, and if they are correctly interpreted as vestigial hair follicles, their occurrence, like the development of conspicuous pads, is an example of recapitulation. Other recapitulations of primitive conditions, superseded in later development, are noted in the brief appearance of secondary pads on basal phalanges and of accessory pads associated with the second and fourth interdigitals.

All fetuses develop pads in conformity to the morphologic plan. There is considerable variation in the time relations of the appearance and regression of pads. This variation is evident in corresponding pads of different fetuses and of right and left hands of the same fetus, as well as

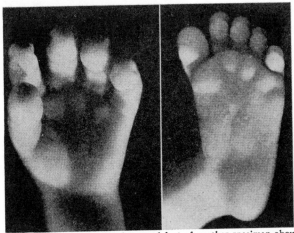

FIG. 126.—Hand of a 10-weeks human fetus and foot of another specimen about two weeks older.

among the several pads of the same hand. There are variations also of contours, of the amount of elevation and shape of individual pads, and of definition of boundaries at their bases.

FOOT. The statements made in reference to the hand apply to the foot as well (Fig. 126), with the following qualifications (159). Pads of the sole are in general more expansive than their homologues in the palm. They develop later and regress later, the onset of general regression being delayed about two weeks as compared to the hand.

COMPARATIVE RELATIONSHIPS. Pads in the human fetus, at first conspicuously elevated and definitely bounded, undergo involution. (The reader might compare his own hand with that of the ten-weeks fetus, figure 126.) This history points to an affinity of man with forms in which pads are permanently retained in full development. Monkeys of the Old World have prominent pads, but even within this group the pads of the adult animal may be relatively lower than in their fetal state (146). In adult great apes the elevation and definition of pads are comparable to conditions in man. In gibbon, pads are even less developed than in man. It may be assumed that the pads of all these higher primates pass through a succession of fetal stages similar to those actually traced in man and the rhesus monkey. There is a positive correlation between pattern intensity and the state of pad development, though in primates whose pads regress only after the dermatoglyphics are differentiated there may be lapses in this correlation.

RIDGES

Differentiation of epidermal ridges has been investigated especially in fingers (153–156) and in palms (165). Except for a casual reference to

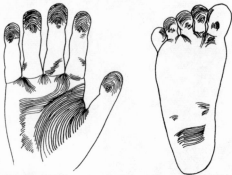

FIG. 127.—The topography of differentiated ridges in hand and foot of a 15-weeks human fetus.

regional differences in the chronology of ridge formation, the following account is confined to fingers.

The critical stages of differentiation occur in the third and fourth fetal months, though ridges are not elevated on the skin surface until about the eighteenth week. The fetal epidermis is at first a thin layer, smooth both on the exposed and deep surfaces. Through continued cellular proliferation the epidermis becomes gradually thicker and the papillary modeling of epidermis and dermis is attained (Fig. 39). This process is not uniformly advanced over the volar surfaces, nor is it uniform even on the ball of one finger. The fingers are the most precocious areas in the differentiation of epidermal ridges, while the sole is the most delayed. Until the differentiation is complete over all areas, the lag of the foot is apparent (Fig. 127).

In a finger, the first region ordinarily presenting papilla-like folds of the deep epidermis is the central portion of the apical pad. Subsequently an independent area of papillary growth arises in the distal and lateral periphery of the finger ball, and another area appears in its proximal region (Fig. 128,A). From these foci ridge differentiation extends progressively until the systems meet. Less frequently, differentiation may be completed by extension from a single focus centered on the finger ball (Fig. 128,B). External pressure on the finger may modify the progress of epidermal differentiation. Bonnevie asserts that the ingrowth of digital nerves may play a part in initiating the differentiation of ridges, and that a blood sinus in the finger ball also may influence the process. Steffens (119), in an attempt to explain the average smaller size of loops and the greater frequency of arches in toes as compared to fingers, does not consider ingrowing digital nerves and the blood sinus as likely regulatory factors.

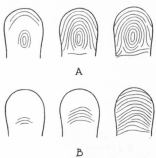

FIG. 128.—Progressive differentiation of ridges on fingers of fetuses. *A*. "Discontinuous" differentiation, with a center and peripheral zones which extend and meet. *B*. "Continuous" differentiation, where the process is completed by extension from a single center on the apical ball. (*From Bonnevie, modified.*)

Developmental disturbances in existence during the period of ridge differentiation may produce imperfect ridges in some areas (313). The defect appears as patches of islands and short ridges (Fig. 129), resembling the effects of some forms of injury to the adult skin.

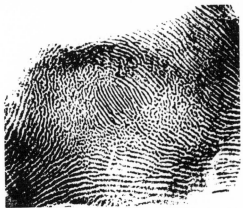

FIG. 129.—Aberrant formation of epidermal ridges: Dissociation of ridges. Enlarged. (*From Abel.*)

Also, though more rarely, the abnormality consists of an extreme narrowing of ridges in the pattern area (Fig. 130). Such disturbances may occur in any region of the dermatoglyphics. In affected cases the faulty ridge formation occurs bilaterally. In its more severe degrees the defect appears on all ten digits of the affected individual, but in the lesser involvements some digits may be spared. The order of decreasing frequency of the defect in individual digits is I (which never is free from defect in the cases studied by Abel)—II—III—IV—V. The expanse of the defective areas follows the same order of diminution. Abel holds that there is no intrinsic fault in the tissues concerned, and he interprets the ridge disturbances as the effect of variations in tension and pressure within the epidermis. The appearance of ridge irregularities in fingers, palms, toes and soles of some cases suggests that abnormal tension and pressure may be widespread in the body. The constitutional aspect of this condition is discussed in Chapter 16.

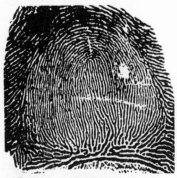

Since developmental disturbances are effective during the period of ridge formation, the regional involvement in a finger may be correlated with the order of formation of ridges. When the factors for abnormality operate after the initiation of ridge development, only those areas not yet active in ridge formation are susceptible. When the factors operate during the phase of union of the originally isolated areas of ridge formation, the defect is localized in the proximal portion of the pattern area and in the regions of triradii. Abel reports that lesser degrees

FIG. 130.—Aberrant formation of epidermal ridges, involving ridge breadth and circumscription of pattern area. Enlarged. (*From Abel.*)

of these disturbances occur in 20 individuals of his series of 4000 criminals, the more pronounced degrees being even less common.

FACTORS WHICH CONDITION ALIGNMENT OF RIDGES

Epidermal ridges differentiate in their definitive character. That is to say, from the very first appearance of ridges the minutiae and configurational arrangements are in their permanent form. The factors determining ridge alignments are identified with two major developmental circumstances, namely, variations in the histology of different regions and differential growth incident to the production of irregular reliefs of the volar surfaces.

Bonnevie observes that variations in progression of ridge differentiation are at least in part correlated with variations in the prospective pattern type. According to her, there are two conditions of the epidermis responsible for variations in pattern type: the thickness of the fetal epidermis at the time of ridge differentiation; a water-logged state of the epidermal cells (the *Polsterung* of Bonnevie, herein termed *cushioning*). Bonnevie states that cushioning predisposes against the development of whorls and loops. This relationship is questioned by three workers (266, 299, 347) who regard the lack of correlation between frequencies of arches in various racial groups and the calculated gene frequencies (Chap. 12) as a sign that arches are not dependent upon cushioning. Karl, however, grants that both epidermal thickness and cushioning might be concerned in the developmental mechanism which produces arches.

Bonnevie also correlates variations in contour of the embryonic finger pads with the presumptive pattern formations, the correspondences indicating the influence of generalized growth processes on the character of configurations, especially as regards the formation of loops and other asymmetrical patterns. Cummins (157) emphasizes the rôle of growth stresses in the developing skin. This source of conditioning of ridge direction, first suggested by Kollmann (136), is now supported by evidence which amounts to an experimental solution of the problem.

The experimental method is commonly applied when it is desired to identify and analyze factors of growth and differentiation. An animal such as the opossum, bearing young which are still embryonic, might lend itself to experimental alteration of the intrinsic developmental environment of the dermatoglyphics. By excising and grafting bits of volar skin or by minute intradermal injections for induction of localized tensions, it might be possible to demonstrate the factors which condition alignment of ridges. This approach never has been attempted, but a natural substitute for experimentation has been utilized (157). The hands and feet are subject to diverse developmental abnormalities such as syndactyly (webbing of digits) and polydactyly (supernumerary digits). Observations of dermatoglyphics in these and other malformations indicate that ridge alignment is conditioned by the stresses and tensions incident to the general growth of the part. Differential growth is obviously a necessity for the production of the characteristic form of any bodily structure. Were it not for the occurrence of unlike rates of growth at different points, the hand and foot would not develop their characteristic form, and pads would not be present as localized elevations. The localizations of greater growth activity, which produce irregularities in the general form of the part, are responsible for variable alignments of ridges. There are no predeterminations of ridge direction other than those which operate through their control of specific contours. The epidermis covering the volar surfaces possesses the inherent capacity to develop ridges, but the dispositions of these ridges are passively determined in the growth of the digit, palm or sole. The evidence for these conclusions, deduced from the dermatoglyphics of malformed hands and feet, may be briefly summarized.

A supernumerary digit, such as an extra toe, may be as fully developed and separate as its normal neighbor. In such cases patterns of the same type may occur on the supernumerary toe and on the normal digit which it duplicates (Fig. 131,A). When the extra digit is imperfectly developed or bound in a syndactyl relation (Fig. 131,B), the pattern of the supernumerary member is dissimilar in type from that of its mate; the dissimilarity is often demonstrably associated with differences in form of the two homonymous digits. Wherever the molding of a palmar or plantar surface is abnormal, and whatever the nature of the .defect, the configurations are partly or wholly unlike the normal, but they conform to the irregularities of the parts (Fig. 131,C). Anomalous eminences, whatever

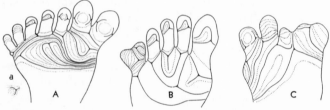

FIG. 131.—*A*. Polydactyly, with patterns of same type on both big toes and on both little toes; the small whorl at the base of the seventh toe is detailed in *a*. *B*. Polydactyly, with the two little toes syndactylous and bearing configurations of unlike type. *C*. Complex malformation of the foot, presenting abnormal dermatoglyphics which conform to the irregular contours.

their nature, may bear distinctive patterns. Occasionally, the form of such an eminence is clearly correlated with the character of its configuration. A symmetrically rounded hillock with a definitely circumscribed base, for instance, has as its developmental correlate a concentric whorl (Fig. 131,a). In this connection cases presenting suppression of distal phalanges are of interest. Fingers so affected bear patterns on the extreme ends of the fingers (162). The placement and aberrant character of these configurations indicate that the patterns are fortuitously developed rather than being apical patterns displaced from their normal position. The various configurations are not determined by self-limited mechanisms within the skin. The skin possesses the capacity to form ridges, but the alignments of these ridges are as responsive to stresses in growth as are the alignments of sand to sweeping by wind or wave.

Triradii, like any other alignments of ridges, are conditioned by growth factors. That their normal disposition is associated with conjunction points of three complexes of growth is demonstrated in developmental defects of the hands and feet (Fig. 131).

Volar pads in the normal fetus are sites of differential growth, each being responsible for production of one of the local configurations comprised in the morphologic plan of dermatoglyphics. If a pad does not completely subside prior to the time of ridge formation, its presence determines a discrete configurational area. Direct observations on the variations in subsidence of pads have been correlated in part with tendencies of the corresponding configurational areas to bear patterns or open fields. The thenar pad of the palm, for example, tends to be precocious in its involution, hence accounting for the infrequency of thenar patterns. Pads on distal phalanges of digits and on the ball of the foot attain more full development and persist longer; in these regions highly expressed patterns occur frequently. While it is difficult to compare the subtile variations in pad contour, such variations may be correlated in some cases with characteristic pattern variants, as are gross contours in abnormal hands and feet.

Abel (151) points out that the elevation of the embryonic pad influences the spacing of the triradius from the pattern center (as determined by the ridge count), the directions of ridge coursing and pattern form. He excludes the possibility of any effect of pad elevation on the number of ridges developed over the distal phalanx as a whole. His evidence consists of ridge counts from the pattern core to the lateral nail fold in two racial groups (Chinese and Germans) which have marked differences in the incidence of whorls, loops and arches. The two groups show approximately the same number of ridges along this line of count. The same author correlates this ridge count with size of the distal phalanx, showing that there is a direct relationship between the two variables, though both are independent of pattern type and pattern size.

Applications

Dermatoglyphics, being differentiated in their final form during the third and fourth fetal months, are significant indicators of conditions existing several months prior to the birth of an individual. During the latter months of pregnancy dermatoglyphics are as unalterable morphologically as they are in postnatal life. The configurations and their component ridges enlarge with the growth of the hand and foot, but all their essential characteristics remain unchanged. The distinctions in adult dermatoglyphics—among races, between the sexes, between right and left hands, or in any other group comparison—reflect the existence of differences dating from the fetal period. This freedom from the effects of environmental influences is shared by few other traits which are accessible to investigation in physical anthropology.

In addition to these general applications, dermatoglyphics may aid in some investigations which call for reconstruction of events in the intrauterine history of an individual.

In studying the inheritance of polydactyly an investigator meets with cases where the supernumerary digits, particularly if they are accessory to the little fingers, have been surgically removed or spontaneously amputated. The former existence of such a digit sometimes is recognizable by a scar, but often no scarring follows the amputation. Nevertheless, it is still possible to prove that there was once a supernumerary digit, since a triradius typically occurring in proximal relation to it remains as a permanent sign.

Often an extra little finger is extremely small and constricted at its base. Such a digit may undergo spontaneous amputation either prior to birth or in infancy. Its former existence may be inferred, however, from a retained small nodule representing the narrowed base, and the nature of the dermatoglyphics on this nodule may be indicative of amputation subsequent to the period of ridge differentiation (160).

Spontaneous amputations of normal digits also may occur in utero, though rarely. Before any specimen presenting the actual early progress of amputation was ever seen, significant chronological evidence was obtained from dermatoglyphics in these cases. Normal ridges cover areas involved in the amputative process, indicating that the process as seen in the newborn is of months standing, its initiation antedating the period of ridge differentiation (158). This is substantiated in later observations of fetal specimens presenting active phases of amputation.[1]

Reference to dermatoglyphics should be profitable also in investigation of the inheritance of webbed digits (zygodactyly, or syndactyly). Observations in families, having one or more members whose second and third toes are webbed, suggest that inheritance may produce variably either actual digital union or a minor expression of zygodactyly evidenced only in certain features of the distal plantar dermatoglyphics (166). These signs have their parallel in the palm (Chap. 11). They indicate that the disturbed embryological processes which produce webbing of the normally free portions of digits extend their influence into the distal zone of the palm and sole. A pedigree of syndactyly which records only the webbed individuals as positive cases is possibly misleading, since cases presenting the dermatoglyphic aberrancy alone would be erroneously classed as normals.

---

[1] Streeter, G. L. Focal deficiencies in fetal tissues and their relation to intra-uterine amputation. Carnegie Inst. of Wash., Contrib. to Embryol., No. 126, 1930.

SYMMETRY AND OTHER ASPECTS
OF SPECIAL MORPHOLOGY

TRANSITIONS OF CONFIGURATION TYPES

INTERGRADATIONS of finger-print types are described and illustrated (Fig. 48) in Chapter 4. Similar transitions are demonstrable in all other morphological areas: middle and proximal phalanges of the fingers, palmar interdigital areas, palmar hypothenar and thenar areas, toes, the several plantar areas.

The essential uniformity of transitions of configuration types in different regions may be illustrated by showing that an area of the palm, interdigital IV for example, duplicates in principle the transitions demonstrated in fingers. The primitive interdigital pattern is a whorl, bounded by three or four triradii and their radiants. Several lines of transition uniting whorls to loops and transitions from both of these to patternless configurations are illustrated in figure 132. The series composing group I traces the degeneration of a typical concentric whorl directly into an open field. In the course of degeneration the three triradii appear to approach simultaneously the center of the whorl, and with obliteration of the pattern there is in its place an open field bounded on the ulnar side by triradius d and line D. Groups II–V show different lines of transition in which central pockets and loops are the intergrades between whorls and open fields.

I W. Wilder traces the transitions in palmar interdigital areas II, III and IV. H. H. Wilder (170) and Cummins (82) deal with transitions of the palmar hypothenar configuration, and Fleischhacker (284) and Bettmann (81) describe the thenar/first interdigital of the palm. The details of transition in different areas vary, because of local morphological distinctions, but all areas exhibit variants which form an orderly series. Again it is to be emphasized that these transitions only reflect gradations in the resultants of growth mechanisms in fetal development (Chap. 10). They are not literally conversions of one configuration type to another.

ASSOCIATIONS OF PATTERNS

The occurrence of like finger-print types in the individual, referred to by Galton (57) as "the tendencies of digits to resemble one another," is termed *association* by Waite. Biologists now designate genetic association of any traits as *pleiotropy*.

Waite finds, in 2000 males, 12% who have patterns of the same type—arches, loops or whorls—on all ten digits. Loosening of the bond of associa-

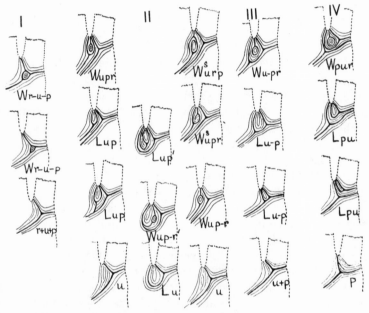

Fig. 132,A.—Types of fourth interdigital patterns of the palm, showing (in vertical rows) lines of transition in reduction of the pattern. Drawn as from prints of right hands. (*From I. W. Wilder.*)

tion, statistically more pronounced in right hands, is evidenced by the occurrence in individuals of different pattern types. Sixteen percent of the persons in Waite's series have nine patterns of the same type, and 10% have eight patterns of the same type. Five percent of the persons bear patterns of all four main types, and of their single hands about one-fourth are thus characterized.

The incidence of complete association in single hands is naturally higher than that in individuals, since there are five instead of ten digits concerned. Volotzkoy (253), who applies the term *monomorphic* to a hand in which all digits bear the same pattern type, reports frequencies of monomorphic hands ranging from 21% to 33% in 11 racially diverse populations. The average is about 25%.

Waite and others more recently report a positive correlation of arches with small loops (loops having counts of 12 ridges or less, and especially those in the lower range), arches being negatively correlated with other pattern types. The bimanuar (Fig. 51) demonstrates the tendency toward

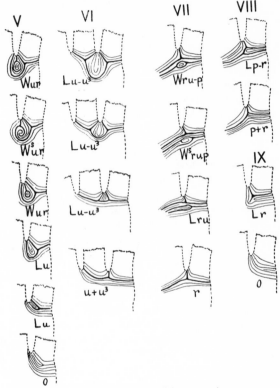

FIG. 132,B.—See legend of figure 132,A.

mutual exclusiveness of arches and whorls. The negative association of arches and whorls is suggested also by the fluctuations in frequencies of the two patterns in different racial series, there being a tendency for arches to increase as whorls diminish (Chap. 15).

It is apparent that toes have at least some associations different from those described in fingers, since the bipedar (Fig. 97) does not disclose the exclusive relationships between arches and whorls which are so noteworthy in fingers.

Steffens (119) makes a study of correlation of pattern type in fingers and toes of the same individuals, reporting that frequent arches on toes are associated especially with arches and loops on fingers. Further, when there are many loops on toes, the fingers bear loops, or loops and whorls. The coefficient of correlation for whorls in fingers and toes of the same individuals is 0.36 ± 0.06, and for arches the coefficient is 0.50 ± 0.05. Newman (118) computes coefficients of correlation for the occurrence of the same pattern type on fingers of both hands and on toes of both feet: whorls, 0.42 ± 0.09; loops, 0.33 ± 0.09; arches, 0.17 ± 0.10.

Associations among patterns in the several areas of the palm have been little investigated. Mass statistics indicate, as in the case of arches and whorls of fingers, a negative correlation in the occurrences of patterns (as distinguished from patternless configurations) in the hypothenar and thenar/first interdigital areas. In general, a racial group presenting few hypothenar patterns has abundant thenar/first interdigitals.

Rife (357) shows by statistical analysis a negative correlation between patterns of the hypothenar and thenar/first interdigital areas within single hands, thus confirming the observation just mentioned. Positive correlations of pattern occurrence exist between the thenar/first inter-digital and second interdigital areas, also among the second, third and fourth interdigital areas. Within individuals, there are positive correlations of pattern frequency between the second and fourth interdigital areas, the second and third, and the third and fourth. An association exists even between the configurations of fingers and palms, since whorls on fingers are positively correlated with the presence of patterns in the second, third and fourth interdigital areas.

Harkness-Miller (105) calculates correlations of pattern occurrences in five homologous areas of palm and sole. There is no significant correla-tion for any area when the left sole is compared with the right palm, or when the right sole and left palm are considered. Even in homolateral comparisons of palm and sole, seven of the ten correlations are much below the level of significance. Only three of these homolateral correlations appear to be significant: thenar areas of right palm and right sole, 0.27; fourth interdigital areas of right palm and right sole, 0.31; third inter-digital areas of left palm and left sole, 0.24.

The positive correlation of arches with small loops and the negative correlation of arches with whorls show that there is a degree of common control of the level of pattern expression in the fingers of individuals. Notwithstanding that the bond among the ten digits is loose, the correla-tions suggest a generalized tendency in the apical volar pads of the fetus to behave in their development and regression as if they were under a common control. Positive correlations of pattern occurrences in areas as remote as fingers and palm, or palm and sole, indicate that all areas are to some extent subject to a common control—rigid enough to determine not only the existence of patterns, as distinguished from open fields, but also to regulate pattern type. The negative correlation of palmar hypothenar and thenar/first interdigital must indicate the existence of superimposed local factors counteracting the effects of the more generalized control.

BILATERAL SYMMETRY

Only in a very general way is the human body bilaterally symmetrical, i.e., equal in the right and left halves. An internal organ which is paired, like lung or kidney, shows unlikenesses of form, size and position between the right and left partners. Most of the unpaired viscera, including organs such as heart, gastro-intestinal tract and liver, are displaced from the midline in an arrangement which conforms to a nearly constant pattern.

The asymmetries evident externally in the lateral body halves comprise many familiar variations in form and size. Differences between right and left sides of the face may be strikingly demonstrated by bisecting two full-face photographs from the same negative, one of them being printed in reverse, and piecing together the halves to construct two full-face portraits. One of these is the combination of the two prints of the right half of the face, the other, of the left half. Facial asymmetry may be so marked that such reconstructed photographs seem to be of two persons, each showing unlikeness to the full face of the original. The right and left arms, though appearing to be counterparts except for the mirrored relationship of one to the other, display anatomical differences and are rarely of equal dimensions. The inequality of size is not dependent merely on use, since asymmetries exist even in the fetal period. It would be pointless to enumerate all the manifestations of structural asymmetry (and functional asymmetry, as expressed in handedness, footedness and eyedness). It is important, however, to approach bilateral symmetry and asymmetry in dermatoglyphics with an understanding that these features are neither exceptional in presenting differences on the two sides nor exceptional in showing frequencies of specific variants greater on one side than the other. Reference to variants of dermatoglyphics does not concern differences in minute characteristics, differences which are taken for granted; the bilateral contrasts under consideration are gross characters of the configurations.

The interrelationships between configurations of right and left members represent one aspect of association, but in considering this bilateral association, or symmetry, interest is more often centered on differences of right and left members rather than on the characters which they possess in common. Distinctive bilateral trends of variation in dermatoglyphics are associated with functional asymmetry. In the palm and fingers certain departures from the usual trends occur in groups of left-handed subjects (Chap. 16).

MIRRORING. In its general conformation each arm is a mirrored counterpart of the other. This applies, within the limits of bilateral variation, not only to the arms but also to the legs and the lateral halves of the head, neck and trunk. The phenomenon of mirroring is an obvious corollary of the plan of construction of a body which in general is bilaterally symmetrical.[1]

Dermatoglyphics exhibit mirroring, a mirroring which is usually partly obscured by factors operating independently of those conditioning basic symmetry. The phenomenon of mirroring will be considered principally with reference to fingers and palms, though it occurs as well in toes and soles.

A prerequisite for the expression of mirroring in finger prints is asymmetry of pattern structure, the asymmetry being referred to the digital axis. A typical plain arch, or a whorl in which all radiants meet, is symmetrical. (For a qualification of this statement, see below.) A typical loop is the extreme of asymmetric construction. As with other variants of dermatoglyphics, there are grades of finger-print asymmetry (Fig. 48). Different series of configurational intergrades connect the completely asymmetric loop to the symmetric arch and to the symmetric whorl. The line of lessened asymmetry leading from the typical loop to an arch is a succession of progressively smaller loops, the ridge count affording a measure of the degree of asymmetry—an asymmetry which has opposed directions, ulnar and radial. The sequence should be regarded as continuous, linking the one extreme of ulnar asymmetry, exemplified in an ulnar loop having a maximum ridge count, to the extreme of radial asymmetry, a radial loop of maximum ridge count. Following this sequence, the ulnar asymmetry is progressively diminished with smaller and smaller ridge counts until the loop is extinguished and the configuration is a symmetric arch. Continuing from the arch, the progression of increasing radial asymmetry is a sequence of larger and larger radial loops. The sequence from the ulnar loop to the meet whorl is composed of central pockets with increasingly larger concentric centers, and these in turn lead to whorls in which non-meeting of radiants on the ulnar side admits outflow of ridges from the pattern area. It is but a step then to the symmetric

---

[1] The term mirroring, or mirror imaging, is used in a different sense in connection with twin comparisons (Chap. 13). When twins show closer resemblance between members of their opposite sides than between members of corresponding sides the resemblance is described as mirrored.

whorl which, as in the case of the arch, can be connected with a series of transitions to maximum radial asymmetry. These sequences of asymmetry may be read descriptively in either direction.

There remains to be characterized another mirroring phenomenon appearing in whorls. The stated symmetry of the meet whorl is in reference to contrast with the asymmetry of a loop, where from one side of the pattern area there is an outflow of ridges to the digital margin. However, both meet and non-meet whorls frequently exhibit asymmetric construction of the pattern area. Whorls may be either twisted, in a clockwise or counterclockwise direction, or distinguished by spiral instead of concentric coursings of ridges. In whorls of right digits the direction of twist or of spiraling is typically clockwise, as viewed in prints, while on the left hand the typical direction is counterclockwise (225). The reversal of direction on right and left hands is an expression of mirroring.

The ideal example of mirroring is the frequent combination of ten ulnar loops, each of the five loops on one hand being the mirror image of the pattern on the corresponding digit of the opposite hand (Fig. 133,A). The palmar main lines and configurational areas are in general mirrored in right and left hands, though, as will be detailed, courses of main lines and occurrences of patterns show unlike statistical trends in the two hands. This bimanual differential disturbs the aspect of mirroring.

Using as a standard of reference the individual who has a complete mirroring expressed in ten ulnar loops, the most extreme reversal of mirroring would be that in which all digits of one hand bear ulnar loops and all digits of the other, radial loops. Such a pattern combination apparently never has been observed, and the drawing of these patterns in figure 133,B is accordingly hypothetical. However, a relation short of complete mirroring, such as a ten-finger set with nine ulnar loops and one radial loop, is common.

In the authors' files there are prints of one individual whose distal palmar configurations are unique in exhibiting a complete reversal of the typical mirrored relationship (Fig. 133,B). The prints of the right and left distal palmar regions appear as if they were two impressions of the same hand (with characteristics typical of right palms). This entails unlikeness of the courses of homologous lines in the two hands: line A in the right hand is identical in course, even to certain sinuosities, to line D of the left; line B of the right hand follows a course equivalent to line C of the left, in enclosing the third interdigital pattern; line C of the right hand is like line B of the left; and line D of the right is like line A of the left hand. It will be seen, therefore, that not only are the right and left distal palms grossly alike, but also that this similarity arises from consistent reversals of the order of coursing of homologous main lines. Notwithstanding this remarkable state of the distal palm, there is nothing unusual in the proximal regions of the palms, and all fingers bear ulnar loops.

Lack of mirrored asymmetries of dermatoglyphics, whether in fingers or palms, may be compared with the rare condition of reversal of visceral asymmetries, *situs viscerum inversus*. When visceral transposition is com-

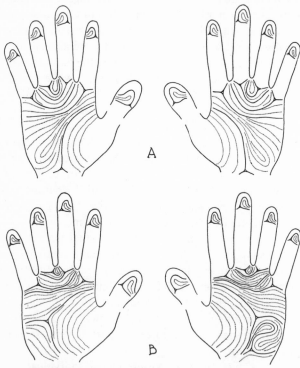

FIG. 133.—*A*. Pair of hands showing typical mirroring of finger prints and palmar features. *B*. A unique case in which the distal palmar features are not mirrored; the finger prints, with all ulnar loops on one hand and all radial loops on the other, are added as an hypothetical illustration of similar lack of mirroring in fingers.

plete, the topography is reversed, as if the normal visceral relationships were viewed in a mirror. The transpositions in dermatoglyphics are manifest as a reversal of mirroring in one of the members.

FINGERS. Right and left fingers display statistical distinctions in ridge breadth, ridge count (quantitative value) and frequencies of the pattern types. In right digits ridges tend to be coarser and quantitative value tends to be higher. Differential trends of pattern type are evident in the total frequencies for the five digits collectively and in the frequencies for individual digits. In mass analysis right digits typically present a larger number of whorls and radial loops than lefts, while arches are more frequent in left hands (though when digits are examined separately, digit II of the right hand generally shows the higher frequency of arches). These trends are evident in table 1. Exceptions, when not due to statistical inadequacy of the collection, are unusual, and are evidences of racial or sexual distinctions.

TABLE 24

FREQUENCIES OF DIGITAL COUPLETS, COMPOSED OF HOMOLOGOUS FINGERS OF RIGHT AND LEFT HANDS, BEARING THE SAME PATTERN TYPE

Germans*.. 74.4%
Dutch—males†... 75.5
Dutch—females†... 76.1
Chilean Spanish—males‡... 77.5
Chilean Spanish—females‡... 76.8
Chilean Indians‡... 77.2
Javanese—males†.. 78.7
Javanese—females†.. 78.4
Liberian negroes—males†.. 82.1
Liberian negroes—females†.. 77.3
Efé pygmies—males†... 75.5
Efé pygmies—females†... 80.4

* Grüneberg.
† Dankmeijer.
‡ Henckel.

Another demonstration of symmetry in pattern type is afforded by comparison of couplets of digits, couplets composed of homologous fingers of right and left hands. Table 24 indicates the degree of bilateral symmetry, the implied percent remainders expressing asymmetry. The essential consistence of findings among races so diverse as those listed in the table suggests that the level of symmetry of pattern type is fairly uniform among all peoples.

The foregoing fails to indicate the degree of symmetry expressed in the individual, since the five digital couplets are dissociated in the mass comparison. Henckel's series (288) of 61,510 Chilean-Spanish males is a representative sample of symmetry relations in individuals. Symmetry is complete in 28.5% of the persons in this series, in whom each of the five digital couplets bears the same type of pattern. The diminishing frequencies of unlike pattern types on one, two, three, four and five digital couplets are, respectively: 40.4%, 22.5%, 7.5%, 1.1%, 0.1%.

The following approximate incidences of symmetry in single digits are from Dankmeijer's data (281) on Dutch and Javanese: Digit I, 75%; digit II, 71%; digit III, 80%; digit IV, 76%; digit V, 84%. Analyses by other authors also show a depression of symmetry in digit II and an elevation in digit V. Distinctions among the digits are explained at least in part by their varying statistical trends of pattern type.

The total frequencies of pattern types and their differential distributions on digits have a bearing on this explanation. In Dankmeijer's series of Dutch males, for example, the level of bilateral symmetry of loops is 54%, whorls, 17% and arches, 4%. Loops exhibit the highest symmetry because they are so abundant. The incidences of these types on particular digits are detailed in Chapter 4. Digit V leads in the expression of symmetry because loops have their maximum frequency on this digit and other patterns are correspondingly uncommon. The high degree of symmetry in digit V is accordingly in part obligative. In contrast, digit II presents the least symmetry because in this digit all the pattern types are commonly represented. Digit II apparently owes its lesser symmetry to the latitude of action of factors responsible for pattern type, the influence of obligative symmetry being thus diminished.

Dankmeijer and Renes determine symmetry of pattern type in several racially different collections. They calculate also the symmetry that might be expected if the pattern distributions on right and left hands were determined by chance. In each of their groups (Dutch, Javanese, Liberian negroes and Efé pygmies—and in the sexes separately, making eight groups in all), the observed symmetry is greater than the computed chance symmetry. Kirchmair (349) also demonstrates this point, both for sym-

TABLE 25

FREQUENCIES OF WHORLS AND ARCHES ON INDIVIDUAL FINGERS

(*Data from Table 1*)

	I	II	III	IV	V
Whorls:					
Right.....................	41.4%	30.8%	16.6%	41.1%	13.8%
Left.....................	29.4	28.2	16.2	27.8	9.0
Arches:					
Right.....................	2.5	10.9	6.1	1.9	0.5
Left.....................	4.5	10.4	8.0	2.7	1.2

metry expressed by occurrences of the same pattern type on couplets of homonymous digits and by the agreement of the numbers of corresponding types in opposite hands irrespective of their digital distribution.

Poll, using the dactylodiagram, emphasizes certain characteristics of statistical distribution of pattern types which occur in the majority of peoples so far studied. The frequencies of arches and whorls on digits I and IV of the same hand are closer numerically than is either frequency to that of the corresponding digit on the opposite hand (Table 25). Each of the other digits, in contrast, presents pattern frequencies closer to those of its homologue on the opposite hand than to the frequencies of any other digit. In recognition of these digital unlikenesses, three couplets (digits II, III and V) are designated as *pairs*, and in each hand digits I and IV form a *group*. The relationships of pairs signify a high degree of bilateral association, or symmetry, and the groups represent an association within the single hand more intimate than the bilateral association.

In a series presenting the relations of pairs and groups just described, there is conformity to the *pair-group rule*, as it is termed by Poll. The pair-group rule obtains in European peoples, Mongolian races, Rwala Arabs, Chilean Indians and the populations of Asiatic Turkey and northern Africa. In some other populations the pair-group rule does not hold. When all five digits display pattern frequencies which couple them as pairs, they are described as conforming to the *rule of all pairs*. The rule of all pairs applies to peoples in the greater part of Africa (Hottentots, Efé pygmies, Bushmen, pygmy peoples of the upper Congo, Negroes of Liberia and the Guinean Gulf), Negroes of Jamaica and Cuba, and North American Indians. In two hybridized populations (Jamaican Browns and Spanish-Americans with evident Indian admixture) the rule of all pairs (characterizing respectively the Negro and Indian components) prevails over the pair-group trait (of the European component).

Further studies of the behavior of groups and pairs doubtless will yield data requiring modification of the foregoing statements. Even now it is known that in certain populations listed among those conforming to the pair-group rule (Chinese, Japanese, Koreans) the females are exceptional in following the rule of all pairs.[2]

PALMAR MAIN LINES. Palmar main lines have distinctive trends of variation in right and left hands, notably: (a) The courses of main lines indicate that general ridge direction tends toward a more transverse alignment in right hands; (b) Line T terminates in a position closer to the thumb in right hands; (c) Line C is more frequently abortive or absent in left hands.

The bimanual distinction in coursing of ridges is shown best by lines A and D. In right hands line A terminates more frequently in the distal levels of the ulnar border, and line D tends to course farther radialward. These distinctions are apparent in any representative sample tallied for main-line terminations (e.g., Table 5).

The contrast is better appreciated when such results are converted into main-line indices. Table 26 carries a listing of the main-line indices in

---

[2] Poll, personal communication, March 23, 1939.

TABLE 26

MAIN-LINE INDICES AND THEIR RIGHT/LEFT RATIOS, GROUPED FOR ILLUSTRATION
PARTICULARLY OF: CONSTANCY, IN EITHER SEX, OF THE BIMANUAL RATIOS IN
DIFFERENT SAMPLES OF WHITE PEOPLES; THE LESSER BIMANUAL DIFFERENCES
IN FEMALES OF THESE SAMPLES

| Group | No. of subjects | Main-line index | | | Right/left ratio |
		Right	Left	Both hands	
European-Americans and Jews, males*.........	200	9.20	7.63	8.41	121
European-Americans, females†...............	150	8.73	7.49	8.11	117
Germans, males‡...........................	1281	9.50	7.82	8.66	121
Germans, females..........................	768	9.17	7.82	8.50	117
Jews, males...............................	496	9.83	8.21	9.02	120
Jews, females.............................	1086	9.79	8.43	9.11	116

* Cummins, 1942.
† Steggerda and Steggerda, 1936.
‡ Data on Germans and German Jews drawn from an unpublished study by Cummins.

several series of White stocks. It is to be emphasized especially that the right/left ratio of the indices is constant in these several series. There is a consistent difference between the sexes, females presenting a slightly lessened bimanual contrast. In the group first listed in table 26 the coefficient of correlation of main-line indices in right and left hands (336) is 0.55 ± 0.03. The numbers of individuals, in that same series, presenting the stated differences of main-line indices in the two hands are: o difference or only 1 unit excess in either right or left hand, 46.5%; excess of 2–7 units in right hands, 49.5%; excess of 2–7 units in left hands, 4.0%.

PALMAR PATTERNS. It is shown in Chapter 5 that the several palmar configurational areas are unlike in the frequencies with which they bear patterns and distinct vestiges. The frequencies (using the sample characterized in tables 7–10) range from 11.7% in the second interdigital area to 60.5% in the fourth interdigital area. Especially in the hypothenar and fourth interdigital, two patterns may occur within one configurational area; these cases are counted as instances of patterning without regard to duplex composition. Each area shows a differential frequency of pattern formations in right and left hands. Combining true patterns of all types and distinct vestiges, the frequencies are: hypothenar—right 36.8%, left 31.7%; thenar/first interdigital—right 9.5%, left 20.2%; second interdigital—right 16.2%, left 7.3%; third interdigital—right 63.9%, left 43.3%; fourth interdigital—right 48.6%, left 72.3%. Both the degree and the direction of bimanual contrast vary to some extent among races. An outstanding reversal of direction, or an approach to it indicated by equivalent frequencies in right and left hands, is noted in hypothenar patterns of some peoples, especially Maya Indians, some samples of North American Indians, Bedouins and Chinese.

In the distal and proximal regions of the palm, there is a reversal with regard to radial and ulnar relationships of the positions of configurational areas showing dextral and sinistral excess of pattern frequency. The areas in the distal palm more frequently patterned in right hands are inter-digitals II and III, and in the proximal palm, the hypothenar. The areas more frequently patterned in left hands are interdigital IV and thenar/ interdigital I.

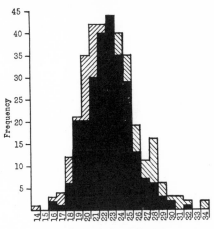

Measurement, millimeters.

FIG. 134.—Frequency distribution of measurements between palmar digital triradii *a* and *b* in 300 young adults. Common distribution of right and left, solid black; right alone ////; left alone, \\\\.

INTERTRIRADIAL MEASUREMENTS. Measurements of distances between digital triradii in 300 young adults (86) yield the following means (milli-meters)—*a-b*: right 22.34, left 23.40; *b-c*: right 14.43, left 14.26; *c-d*: right 20.57, left 20.74; *a-d*: right 52.49, left 53.08. With the exception of the *b-c* measurement, these intervals are slightly larger in left hands. However, only the excess in left hands of the *a-b* measurement (Fig. 134) is statis-tically significant.

RIDGE BREADTH. In all digits ridges are finer in left hands (Fig. 135). Digit IV presents the least bimanual difference in this respect. The reported bimanual differences in individual palmar areas are not statis-tically significant, though concordant findings in two independent investi-gations (24, 30) indicate that the following regional comparisons are valid. Interdigital III presents maximal difference between right and left hands, and is the site of the most pronounced tendency to present finer ridges in right palms. Digit IV exhibits the same tendency though in lesser degree. This agreement of digit IV and interdigital III, with regard to the bimanual differential in ridge breadth, parallels findings in other features indicating an intimate relation of digit IV and interdigital III to the anatomical axis.

PLANTAR MAIN LINES. Bilateral distinctions of ridge coursing in soles are comparable to those of palms. Unlike trends on right and left soles are exhibited by all main lines (105), the radiants of triradius p (Table 12), and ridge directions in proximal regions not entered by main lines (Table

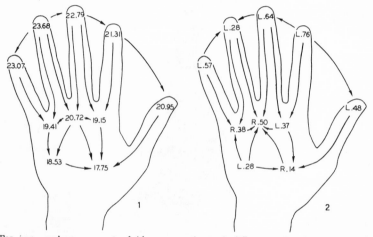

FIG. 135.—1. Average counts of ridges per centimeter in different regions (200 young males). 2. Differences of average regional counts in right and left hands, R and L denoting the hand in which the count is larger—and hence the ridges narrower.

13). In the distal sole there is a tendency for the fibular and distal radiants of triradius p to terminate farther tibialward in right soles than in lefts. This matches the behavior of line D of the palm, and other plantar main lines agree with the trends distinguishing the main lines of right and left palms. A new trend is introduced in the middle and proximal regions of the sole. In right soles there is not only a larger frequency of transverse alignments, but a greater tendency toward fibulo-proximal alignment (symbols 1 and 2, Fig. 83,B), contrasting with the sinistral trend of more frequent tibio-proximal alignment.

PLANTAR PATTERNS. The sole shows less asymmetry of pattern frequencies than the palm. In a diverse assemblage of racial material (Table 27) the hallucal area (Th/I) and interdigital II present slight, though fairly consistent, trends toward greater pattern intensity (here used in preference to percent frequencies of patterns) in left soles. Other areas tend toward right superiority or equality of pattern intensities. The sinistral excess of patterns in interdigital II is less consistent among various racial samples than that of the hallucal area. There are suggestions that in certain races (e.g., Chinese and American Indians) the bipedal differences of interdigital II are the reverse of those just stated. Such reversals are a suggestive parallel to conditions in the palmar hypothenar area of the same and related peoples, noted above.

TABLE 27

BIPEDAL COMPARISONS OF PATTERN INTENSITY AND PATTERN FREQUENCIES IN MAN

(*Data from several publications of the present authors*)

Series	Number of individuals	Hallucal (Th^d/I)		Interdigital II		Interdigital III		Interdigital IV	
		R	L	R	L	R	L	R	L
European-American	200	.83	.86	.20	.26	.62	.56	.21	.14
European-American	100	.82	.82	.22	.23	.64	.59	.16	.16
European-American	100	.84	.85	.24	.25	.64	.60	.14	.06
Jew	100	.82	.85	.38	.38	.78	.75	.21	.15
Spanish-American—Bernalillo	96	.75	.77	.23	.30	.58	.52	.08	.07
Spanish-American—Chamita	110	.81	.83	.24	.23	.65	.57	.08	.05
Hopi	59	.67	.72	.37	.30	.39	.44	.03	.06
Navajo	95	.78	.83	.19	.15	.53	.50	.06	.06
Pueblo	131	.74	.76	.17	.12	.50	.48	.11	.12
Maya	124	.78	.76	.19	.19	.52	.50	.16	.10
Eskimo	31	.57	.63	.24	.21	.44	.55	.05	.00
Negro	98	.87	.88	.25	.28	.58	.63	.30	.26
Weighted average	1244	.79	.81	.23	.24	.59	.56	.15	.11
Frequencies of patterns and vestiges	1244	93%	94%	28%	29%	71%	68%	18%	14%

TOES. Bilateral trends of pattern-type frequencies are different in toes and fingers. Table 21 is a compilation of all the available data on toes. Though only European stocks and Japanese are represented, the likeness among them of bilateral distinctions suggests that the trends may prevail as generally among races as the bilateral distinctions of finger patterns. In toes, except toe III, whorls are more abundant on the left side than on the right (Table 20), the reverse of the bilateral distinction characterizing fingers. (See table 1, noting that in fingers the dextral excess in whorls is at its minimum in digit III.) Tibial loops likewise are more frequent on left toes, which is a reversal of the trend noted in radial loops of the fingers. Arches are more frequent on left toes. This is the same trend as in fingers, with the exception that the index finger presents a slightly higher frequency on the right side.

Variation in Reference to the Anatomical Axis

In descriptive anatomy the axis of the hand or foot is usually considered only with reference to the relationships of certain muscles which have their attachments confined to the skeleton of the hand or foot. These

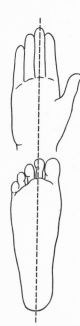

muscles are the interossei, the name literally describing their situation between the metacarpal (or in the foot, metatarsal) bones. The interossei are so inserted on the phalanges that they participate in the acts of spreading and apposition of the digits. Their centering with respect to the anatomical axis of the hand is illustrated by spreading the fingers. In this act the index moves away from the middle finger in one direction and the ring finger and little finger move in the other. The axis of the system of muscles concerned in these movements, the anatomical axis of the hand, is a line through the middle finger and third metacarpal. The axis of the foot differs, being in line with the second toe and second metatarsal (Fig. 136). Characteristically in primates the axis of hand and foot alike passes through the middle digit; the human foot presents one of the few exceptions.

Many structural features are correlated with the anatomical axis. In most primates the longest finger or toe is in the axis. Serial alignment of the human digits, so arranged that digits of maximum length in hand and foot

Fig. 136.— Anatomical axis in the human hand compared with the axis in the foot.

coincide, leaves unpartnered the digits having the least distal reach, thumb and little toe (Fig. 137,A). The distribution of hair on the digits also is associated with the anatomical axis. All digits are devoid of hair on terminal phalanges, and all have hair on their proximal phalanges. The middle phalanges are variable in the amount of hair and in its distribution among the digits. The greatest frequencies of hair retention on middle phalanges are on fingers III and IV and toes II and III.[3] Accordingly, and in agreement with the localization of maximal digital lengths, the serial comparison of fingers and toes involves a shifting by one digit (Fig. 137,B). Zygodactyly, or webbing, is localized most commonly in

---

[3] Danforth, C. H. Distribution of hair on the digits in man. Am. J. Phys. Anthropol., vol. 4, pp. 189–204, 1921.

digits III and IV of the hand and II and III of the foot. Some dermatoglyphic variations are similarly referable to the anatomical axis; data for the following account of such variations is obtained from non-human primates (141) as well as man.

APICAL PATTERNS. The digital distributions of pattern types yield four generalizations relevant to the anatomical axis.

.90	.85	.80	.91	.84	Fingers
1	II	III	IV	V	
	.80	.78	.91	.77	45
Toes					
	I	II	III	IV	V

A. *In man*: digital lengths; pattern intensity in apical patterns, localization of maximal frequency of radial (*tibial*) loops; and common localization of syndactyly. (The numbers inserted represent pattern intensities in Newman's series of fingers and toes.)

3.8	30.8	44.2	21.2	Fingers
II	III	IV	V	
	32.6	45.4	20.5	1.5
Toes				
	II	III	IV	V

B. *In man*: retention of hair on middle segments of digits (Danforth.)

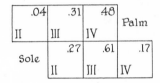

.04	.31	48	Palm
II	III	IV	
	.27	.61	.17
Sole			
	II	III	IV

C. *In man*: pattern intensities of interdigital areas.

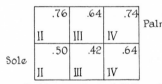

.76	.64	.74	Palm
II	III	IV	
	.50	.42	.64
Sole			
	II	III	IV

D. *In non-human primates*: pattern intensities of interdigital areas.

FIG. 137.—Serial comparisons of digits and of interdigital areas of hand and foot.

(a) Radial loops are most frequent on finger II, and tibial loops, the equivalent pattern type of toes, are chiefly concentrated on toe I. In the foot the factors conditioning such loops shift their operation by one digit, the direction of shifting being in accord with that demonstrated for other variables. Whether the axis is directly concerned in this unlikeness of hand and foot might perhaps be questioned. The distribution of arches does not conform to this relationship between hand and foot. Arches occur most frequently on fingers II and III, while toes V and IV have the maximum frequencies. It is possible, since arches are more common in toes than in fingers, that both increased frequency and altered digital distribution in the foot are due to factors unrelated to the axis. That this may be the case is suggested by the order of arch frequencies on fingers and toes. In the hand, digit II is the center of reference not only because it bears the maximum frequency of arches but also because there is progressive diminution in arch frequencies in the natural order of digits on either side of the index. In the foot, where the greatest frequency of arches is on digit V, a quite different but still orderly seriation is evident. Arches are at a minimum on toe III and they increase in frequency from toe II to I and from IV to V. The unlike distributions of arches on fingers and toes are difficult to explain in any relation to the anatomical axis which would be comparable in hand and foot.

(b) Pattern intensities of digits vary in conformity to relations with the anatomical axis. Pattern intensities of fingers and toes of the same individuals (118) are shown in figure 137,A. There is nearly exact serial agreement of digits II through V in the hand with digits I through IV in the foot. Parallelism between fingers and toes is thus demonstrated by shifting the toe series in the same direction as the shifted anatomical axis of the foot. As in other comparisons this isolates the thumb and little toe from partnership with other digits. It may be significant that in neither hand nor foot does the peak of pattern intensity coincide with the digit lying in the axis. Instead, the digit adjoining the anatomical axis, toward the little finger or toe, has the maximum intensity. The same relationship exists in hair distribution (Fig. 137,B).

(c) Pattern form, especially when determined by the method of Bonnevie or of Geipel, exhibits digital variations which may be referred to the anatomical axis. Fingers III and IV represent a zone in which patterns tend to be more elongated. The patterns become progressively broader in the fingers on either side of III or IV. Comparable statistics for toes are lacking.

(d) Whorls showing monocentric construction—which excludes twin loops, lateral pocket loops and accidentals—have peak frequencies differently localized in fingers and toes. Among fingers, the highest frequency is in IV, and next in II. In toes the maximum frequency is in I, and next in III. Finger IV and toe III therefore have in common an abundance of monocentric whorls.

Reference is made earlier to the possibility that the concentrations of radial (tibial) loops on finger II and toe I may not be truly explained in terms of axial relationships. The abundance of radial loops on the index finger has been the object of much speculation. Wilder (262) was at first misled by the occurrence of radial loops in some pairs of identical twins. He originally considered this reversed asymmetry a correlate of twinning, perhaps akin to the transposed visceral asymmetry occurring frequently in one member of joined twins. In a later paper (101) he is more reserved in judging the significance of radial loops in twins, and since then it has been shown conclusively "that radial patterns have nothing whatever to do with monozygotic twinning" (225).

Bonnevie (44) explains these patterns on a functional basis:

> Remembering the position of the second finger when working alone in opposition to the first one, it seems evident that the radial side of digit II and its papillary pattern should be of great importance whether the function of those lines be of a mechanical or of a sensory nature. Among the different pattern-types, therefore, the ulnar loop will be the one least useful, its ridges running away from the radial side of the finger. Whorls and arches, the peripheral ridges of which patterns run out parallel on both sides of the finger, seem here to be of equal use as compared with each other. But no other pattern would, for the special use of the second finger, serve better than the radial loops, the ridges on the radial side of the finger here being combined into pairs as arms of one and the same loop.

This argument is hardly tenable (225), and Newman proposes another interpretation of radial patterns. He considers the hand to be bifid, an organ that has undergone a sort of twinning, the thumb representing one member and digits II-V the other. As thus viewed, Newman would expect asymmetry of the thumb to be mirrored as compared to asymmetry of the other digits. The prevailing asymmetry of digits II-V is an ulnar asymmetry. Since the thumb usually has an ulnar asymmetry, he postulates that its expected radial asymmetry, incident to "twinning" of the hand, is commonly cancelled by the ulnar asymmetry of the hand as a whole.

Radial asymmetry is most common in the index finger, which Newman regards as a component of the twin of the thumb. It is obvious that the thumb is anatomically largely independent of the other digits, but whether bifidity of the hand predisposes to radial loops on index fingers seems questionable, particularly when conditions in the foot are examined. The foot is not distinctly bifid and, even if it were, the distribution of tibial loops does not fit the interpretation advanced for the hand. The toes collectively present a much lower incidence of tibial (radial) loops than do fingers. The prevailing fibular (ulnar) asymmetry in toes is thus even more intense than in fingers. The toe presenting the maximum frequency of tibial (radial) loops is the big toe, a marginal digit and hence lacking a twin partner on its tibial side (Table 20). Moreover, the next highest frequency of tibial loops occurs on toe IV, a digit so situated that it hardly can be considered a "twin" partner of any toe.

Another line of evidence against the "twinning" origin of reversed pattern asymmetries is obtained from the dermatoglyphics in polydactyly (157). In such cases a couplet of twin digits is represented by two big toes, two thumbs, or combinations of other digits with their supernumerary mates. If the twinning process were an agency producing asymmetry reversals, then such couplets surely should evidence the effect. Actually, however, reversed asymmetry in such couplets is the exception rather than the rule.

PROXIMAL AND MIDDLE PHALANGES. The configurations of proximal and middle phalanges (Chap. 4) are of some interest in connection with the anatomical axis. In the human hand, the ridges over these portions of the digits are characteristically slanted. Commonly the slant is in the proximo-radial direction on digits I, II and III, and on digits IV and V the slant is reversed, the ridges here coursing proximo-ulnarwards. Though the digital distribution of these systems is individually variable, the general tendency may be appreciated by considering digits I-V as one system. Collectively, the opposing slants form a broad chevron, the distally directed apex being most commonly in the third, or axial, digit. The same relations exist in the hand of chimpanzee (129).

PATTERN INTENSITY OF PALM AND SOLE. Consideration of palmar and plantar configurations with respect to the anatomical axis will be limited to interdigital areas II, III and IV. Recalling that the axis in non-human primates generally lies in the line of digit III in both members, it is noteworthy that interdigital area III, both in palm and sole of non-human primates, presents the least pattern intensity of the three regions (Fig. 137,D). In man, also, where the axis of the foot is shifted, pattern intensity is depressed in areas related to the axis, i.e., palmar III and plantar II (Fig. 137,C). It is therefore suggested that factors which are associated with the anatomical axis reduce pattern intensity in the distal palm and sole.

The extreme reduction of pattern intensity in plantar interdigital IV, and palmar interdigital II, indicates that still other factors may depress pattern intensity. A parallel exists in the distribution of hair, finger II and toe V being the digits having the least hair on middle phalanges. These digits, significantly, are topographically related to the interdigital areas presenting minimum pattern intensity, i.e., palmar II and plantar IV.

EXPRESSIONS OF ZYGODACTYLY IN PALM AND SOLE. A common malformation of the foot is the condition of syndactyly (zygodactyly). Of the different varieties of this defect, special interest is attached to that in which the second and third toes are firmly and closely joined by a cutaneous web. The web may extend to the very tips of the digits, but more frequently it is confined to their proximal portions. In all these cases the volar surface of the web presents transverse alignment of ridges, though in instances of complete webbing the apical patterns introduce deviations of ridge courses. When the web does not reach the distal ends of the digits (Figs. 138,B and C) it bears characteristically a triradius in close relation to the interdigital interval. Such a triradius is termed an *interdigital triradius* in recognition of its position. Interdigital triradii may occur in the absence of any real digital union both in the palm (Fig. 73) and in the sole (Fig. 90). When an interdigital triradius is present in a palm its usual location is between the middle and ring fingers. In the sole the most common site is in the second interval, between the second

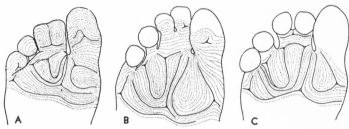

FIG. 138.—Dermatoglyphics in three cases of syndactyly of the second and third toes. *A.* Complete webbing. *B* and *C,* Partial webbing.

and third toes. This localization of interdigital triradii conforms to the typical foci of zygodactyly.

Interdigital triradii signify an intimate developmental relationship between neighboring digits. An interdigital triradius may be considered as a minor expression of the zygodactyl relationship. An interdigital triradius seated at the free margin of the web (as in figure 138,C) might be imagined, in a series of cases which present progressively shorter skin webs, as migrating proximally with the web. Finally, when there is no actual union of the digits, the interdigital triradius remains as a mark of zygodactyly.

The origin of an interdigital triradius may be traced descriptively from an approximation and blending of two digital triradii. This process will be discussed with reference to the palm alone, metric data not being available for the plantar digital triradii. Measurements between consecutive palmar digital triradii (86) show that the interval *b-c* tends to be considerably shorter than either *a-b* or *c-d*. This indicates that the tendency toward approximation of triradii *b* and *c* (Fig. 139) is a step toward the substitution of a single interdigital triradius for these two digital triradii. Triradii *b* and *c* lie in the zone of common localization of major expressions of zygodactyly, and the relative contraction of the interval *b-c* may be justly interpreted as a minimal expression of zygodactyly. The relatively higher variability of the interval *b-c* indicates that this zone is the focus of an active evolutionary trend. (The coefficients of variation of the intertriradial intervals are: *a-b*, 12.5; *b-c*, 21.5; *c-d*, 14.7.)

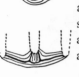

Fusions of digital areas, whether in the sole or palm, accompany zygodactyly (Fig. 138). Such fusions may occur also in the absence of digital union, either in association with interdigital triradii or with some form of displacement or suppression of digital triradii. Fusions of digital areas are very common in the sole, occurring in about 35% of subjects selected at random (193). The second and third interdigital areas are chiefly involved, and usually digital triradii in these areas are suppressed or apparently displaced.

Reduction or suppression of line *C* in the palm is perhaps related to the phenomenon of zygodactyly. The digital triradius (*c*) from which line *C* arises is at the base of digit IV. Triradius *c* does not lie in the anatomical axis, but proximity may render the region susceptible to agencies of variation associated with the axis. The neighboring digit, IV, rather than II, is the one more commonly involved with digit III in zygodactyly, and there is similar behavior in other variations, such as retention of hair on middle phalanges. The variable degrees of involvement of the main lines are illustrated in figures 65–69. As shown in table 5, such involvements are practically confined to line *C*. The line is more commonly reduced than completely suppressed, and all degrees of its zygodactyl expressions are more common in left hands than in rights. Figure 140 illustrates an extreme example of "minor zygodactyly."

FIG. 139.—
Trends of zygodactyly exhibited in reduction of the palmar third interdigital pattern: approximation of digital triradii *b* and *c*, culminating in the appearance of an interdigital triradius. (*From I. W. Wilder.*)

Triradii *a*, *b* and *c* of the sole often are absent, the following absolute frequencies of their lack in 200 soles being reported (105): *a*, 23; *b*, 13; *c*, 16; *d*, 0. Heightening of the tendency to suppress digital triradii is localized farther tibialward (radialward) than in the palm, where triradius *c* is the one most frequently involved, other digital triradii being only rarely absent.

RIDGE BREADTH. Regional differences in breadths of epidermal ridges may be correlated with the anatomical axis. Figure 135 shows average counts of ridges per centimeter for all fingers and five palmar configurational areas. The following regional unlikenesses merit emphasis. The finest ridges of the fingers are those of digit IV; radialward from it, digits III, II and I exhibit a progressive increase in ridge breadth, and ulnarward, digit V likewise displays an increase. Thus digit IV may be regarded as a center of reference for variations in ridge breadth. The narrowest ridges of the palm occur in the region of interdigital III. It may be added that

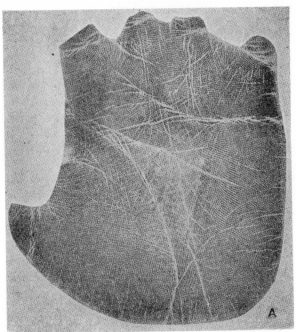

FIG. 140.—A right palm showing dermatoglyphic signs of zygodactyly of the middle and ring fingers. (*From I. W. Wilder.*)

interdigital III is also the site of minimum variability in ridge breadth of the palm. This area, previously identified as the site of reduced pattern intensity, has a proximate relation to the anatomical axis.

A gradient of increasing ridge breadth (Fig. 135) passes proximally in the palm, i.e., lengthwise in the anatomical axis. Ridges are narrower on the distal phalanges of fingers than on the middle and proximal phalanges (72), and ridges here in turn are narrower than on the palm. Ridges in the distal region of the palm are narrower than those in the thenar and hypothenar zones (24).

>>>>>>>>>>>>>>> *12* <<<<<<<<<<<<<<<<

INHERITANCE

Perspectives

GALTON, 1892, opens his discussion on the heredity of finger prints with this comment: "Some of those who have written on finger marks affirm that they are transmissible by descent, others assert the direct contrary." Few writers of Galton's time or since express doubt as to the hereditary transmission of finger-print traits. Forgeot, in 1892, maintains that there are no indications of inheritance even when families are traced through three generations. Locard, in 1906, and Senet in the same year, report on families composed of several generations, and both deny that inheritance plays a rôle in determining finger-print patterns. Stockis, in 1908, declares flatly that the idea of inheritance of finger-print traits is a myth. These and other authors who deny the fact of inheritance have the mistaken notion[1] that identical patterns would be transmitted, if inheritance operates, from parent to offspring. Their opinions, therefore, may be ignored.

Abundant evidence now is at hand to prove that some characteristics of finger prints and of other dermatoglyphic areas are inherited. In preview of this evidence, it may be pointed out that genetic factors have a large share in determining variations of dermatoglyphics, as instanced especially by gradations of similarity observed among individuals having different degrees of relationship. The closest possible genetic relationship is that of monozygotic twins. In their dermatoglyphics, as in other features, the members of monozygotic twin pairs typically present similarities of higher degree than those found in any other comparisons of individuals. A pro-

---

[1] This notion is not confined to the earlier writers. In a recent series of lectures on criminology it is emphatically restated: Mühl, A. M., The ABC of Criminology (p. 174), Melbourne University Press, 1941. The Civil Service Commission of New York City gave in 1936 an examination for finger-print experts in the form of completion questions; one of the 100 questions concerns this point. The question reads: "Practically all fingerprint experts believe that patterns are _____ [sometimes inherited, never inherited, always inherited, inherited as Mendelian characteristics]," the answer accepted as correct being "never inherited."

gressive reduction in degree of similarity is demonstrable in comparisons involving lessening relationships. Thus paired siblings and the members of fraternal twin pairs are rarely as similar as the members of monozygotic twin pairs. Parent and child on the average show less resemblance than siblings, unrelated individuals of the same race show still less, while maximum differences are found in comparing persons of different races. Further, paired siblings show associations between certain dermatoglyphic features and functional handedness which are explainable only on the basis of autosomal linkage of genes responsible for these traits (357). The genetically prospective qualities are termed the *genotype*. Because the genetic control is not a rigid one, these qualities may be expressed (*phenotype*) in an incomplete or altered fashion. Such non-genetic variations are *paratypic* in origin, produced during the process of ridge differentiation and prior to it by modifying influences of the developmental environment. MacArthur (215) measures these effects in terms of the standard deviation (20.8%) for the distribution of homolateral differences in monozygotic twin pairs.

It would be surprising if the traits of dermatoglyphics were not inherited, since there is reason to expect that dermatoglyphics are subject to the same biological laws which determine inheritance of other characteristics, whether structural, physiological or psychological. No student of inheritance, however, has claimed that the totality of pattern characteristics is transmitted. The studies have disclosed only transmission of grades of resemblance which invariably fall short of complete likeness. Newman, who through many years has investigated dermatoglyphics and other characters of twins, relates (225) that once he had been misquoted as stating in a public lecture that the finger prints of twins are "often alike." As a result, he was besieged with requests from identification workers for proof of this statement. He was, of course, in a position to assure the inquirers "that, even in identical twins, *no two finger prints of different individuals are ever exactly alike.*" Findings in these "identical" (or better, monozygotic) twins are of crucial importance; if ever there could exist two identical finger prints, prospects for their production would be most favorable in such twins.

Newman, in the reply quoted above, reaffirms a fact which has been repeatedly emphasized by reliable investigators of his own period and of the generation before him. Galton made the point clear in his statement that "it would be totally impossible to fail to distinguish between the finger prints of twins." If this were not sufficient to settle the issue once and for all, the pronouncement of Wilder, in 1902, should have done so: "The completeness of identity in these cases is, however, not so great but that, both in the finger tips and on the surface of the palms and soles, *there are differences sufficiently marked to render impossible the mistaking of one print for another.''* The question is of obvious importance to finger-print identification, and it is unfortunate that an elementary fact has been so frequently misunderstood, especially by writers of "newspaper science." Erroneous views occasionally make their way into reputable scientific journals, as in the instance now to be cited.

Thirty years ago there appeared in a newspaper (Strassburger Neue Zeitung, Dec. 15, 1912) a sensational article dealing with a case of questioned paternity in which, among other traits, finger prints allegedly established the relationship of the child and putative father. According to the reported expert testimony: "It is very remarkable that not only the prints of the father but those of the grandfather may appear in the child. . . . In twins equivalent patterns of ridges may occur, and they agree so well that a differentiation is impossible." Another curious phase of this case appears in the sequel. Boas reprinted the press article in the *Archiv für Kriminologie*, and added his own commentary. Though his remarks are in a facetious vein, they were taken seriously by Harster, who writes:

> Year in and year out there is waged by the representatives of finger-print science an untiring and often thankless battle, in order to bring recognition of this means of identification before the courts, legal profession and laymen. . . . This recognition it deserves and is in process of attaining. What should we then say in our own camp, when friends appear with the best intentions to further our work and are not aware that they shake our position at the very foundation. How can we in the future stand before the judge and show that the accused is not the actual miscreant, but another? How can we show that the finger prints found at the scene of a serious crime belong to a certain person—when we would be confronted with statements printed in our most outstanding professional journal, statements from a disciple of finger-print procedure affirming the possibility even though conditionally that parents and their children or siblings can have the same prints? Our assurances that there is nothing to it, and that innumerable investigations have shown the opposite will pass unheard, and we will not need to wonder when the accused is set free because finger prints do not furnish sufficient proof. When even the possibility that finger prints are inherited is stated, then the basis of all dactyloscopy, namely that two different fingers never can furnish the same prints, is shattered. . . . Let us not be confused in our work by newspaper articles.

Harster, ignoring published proofs of inheritance which should have been known to one writing as late as 1913, is fearful that the security of the science of identification would be jeopardized by the admission of inheritance. Had Harster been familiar with the reports then available, he would have granted the fact of inheritance, and he might have seen in the twin observations a strengthened support for finger-print identification.

QUALIFICATIONS OF DERMATOGLYPHICS FOR GENETIC STUDIES

As objects for the study of inheritance, dermatoglyphics present certain advantages: (a) It was Galton's opinion that the minutiae, in monozygotic twins, are suitable for determination of "the minutest biological unit that may be hereditarily transmissible." A forking, termination or other ridge detail may not be an ultimate anatomical unit, yet these features are at least among the smallest characteristics readily accessible for testing the limits of hereditary control. (b) The configurations are widely variable, hence they are favorable for comparison among members of families. (c) Unlike many other bodily traits, dermatoglyphics are age-stable. Postnatally, the configurations persist unchanged in all respects except dimensions, and it is justified to assume that no alterations except dimensional increase occur during the prenatal months following their differentiation. It is therefore feasible to compare parents and children, or to compare siblings, with confidence that none of the configurational differences encountered is due to their unlike ages. (d) Dermatoglyphics are environment-stable also. Environment-stability dates from the fifth fetal month, when the dermatoglyphics are completely differentiated.

There are, on the other hand, some working disadvantages in genetic analysis of the dermatoglyphics: (a) The genetic process is exceedingly complex. (b) In comparing apical patterns of corresponding digits, for example, one deals especially with pattern type (including the tendency to "twisting") pattern direction (radial or ulnar), pattern size (quantitative value) and pattern form (breadth/height proportion). Each of these characteristics is in part dependent upon a genetic foundation more deeply seated than that which gives rise to individual distinctions. Statistically there are characteristic trends of unlikeness between the two sides of the body and among different digits, between the sexes, and among racial stocks and constitutional types. To extricate the more immediate manifestations of inheritance in the individual or family from the generic human qualities and distinctions of sex and race is a major problem confronting the investigator. (c) Extensive paratypic variation introduces a handicap in recognizing the genotype. The genes which determine the capacity to form ridges operate as independent conditioners of this fundamental trait. The determination of specific configurational character is indirect. Configurational character depends upon developmental circumstances (Chap. 10) such as stress and tension in the growth of the part, the thickness of the embryonic epidermis (whether under primary genetic control, as conceived by Bonnevie, or secondarily induced by stresses of the underlying tissues, as suggested by Abel) and the distribution of cushioned areas, i.e., areas of thickening due to increased fluid content of the epidermis. These several conditioners of specific configurations are themselves under the control of genes, hence the genetic regulation of ridge alignment is accomplished indirectly through them.

Selective mating on the basis of dermatoglyphics is practically excluded. It is hardly probable that features so inconspicuous as these patternings would be concerned in sexual selection, though it is conceivable that dicta regarding finger patterns and marriage might be embodied in the folk teaching of some peoples, inasmuch as the Chinese have included the patterns in their fortune-telling lore.

MATERIAL AND METHOD OF STUDY

Investigation of the inheritance of dermatoglyphics, as of other normal human characteristics, is hampered by limitations which are thus described by J. Weninger (258):

> Man is difficult to study genetically, more so than plants and animals. Children are few, the development of the individual is slow, and the span of life and of generations is long. Counting a generation as 33 years, there are three generations in a century and 30 generations in a millenium. From the present time to the recent Stone Age there would be 200 generations; in Drosophila 200 generations may be studied in ten years.

Furthermore, the investigator has no selective control of breeding. Despite these handicaps, which are avoided when genetic research concerns organisms so favorable as Drosophila (the fruit-fly), it is still possible to assemble materials for the elucidation of the genetic process in man.

Three classes of material have been utilized in investigations of inheritance:

(a) *Random collections of individuals from the general population* are used as control for comparison with the occurrences of traits within family groups; they are necessary also if gene frequencies are to be calculated. References to "general population" apply to such control series. The existence of racial distinctions in dermatoglyphics (Chap. 15) requires that these series be appropriately selected. Racial homogeneity, insofar as that may be attained in the collection of material, is a first requirement.

Due attention must be paid to the known sexual variations which occur within a race. Specially chosen racial collections may be of value in examination of the genetic process en masse. Two racial stocks which present dermatoglyphic distinctions may be supplemented by a series in which these stocks are hybridized, as in the Jamaican "Blacks," "Browns" and "Whites" studied by Davenport and Steggerda (Chap. 15). Finally, statistics drawn from mass collections are indispensable as a standard of reference for any inquiry involving variation.

(b) *Family groups* provide material for tracing the genetic transmission of dermatoglyphics. The family groups may be large or small and they may embrace more than two generations, with or without collateral lines. The examination of paired siblings is of value in certain analyses; twin pairs (or other sets of multiple births) are segments from family groups which call for separate characterization (see below). Several writers dealing with the subject of questioned paternity stress the importance of "purity" of family material for genetic study. The special interest of these writers makes them keenly aware of the uncertain paternity in some families, especially in certain racial groups and at some social levels. Metzner supplies an interesting sidelight on this question. In an analysis of the genetic formulae embracing a large material he divides the families into two groups. In the first, including 50 families with 198 children, there is no doubt of true paternity. For the second group, consisting of 50 families with 233 children, there was no information by which paternity could be validated. In the latter group the number of instances in which offspring do not conform to the genetic expectation is three times as great as in the first group, the respective totals being 23 and 7.

(c) *Twins* are either dizygotic or monozygotic. Dizygotic pairs, which may be same-sexed or opposite-sexed, are siblings of the same age, not differing in limits of heredity from siblings born at different times. Monozygotic twins, on the other hand, are probably equivalent genetically. The members of a monozygotic pair always are of the same sex, and generally they resemble each other more closely than do the members of a dizygotic pair, their likeness being in some cases so extreme that they are often mistaken for each other. The two individuals are of the same genotype, that is to say, they have the same genetic composition. Multiple births in which there are three or more members are classifiable just as are twins in the stricter sense. A set of triplets, for example, might be trizygotic, dizygotic—two individuals being monozygotic twins—or monozygotic. With increasing numbers in a set the number of possibilities as to zygotic origin is increased, but even with a number as high as five, as in the Dionne set (216), there is still the possibility of monozygotic origin of the several members. The phenotypical expression of germinally prospective traits may be incomplete or altered, owing to early intra-uterine influences. Observations in monozygotic twins provide a measure of the limits of freedom of the genetic process. Against this standard, comparisons may be made with other paired individuals such as siblings or unrelated persons selected at random. It is usually but not always possible to diagnose zygosity with reasonable assurance, and if twins are to serve as a standard of reference in genetic analyses the diagnoses must be valid (Chap. 13).

Any characteristic or zone treated in the descriptive section (Chaps. 4–7) is open to genetic investigation, though fingers and palms figure mainly in the literature. It is apparent that hereditary regulation is not uniformly rigid throughout all zones of the dermatoglyphics. Toe patterns are less rigidly controlled than finger patterns (119), suggesting that lag in differentiation of the foot may admit a larger parakinetic influence.

EARLY STUDIES ON INHERITANCE

The earlier students of dermatoglyphics first had to establish the fact of inheritance, leaving for later investigation the mode of transmission and the developmental vehicle of its expression.

Galton (57) undertakes a preliminary examination of the inheritance of pattern type in the right index fingers of 105 paired siblings. Noting the pattern types occurring in each couplet, he counts the instances in which each of the nine possible combinations of patterns occurs. Comparisons are made against a control series of unrelated persons, their right index fingers being paired at random into couplets. In this control series the observed frequency of each of the nine possible combinations of pattern types agrees very closely with the calculated chance of such combinations in random selection, while the number of agreements of pattern type in the paired siblings is greater than would be expected on the basis of chance. The increased concordance, Galton explains, is due to inheritance of pattern type. On a similar basis he proceeds to other analyses, including observations of twins, all of which point to hereditary determination of pattern type.

Wilder's early studies on twins extend the evidence of inheritance, and he adds to the literature two family trees demonstrating the transmission of patterns, patterns as opposed to patternless configurations in the areas concerned. One family illustrates especially the transmission of patternings of the thenar eminence of the palm (Fig. 141). This family is represented by six children, their parents, and the three sisters of the father. Both hands of the father carry conspicuous thenar patterns, and his three sisters have thenar patterns. Every one of the six children bears thenar patterns, bilaterally in four of them and unilaterally in two. Neither hand of the mother shows any indication of thenar or first interdigital patterns. Among White stocks, such as would be representative of this family, thenar patterns occur in not more than 15–20% of individuals. The family is therefore a strik-

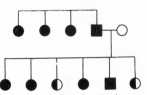

FIG. 141.—A family demonstrating inheritance of palmar thenar patterns. Squares represent males and circles, females. Solid black indicates occurrence of patterns on both hands; half-solid symbols signify presence of the pattern in one hand only, the left hand in both cases. (*Data from Wilder.*)

ing illustration of direct transmission through the father of the factors underlying production of thenar patterns. In connection with the same configuration, a set of monozygotic triplets reported by Gardner and Rife is of interest, not only in that all six hands bear thenar patterns but also because their configurational variations afford a measure of parakinetic influences.

Even more striking than these examples is another family recorded by Wilder, in which several members present the rare calcar pattern.

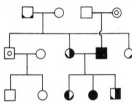

FIG. 142.—A family demonstrating inheritance of the rare calcar pattern. Squares represent males and circles, females. Two members of the family who were not examined are indicated by the symbols with enclosed circles. Solid black indicates the occurrence of a pattern, on left or right foot corresponding to the black halves of the symbols, or on both feet if the symbol is entirely filled. The occurrence of ridge convergences which suggest vestigial patterns is shown by small black areas. (*Data from Wilder.*)

The pattern occurs in no more than 1% of individuals of the general population, yet in this family (Fig. 142) calcar patterns or their rudiments appear in seven of the twelve persons examined. The occurrence of calcar patterns in both man and wife is a noteworthy coincidence. All three of their children present calcar patterns. Again there is provided an illustration of the fact of inheritance, and one which suggests a dominance of patterns over patternless configurations.

Another family group composed of six individuals of three generations, reported by Cevidalli (Fig. 143), illustrates inheritance of the palmar hypothenar pattern in its unusual form as a whorl. Hypothenar whorls are present in two siblings, their father and the paternal grandmother.

Similarly, Carrière records a Lapp family in which the members show varying degrees of reduction of palmar main line C, occurring with such frequency in this family as to indicate that the condition is hereditary.

Numerous isolated finger-print family trees are available in the earlier literature. As an example, a family described by Heindl (60) is selected, its importance being that the eleven individuals composing it had been independently studied by two investigators, one of them examining finger prints alone, and the second concerning himself only with general bodily traits. Neither was informed of the observations of the other until the results were finally assembled, when it became apparent that those mem-

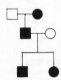

bers who show close finger-print resemblances are likewise the more similar in other bodily traits. Heindl does not attempt to formulate rules of inheritance but merely analyzes the distribution of pattern types. He notes, in the single available member of the third generation, a much reduced ulnar loop on the left index, the reduction being traced to the mother, who shows a related condition in three digits. Tirelli reports on finger-print pattern types in two families. One of them is significant for the occurrence of all arches in the mother, and the tendency to pattern reduction in her two siblings and the majority of her six observed children.

FIG. 143. —A family demonstrating inheritance of whorls on the palmar hypothenar area. (*Data from Cevidalli.*)

Reports of isolated family lines, and casual observations such as close resemblance of finger prints in a father and son or occurrence of arches alone in two brothers, are not productive of great advance in the knowledge of heredity. It remained for Bonnevie to create a more fruitful approach. Her work forms a central structure of the body of information now available on inheritance of dermatoglyphics.

THE GENETIC PROCESS

Bonnevie's study of 1924 opened the way for searching analysis of the genetic process, carried out in a series of studies (44, 153, 154, 155, 156, 174, 175). Her first observations are confined to finger prints in family material amounting to about 200 individuals and in a small series of twins. She concludes that in the phenotypic expression of the patterns at least three different characters are transmitted independently of each other. These characters are: (a) Quantitative value of the pattern, or ridge count from triradius to core; (b) Breadth/height proportion, the variants composing three general classes of pattern form—circular, intermediate and elliptical; (c) Tendency to "twisting"—indicated by lateral pockets and twin loops as well as certain true whorls with interlocked double cores. It is shown also that some minor characteristics of pattern construction and pattern direction (radial loops) are possibly inherited. Subsequent studies by the same author are based upon a larger material, 100 families with 321 children. The results are of fundamental significance, the conclusions of the earlier study being extended and modified largely through interpretations gained from the new viewpoint of her observations of pattern formation in the fetus.

In the following discussion each of the finger-print traits is treated separately, and a representative selection of observations in other dermatoglyphic zones is included. Much of the material presented in Chapters 13 and 14 also is applicable as demonstration of the nature and limits of hereditary control.

PATTERN TYPE. Bonnevie remarks that the affinities among transitional patterns are demonstrated by series assembled from different fingers of one person, from persons closely related to each other, or from unrelated persons who carry the same general types of patterns. It is her opinion that each such series of transitions "represents in the main one and the same genotypical design." Bonnevie later emphasizes that the distinctive pattern-type trends of different digits suggest that individual fingers are not independent, but that each digit represents one part of a common genetic complex.

Grüneberg (202) offers observations in twins and in families. He does not agree that there is a genetic control of the digits collectively, whether concerned with pattern type, quantitative value or any other characteristic. Tracing pattern types without reference to ulnar and radial direction, he compares homologous fingers in 390 pairs of monozygotic twins. Pattern types agree in 80% of the digital couplets (substantiated in MacArthur's finding of 81%). In contrast, there is a significantly lower frequency in dizygotic twins, 63.4%. His family trees show that where parents have loops, in corresponding couplets, 80.9% of the patterns in children are loops, and that when whorls occur in parents, 70.8% of the children possess whorls. Grüneberg concludes that these observations afford positive evidence of the inheritance of pattern type.

Grüneberg assumes that pattern type is conditioned by two pairs of factors $XX(xx)$ and $YY(yy)$, with nine possible genotypic combinations:

$$XXYY........ \text{loop}$$
$$XXYy........ \text{whorl}$$
$$XXyy........ \text{whorl}$$
$$XxYY........ \text{loop}$$
$$XxYy........ \text{loop}$$
$$Xxyy........ \text{whorl}$$
$$xxYY........ \text{loop}$$
$$xxYy........ \text{loop}$$
$$xxyy........ \text{arch.}$$

According to his interpretation, Y is epistatic over X, YY is epistatic over XX, and XX is epistatic over Y. If the dominant factor of one factor-pair is absent, the dominant factor of the other pair expresses itself, and if dominant factors are all absent, the arch appears as a double recessive.

Essen-Moller (190) investigates the presence or absence of whorls in twins. Counting those instances in which both members of a twin-pair have no whorls, or both have one or more, he reports that 65.8% of a dizygotic series are thus characterized, while in monozygotics the frequency rises to 85.7%.

Böhmer and Harren, studying 100 families with 436 children, emphasize the extreme variability of pattern type among siblings. This variability, they observe, indicates that pattern type is not inherited, but their further comments and tabulated data show the actuality of heredi-

TABLE 28

INHERITANCE OF THE TENDENCY TO BEAR THREE OR MORE WHORL PATTERNS (W 3-10) AS CONTRASTED WITH THE PRESENCE OF NO MORE THAN TWO WHORLS (W 0-2)

(*Böhmer and Harren*)

Parental combinations	Children	
	W 3-10	W 0-2
16　W 3-10 × W 3-10..	57	15
42　W 3-10 × W 0- 2..	76	100
42　W 0- 2 × W 0- 2..	41	147

tary transmission. Their observations on whorls (Table 28) demonstrate, in keeping with the conclusions of most other authors, that in spite of obscurity of the genetic process there is a definite hereditary tendency in the expression of whorl patterns. Their characterization of whorl-bearing individuals makes allowance for the fact that whorls are common in digits I and IV; individuals having no whorls at all, or not more than two, form one group, and those with three or more whorls form another.

Ennenbach stresses the parakinetic origin of differences of pattern type in monozygotic twins. He believes further, as Bonnevie suggested earlier, that there is a causal relation between epidermal thickness and pattern type.

Elderton, confining attention to patterns of the index fingers, and considering rights and lefts separately, tabulates the parental combinations and patterns in offspring (about 650 children) and notes that: (a) Neither *arch* × *arch* nor *arch* × *composite* yields whorls; (b) Neither *whorl* × *whorl* nor *whorl* × *composite* yields arches; (c) *Arch* × *loop*, *arch* × *whorl*, *whorl* × *loop*, *composite* × *loop* and *loop* × *loop* produce all types of patterns; (d) Possibly *composite* × *composite* yields no arches. (Whorl, in Elderton's usage, refers to true whorls.)

DOUBLE-CORED PATTERNS ("TWISTING"). The twisting tendency is considered a character of an individual having even one double-cored pattern. Bonnevie suggests that though the mode of inheritance cannot be definitely established in her material, the indications are that twisting is dominant over the single-cored condition. Mueller (221) insists that if dominance is present it is incomplete. He points out, however, that

TABLE 29

INHERITANCE OF THE TENDENCY TO BEAR ONE OR MORE DOUBLE-CORED PATTERNS (*T*)
AS CONTRASTED WITH THE LACK OF SUCH PATTERNS (*R*)
(*Data from Bonnevie, Mueller, and Böhmer and Harren combined*)

Parental combinations	Children	
	R	T
90 *T* × *T*..	36	129
170 *R* × *T*..	255	178
97 *R* × *R*..	262	37

parents without twisting tendency have children usually lacking double-cored patterns, and that when both parents bear twisted patterns the children will in general have one or more such patterns (Table 29). Even when he excludes those digits in which double-cored patterns are most common (Table 2), the results obtained are comparable. Böhmer and Harren, while conceding inheritance of the twisting tendency, emphasize that dominance has not been proved. Karl (347) regards the character as probably recessive. Steffens (119) considers that with present information, hereditary tendencies have not been established.

The genetic process thus remains obscure, yet the data in table 29 conform to the rules of Mueller and to the generalizations of Nürnberger: (a) When both parents have double loops, the children as a rule also have them; (b) When double loops are lacking in both parents, they are as a rule lacking in the children; (c) If double loops are present in only one parent, some children will carry them, others not.

PATTERN FORM. Bonnevie proves that variations in pattern form, or breadth-height proportion, are hereditary. She suggests that elliptical and circular patterns represent a pair of alleles (factors or factor-groups) and that the elliptical form is dominant.

Geipel (197) investigates pattern form in a large family material and in an extensive series of twins. His groupings of the indices into classes (large, medium and small) are listed in Chapter 4. Of 208 pairs of mono-zygotic twins, the members of each of 200 pairs are in the same index class, and in the small remainder the combinations invariably are in adjoining classes—large and medium, or medium and small—and the differences of the numerical values in these cases are slight. Of his 237 pairs of dizygotic twins, 40% of the pairs have members in different index classes.

Geipel's family material (113 pairs of parents with 386 children) yields these generalizations: (a) From the parental combination *large* × *large*, 75% of the children are in the class *large;* (b) From the parental combination *small* × *small*, 71% of the children are in the class *small;* (c) From the parental combination *medium* × *medium*, the children, in the respective proportions 1:2:1, are in the classes *large, medium* and *small;* (d) From the parental combination *medium* × *large*, the children are mainly in the classes *medium* and *large;* (e) From the parental combination *medium* × *small*, the children mainly are in the classes *medium* and *small*, about equally divided between them; (f) From the parental combination *large* × *small*, the children are mainly in the class *medium*. Geipel concludes that the ten-finger index is associated with a single gene, though he grants the possibility of an allelic series. The individual who has a large or a small index is a homozygote, while one with a medium index is a heterozygote.

Mueller (222) supplies similar statistics on the form index in families. He refers, as do Bonnevie and others, to circular, elliptical and medium patterns, but in characterizing an individual he does not use the ten-digit set in all cases. An individual is placed in the class *circular* when all ten patterns are circular, but the presence of one or more elliptical patterns would transfer this individual to the *elliptical* class; to the *medium* class he assigns the remaining cases—all ten patterns medium or some patterns

TABLE 30
INHERITANCE OF PATTERN FORM
(*Mueller*)

Parental combinations	Number of children	Pattern form in children		
		Circular	Medium	Elliptical
73 C × C	119	98.3%	1.7%	0.0%
56 C × M	99	57.6	35.4	7.1
44 C × E	85	37.6	34.1	28.2
19 M × M	29	55.2	34.5	10.3
20 M × E	44	20.5	29.5	50.0
9 E × E	23	0.0	13.0	87.0

medium and some circular. When these results (Table 30) are compared with the generalizations of Geipel, attention must be given to the difference of classification. Mueller does not agree with Bonnevie that elliptical pattern form is dominant over circular, holding that the genetic process is much more complicated and possibly similar to that regulating pattern size. He resolves the following rules from his material: (a) Parents who possess at least one elliptical pattern on each hand have children who carry at least in one hand an elliptical pattern; (b) Children who bear at least one elliptical pattern on each hand are from parents who have at least one elliptical pattern; (c) Parents who have only circular patterns produce offspring who in the majority of cases have only circular patterns; in less than 2% of the children elliptical patterns or closely related intermediate patterns occur, but only in one hand.

Nürnberger formulates a scheme of inheritance of pattern form adapted for application in paternity cases (Chap. 14).

PATTERN DIRECTION. Bonnevie does not find extensive evidence for heredity of the direction of finger patterns (radial or ulnar), though she notes that certain families present a concentration of radial patterns on digit III. This suggests inheritance of pattern direction since radial patterns are rare on this digit. Karl, like Bonnevie, observes that there is little evidence supporting hereditary transmission of pattern direction.

Grüneberg (202) investigates radial and ulnar direction in asymmetric whorls as well as in loops. In monozygotic twins 91.8% of homologous finger pairs show the same asymmetry of patterns, in dizygotic twins 84.7%, and in unrelated individuals 73.4%. Though the difference between monozygotic and dizygotic twins is of questionable statistical significance, the large difference between monozygotic twins and unrelated persons demonstrates that pattern direction is inherited. He postulates, in a scheme similar to that which he proposes for pattern type, a series of paired factors responsible for pattern direction.

The question of possible relationship between pattern type and pattern direction is raised by Grüneberg. In his material 18.6% of whorls are radial in direction, as contrasted with an incidence of only 5.3% radial direction among all loops. He interprets the correlation as an expression of "coupling." Whether these figures prove the point may be questioned.

Mueller (222), whose results agree with those of authors mentioned above, points out that if both parents have radial patterns the children commonly have them.

It is Poll's opinion that patterns of the same type but of reversed direction (ulnar and radial loops) should be considered similar from the genetic standpoint.

Mueller (221) imposes a restriction on the characterization of an individual with respect to radial patterns. Believing that the frequency of radial patterns on digit II precludes use of this digit in genetic studies, he defines a "radial person" as one who has at least one radial pattern on any digit other than the index. He finds (Table 31) no evidence that the radial character is inherited, though he admits that the material is very limited.

TABLE 31

INHERITANCE OF RADIAL PATTERNS (R) OCCURRING IN DIGITS OTHER THAN THE INDEX, AS CONTRASTED WITH THE ABSENCE OF SUCH PATTERNS (O)

(*Mueller*)

Parental combinations	Children			
204 $O \times O$	R	15	O	301
16 $R \times O$	R	5	O	20

Newman (225) points to evidence drawn from twins on the inheritance of radial patterns (including not only radial loops but also radial whorls). Among 50 pairs of identical twins radial patterns occur in both members of 21 pairs, and of these, all four index fingers are so distinguished in seven pairs.

Walker, confining attention to radial loops on right index fingers, concludes that the transmission is by a sex-linked recessive gene. This conclusion is difficult to reconcile with nearly equal incidences of such patterns in the sexes. Walker's material is small and the agreement of findings with a mathematical formula indicating recessiveness is doubtless only a matter of chance.

QUANTITATIVE VALUE. Bonnevie's original determination of quantitative value was later superseded by a procedure in which only the larger of the two counts in whorls is considered. Class groupings are discontinued, and the quantitative value of the individual is the average of ridge counts of the ten digits.

Proof of the inheritance of quantitative value is furnished by determining the correlations between pairs of individuals of different degrees of relationship. Several workers present such data. The following coefficients of correlation (44) illustrate that monozygotic twins are more closely related to each other than are fraternal twins or single-born siblings: monozygotic twins, 0.92; dizygotic twins, 0.54; siblings, 0.60; unrelated individuals, 0.27. Single-born siblings are, of course, closer to each other than are randomly paired unrelated individuals. In the latter, similarities depend on a generic human inheritance rather than on a specific familial inheritance.

Bonnevie (175) later revises her ideas on the inheritance of quantitative value, making use of her embryological studies of epidermal thickness and of the distribution of cushioning. She concludes that there are three independent factors responsible for quantitative value of a pattern, instead of the five originally assumed: V, expressed in the general thickness of epidermis over the digital pads of the embryo; R, which produces cushioning in the more radially placed digits, II and III; U, responsible for cushioning in the more ulnarward digits, IV and V.

The measure of epidermal thickness, the factor V, is the highest ridge count obtained in any one of the ten digits of the individual, higher counts indicating thinner epidermis. One source of error in investigations of the V factor is depression of ridge counts by cushioning, with the result that recessive individuals would be erroneously considered as heterozygotes, and heterozygotes as dominant homozygotes. Bonnevie discusses the problem of defining borderlines between genotypes, a matter which is further emphasized by Metzner. The highest values, about 22 ridges or more, are recessive (vv) to lower values, the boundary between heterozygotes and dominant homozygotes being at about 14–16 ridges (Table 32).

TABLE 32
INHERITANCE OF EPIDERMAL THICKNESS (V)
(*Data from Bonnevie and from Metzner combined*)

Parental combinations	Children		
	VV	Vv	vv
0 $VV \times VV$...............................	46	54	1
27 $VV \times Vv$...............................	33	.74	33
37 $Vv \times Vv$...............................	1	34	6
12 $VV \times vv$...............................	5	171	158
85 $Vv \times vv$...............................	2	8	126
39 $vv \times vv$...............................			

Heterozygotes (Vv) have maximal digital values of approximately 16–21 ridges, and dominant homozygotes (VV) present maximal values of 6–15 ridges. Counts of 0–5 ridges (arches and very small patterns) probably result from cushioning, produced by factors R and U.

Grüneberg (202), on the basis of the frequency distribution of quantitative values, assumes that epidermal thickness is regulated by four to six pairs of polymeric factors. Like other authors who have dealt with twin material, he contrasts monozygotic and dizygotic twins with respect to this feature. His data, rearranged in table 33, show a distinct trend of lesser difference in monozygotic twins. This distinction is illustrated also in the average differences of quantitative value (class values, not absolute ridge counts): 1.61 in monozygotics and 4.15 in dizygotics.

TABLE 33

DIFFERENCES OF QUANTITATIVE VALUE (FOR LOOPS ONLY) IN HOMOLOGOUS FINGERS OF MONOZYGOTIC AND DIZYGOTIC TWINS

(*Grüneberg*)

Difference in ridge count	Number of cases	
	Monozygotic, 141 pairs	Dizygotic, 144 pairs
0– 1	95	49
2– 3	25	26
4– 5	10	22
6– 7	7	17
8– 9	4	13
10–11	..	7
12–13	..	2
14–15	..	4
16–17	..	3
18–	..	1

Galton's law of filial regression, to the effect that persons who deviate much from the average of the general population most commonly have children who deviate less, has been tested by Mueller (221) from the standpoint of quantitative value (determined according to Bonnevie's 1924 method). Mueller believes that the results (Table 34) indicate conformity

TABLE 34

DEVIATIONS (FROM THE MEAN OF THE POPULATION) OF QUANTITATIVE VALUE IN PARENTS AND THEIR CHILDREN, IN POSSIBLE CONFORMITY TO GALTON'S LAW OF FILIAL REGRESSION

(*Mueller*)

Deviations from the mean quantitative value of the population, 46.0	Number of parental pairs					
	7	20	19	12	9	3
Parental groups..........	−25.3	−16.1	−3.4	3.9	15.6	21.3
Their children............	−29.0*	−11.9	−1.1	3.6	15.1	19.4
Number of children.......	15	36	39	21	13	6

* Mueller explains this discrepancy by the small number of cases in this group.

of quantitative value to Galton's law. It would be important to test the question with the use of Bonnevie's revised method and with larger material.

Both Mueller and von Wehren stress that parental combinations with low values yield low values, and that when the parental values are high, those of the children are high. Thus the children have values which lie within the variational limits of their parents. Von Wehren, combining his own family material with that available to him in the literature, notes in the 266 families only two exceptions to this rule, the exceptions being the same cases which Bonnevie had reported as such. The same author brings out a striking contrast to this evenness in the family groups by dissociating parents and children and recombining them in 32 different "family" groups. The exceptions to rule range from 0 to 32 in these arbitrarily composed "families."

Geipel (199), employing the total ridge count of the individual, reports on 469 pairs of monozygotic twins, 405 pairs of same-sexed dizygotics, and 107 pairs of opposite-sexed dizygotics. The frequency distributions of the differences of ridge counts in these three groups are shown in table 35. The mean differences in the groups are: monozygotics, 11.1 ± 0.4

TABLE 35
DIFFERENCES IN TOTAL RIDGE COUNTS IN TWINS
(*Geipel*)

Difference in ridge counts	Monozygotics (469 pairs)	Same-sexed dizygotics (405 pairs)	Opposite-sexed dizygotics (107 pairs)
0– 10	60.8%	19.3%	17.8%
11– 20	24.3	13.8	15.9
21– 30	11.1	12.6	14.0
31– 40	3.0	12.3	11.2
41– 50	0.6	9.9	3.7
51– 60	0.2	10.9	8.4
61– 70	......	5.9	3.7
71– 80	......	5.7	8.4
81– 90	......	3.5	5.6
91–100	......	2.2	4.7
101–110	......	1.0	3.7
111–120	......	1.7	0.9
121–130	......	0.25	0.9
131–140	......	0.25	0.9
141–150	......	0.25	
151–160	......	0.25	
161–170			
171–180	......	0.25	

ridges; same-sexed dizygotics, 39.3 ± 1.4; opposite-sexed dizygotics, 42.3 ± 4.8. These figures are closely matched in the work of Lehtovaara (cited by Geipel), who reports in monozygotics a mean difference of 11.1 ridges, and in dizygotics, 35.5.

The question of penetrance is considered by von Verschuer (251) in reference to epidermal thickness and cushioning. The gene or genes conditioning these characteristics may vary in penetrance (the ability to become manifest in the phenotype), owing to paratypic influences and the existence of accessory genes which may promote or inhibit action of the primary genes. Calculations based on 205 pairs of monozygotic twins indicate, in his opinion, that penetrance of factors for epidermal thickness is much greater than penetrance of factors for ulnar and radial cushioning. This finding, according to Weninger (260), is in harmony with the unlike developmental mechanisms associated with epidermal thickness and cushioning. Weninger presents a theoretical consideration of epidermal thickness, radial cushioning and ulnar cushioning, with particular reference to their phenotypic variants and the principle of penetrance. The details do not lend themselves to condensation, and the reader must be referred to the original publication.

Böhmer and Harren supply data on epidermal thickness from material consisting of 100 families with 436 children. They do not accept Bonnevie's conclusion that thin epidermis (expressed by ridge counts above 21) is recessive (to thick epidermis, counts of 15 or lower). They agree, however, that there is some hereditary influence, since ridge counts below 5 occur in children only when the average parental value is at least below 15; but it is impossible to set a generally valid rule, since even among such families there are some children with counts as high as 20.

CUSHIONING. Bonnevie asserts that cushioning depresses the quantitative value which is potential in the V factor. Cushioning is lacking when all digits of one or both hands of an individual have counts greater than 15 ridges. Uniformity in low values, 0–5 ridges, indicates that thick epidermis and cushioning are both present. (When the values are intermediate, 6–15 ridges in many or all of the digits, clues to the genotype may be obtained through examination of the parents or the children of such individuals.) The degree of cushioning is expressed by the difference between the highest digital value of a hand and the lowest value of digits of the radial or ulnar groups. The two hands are investigated separately to avoid confusion due to asymmetric distribution. Cushioning is absent when the difference is 0–4, this condition being recessive to its presence. In heterozygotic cushioned individuals the difference amounts to about 5–10 ridges, while in dominant homozygotes the difference is usually greater than 10 ridges. Cushioning is heritable both as to presence or absence and localization on either the radial or ulnar digits (Tables 36 and 37); the respective factors, R and U, are independent of each other.

There are two sources of error in the results on cushioning. First, the boundaries between heterozygotes and homozygotes, as well as the distinction between dominant and recessive homozygotes, are uncertain.

TABLE 36
INHERITANCE OF RADIAL CUSHIONING (*R*)
(*Data from Bonnevie and from Metzner combined*)

Parental combinations	Children		
	RR	Rr	rr
66 *RR* × *RR*	223	19	3
110 *RR* × *Rr*	226	193	1
17 *Rr* × *Rr*	18	31	11
4 *RR* × *rr*	3	11	
3 *Rr* × *rr*	...	10	3
0 *rr* × *rr*			

TABLE 37
INHERITANCE OF ULNAR CUSHIONING (*U*)
(*Data from Bonnevie and from Metzner combined*)

Parental combinations	Children		
	UU	Uu	uu
15 *UU* × *UU*	41	13	
78 *UU* × *Uu*	132	171	10
69 *Uu* × *Uu*	79	134	57
11 *UU* × *uu*	1	29	4
24 *Uu* × *uu*	...	46	29
3 *uu* × *uu*	...	1	5

The second difficulty is that cushioning is manifest in the ridge counts only when it extends into the pattern area. In consequence, some of the individuals classed as non-cushioned recessives may be cushioned. Likewise the degree of cushioning may not be expressed. Bonnevie considers that in her material some cushioned individuals identified as heterozygotes are really dominant homozygotes.

Böhmer and Harren question the heritability of cushioning.

GENE FREQUENCIES. Abel (265) points out that racial differences in gene frequency exist, especially for the factor of epidermal thickness (*V*). This question is later elaborated by Piebenga (299). In Eskimos of Eastern Greenland the factor *V* is practically non-existent. It is rare in Chinese, and infrequent, though at its maximum, in European stocks, Hindus, South Melanesians and Formosans—reaching a maximum in Bushmen (Table 38). The gene frequencies for epidermal thickness differ not only among widely separated racial groups but also among Central and North European peoples. The factors for radial and ulnar cushioning (*R* and *U*) exhibit less variation among different peoples. Abel interprets the relative stability of the factors of cushioning as an indication that they are more ancient properties than the factors of epidermal thickness.

TABLE 38
GENE FREQUENCIES IN VARIOUS RACIAL GROUPS

Racial group	VV	Vv	vv	RR	Rr	rr	UU	Uu	uu
395 Danes (Bonnevie)....	9.8%	45.6%	44.6%	70.0%	26.5%	3.5%	26.8%	45.9%	27.3%
1300+ Austrians (Geyer*)	10.0	43.9	46.1	61.8	37.1	1.1	30.4	51.0	18.6
214 Germans (Abel)......	11.0	48.2	42.2	54.0	36.0	8.0	21.0	53.0	24.0
93 Germans (Piebenga)...	11.0	35.2	53.8	51.6	40.7	7.7	29.7	42.9	27.7
200 Belgians-Walloons (Piebenga)............	11.0	27.5	61.5	63.0	32.5	4.5	32.0	45.5	22.5
521 Norwegians (Bonnevie).................	12.5	50.5	37.0	59.3	38.4	2.3	29.5	53.5	17.0
161 Germans (Abel)......	13.0	39.7	47.2	62.8	31.4	5.6	31.5	54.3	14.1
200 Flemish (Piebenga)...	13.5	38.5	48.0	62.5	31.5	6.0	30.0	46.5	23.5
450 Germans (Karl)......	15.7	44.5	39.8	54.8	38.5	6.7	28.0	55.0	17.0
400 Dutch (Piebenga)....	18.0	46.3	35.7	64.5	31.5	4.0	31.0	48.0	21.0
40 Hindus (Biswas)......	10.0	27.5	62.5	40.0	57.5	2.5	7.5	75.0	17.5
35 Melanesians (Karl)....	......	53.0	47.0	26.5	61.8	11.7	11.7	79.5	14.8
68 Eskimos (Abel†).....	......	1?	98.0	32.2	42.3	25.4	23.0	57.0	18.0
70 Chinese (Abel)........	4.2	21.4	74.2	52.8	44.2	2.8	31.4	54.2	14.2
400 Formosans (Okuma)..	12.3	40.0	47.8	44.3	50.3	5.5	30.5	58.8	10.8
450 Chilean Indians (Schaeuble)............	16.4	35.8	47.8	61.1	33.4	5.5	35.6	52.0	12.4
27 Bushmen (M. Weninger).................	48.1	48.1	3.7	50.0	50.0	......	37.5	54.2	8.3

* To make these figures comparable to those reported by other authors the observed values only are included in the table; Geyer reports also percent values adjusted by the genetic numbers according to Wellich.

† Abel's series of Eskimos comprises family groups, and hence may not be representative of the general population.

MINOR CHARACTERISTICS OF PATTERNS. Bonnevie demonstrates the inheritance of "minor" characteristics of patterns, these including not the ultimate minutiae but various local configurational features. As to the mode of inheritance, no suggestions are offered by Bonnevie, Siemens or Leven.

MINUTIAE. Grüneberg (202) selects homologous fingers of twins having the same pattern type, pattern direction and ridge number, expecting that ridge details might be in closer agreement in such patterns than in those presenting coarse differences. Even here there is no identity in minutiae, a finding which has been repeatedly mentioned since Galton's observations on twins. Grüneberg concludes that the minutiae are accordingly conditioned paratypically, and emphasizes further that differences in quantitative value may be brought about by these variations of paratypic origin. He and others stress that ridge counts presenting differences of one, two or possibly three ridges may thus not be genetically different, since such discrepancies are introduced by differences of ridge detail that may influence the count to this extent.

Newman (225) observes that in twins minor configurational details and minutiae of homologous fingers often show close resemblances (Fig. 144). Occasionally there is similar close resemblance in ordinary siblings and in parent and offspring.

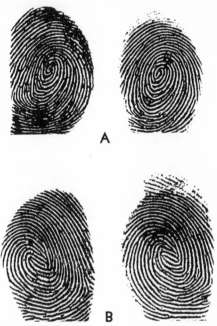

Fig. 144.—Close resemblance in prints of corresponding fingers in twins. Two pairs of twins, marked respectively A and B, are illustrated. (*From Newman.*)

RIDGE BREADTH. Karl (347) suggests the possibility of inheritance of ridge breadth. According to Ennenbach the ten-digit average (of ridge counts on a 1-cm. line) shows intra-pair differences in monozygotic twins ranging from 0.2 to 1.5 ridges, the average difference being 0.7; the average difference in dizygotics is 1.4, the range being 0.1–2.7 ridges.

TOES. In toes, according to Steffens (119), the range of variation of ridge number is greater than in fingers. The frequency distribution of ridge counts on toes shows neither a distinct cleft between counts 15 and 16, nor one between 21 and 22. Steffens does not find it possible to differentiate in toes the three genotypes *VV*, *Vv* and *vv*, unless there be some modification of the border lines (as suggested: *VV*, 0–15; *Vv*, 16–24 or 16–25; *vv*, 25 or 26 and above). In evaluating epidermal thickness in toes, the same author advises exclusion of those cases of monozygotic twins which present wide discordances. With the suggested modification of the genotypes, there are among her 50 pairs of monozygotic twins but two instances of discordance in fingers and none in toes.

Steffens has no instance in which embryonic epidermal thickness is less in the foot than in the hand. In 85% of the subjects the relationship between fingers and toes is about the same. The outstanding contrasts between toe and finger patterns are indicated in table 39.

TABLE 39
FREQUENCIES OF CUSHIONING FACTORS IN FINGERS AND TOES OF THE SAME SUBJECTS
(*Steffens*)

Cushioning factors	Fingers	Toes
rr	4	11
Rr	79	46
RR	117	143
uu	42	2
Uu	101	23
UU	57	175

It is suggested that toes are more frequently cushioned than fingers. For the study of cushioning, Steffens combines toes I and II as the tibial group, and III, IV and V as the fibular (though it is immaterial whether toe III is grouped with the tibial or fibular set). The results indicate that cushioning in toes probably is not regulated on the same basis as in fingers.

PALMS. Wilder's observations, noted briefly and illustrated in the introductory section of this chapter, suggest a dominant inheritance of thenar/first interdigital patterns. Weninger (259) also devotes attention to the thenar/first interdigital areas. Her material comprises 290 families with a total of 562 children. She regards the inheritance as too complex to be explained on the basis of a single factor. There is some indication that presence of the pattern in fathers has a greater influence in producing patterns in the offspring than does presence of the pattern in mothers. The data in table 40 show that not only the presence of patterns but also the degree of pattern elaboration is determined by genetic factors.

Weinand supplies information on palmar patterns and on palmar main lines. In palmar interdigital II it appears that the presence of a pattern is dominant over open field. Of 13 offspring from parents *O* × *D*, 5 show patterns in interdigital area II. This is in marked contrast to the rare occurrence of this pattern in the general population. Further, among 44 families wherein parents are *O* × *O*, only 7 of the 197 children have these

TABLE 40

INHERITANCE OF PALMAR THENAR/FIRST INTERDIGITAL PATTERNS

(*M. Weninger*)

Presence or absence of patterns			Degree of development of patterns		
Parental combinations	Number of children	Children with thenar patterns	Parental combinations	Number of children	Children with thenar patterns
O × *O*....................	374	9.9%	*O* × *O*....................	374	9.9%
O × unilateral.............	95	25.3	*O* × incomplete...........	71	26.8
O × bilateral..............	72	37.5	*O* × complete.............	96	33.3
Unilateral × unilateral.....	11	54.5	Incomplete × incomplete...	3	33.3
Unilateral × bilateral......	8	62.5	Incomplete × complete.....	9	22.2
Bilateral × bilateral.......	2	0.0	Complete × complete......	9	88.9

patterns. Similar observations are recorded for interdigitals III and IV and for the hypothenar. The hypothenar, however, presents a discrepancy. Parental combinations *O* × *O* and *O* × *unilateral presence* produce equal numbers of hypothenar patterns in the offspring. Weinand assumes that there is a particular susceptibility of this palmar area to parakinetic influences. He offers the alternative explanation that patterning is transmitted recessively. Except for interdigital III, as illustrated in the thenar/ first interdigital from Weninger's data, the number of children with bilateral patterns is greater from *O* × *bilateral presence* than from the combination *unilateral* × *unilateral*. *Unilateral* × *unilateral* produces children who, if patterned, are predominatingly patterned on one hand only, and *bilateral* × *bilateral* gives rise to children who are predominatingly bilaterally patterned.

It is definite that the directions of line *D* and the associated line *C* are heritable. Abundant evidence from twins is available from other sources, but Weinand's data on 52 families with 230 children supply clues to the mode of inheritance. When the parental combination is *11.11.—.—* × *11.11.—.—* about three-fourths of the children have similarly high terminations of the main lines. If parental instances of the topographically similar *11.9.—.—* be added to this group, then over 90% of the children present high terminations. The parental combination of *high termination* (*11.11.—.—*) × *low termination* (*9.7.—.—*) yields children who have preponderantly high terminations. The offspring are about equally apportioned between high and low terminations when the parental combination is *11.9.—.—* × *9.7.—.—*, but they are preponderantly low from the combination *11.9.—.—* × *7.7.—.—*.

Czik and Malan report on the palmar main lines and palmar patterns in carefully diagnosed series of monozygotic and same-sexed dizygotic twins. As an illustration of the results, and of the influence of heredity in determining the main lines, it may be noted that 77.9% of the monozygotic pairs agree in the position of termination of line A, while for dizygotics the concordance is only 25.7%.

TWIN DIAGNOSIS

OBJECTIVES AND GENERAL METHODS

KNOWLEDGE of the inheritance of dermatoglyphics prepares the way for practical applications. Many basic problems in biology, psychology and medicine are approachable through studies of twins. Inasmuch as twins are being used to determine, for example, the rôle of inheritance in susceptibility to a disease, sound diagnostic procedures for distinguishing the monozygotic and dizygotic types are essential. Dermatoglyphics are included among the items generally accepted as valid diagnostic criteria. Another application (Chap. 14), as yet not on as secure a foundation, is concerned with the determination or exclusion of parentage under circumstances when there is question of the paternity of a child or, more rarely, of the maternity.

Differentiation of monozygotic and dizygotic twins ordinarily is accomplished by the "similarity method." Siemens, Newman, Komai, von Verschuer, Rife, Meyer-Heydenhagen, Geipel, MacArthur and others have sought to establish methods leading to diagnoses that are reasonably dependable. The principle of diagnosis in the similarity method is the assembling of observations on a variety of traits, which preferably are non-linked in inheritance. For instance, Rife (235) presents a test of a diagnostic formula comprising four qualitative and four quantitative items, the exact mode of inheritance of each qualitative trait being known: (a) blood types *A*, *B*, *AB* and *O*; (b) blood types *M* and *N*; (c) presence or absence of hair on the middle segments of fingers; (d) ability to taste phenyl-thio-carbamide; (e) iris pigmentation; (f) intelligence quotient; (g) quantitative values of finger prints; (h) stature. A twin pair showing correspondence in the eight traits is diagnosed with fair assurance as monozygotic. The chance of error may be as low as 27 out of 1,920,000 if the parents are heterozygous for each of the qualitative traits.

Possibilities of error are inherent in the similarity method. However small the chance of error may be in a properly executed diagnosis, the close resemblances sometimes observed in individuals who are not mono-zygotic twins illustrate how a mistaken diagnosis might be made if the comparison is not exacting. Wilder (264) mentions three sisters, two of whom are fraternal twins; the single-born sister so closely resembles one of the twins that she is commonly taken to be the twin partner.

As a supplement to the similarity method, the character of the after-birth (a single chorion or two chorions) has been considered by many workers a reliable diagnostic aid. Some recent students of twins, however, find instances of conflict between the results of the similarity method and the diagnosis based on fetal membranes, and they question the validity of the latter criterion. Essen-Moller (190) considers that 17% of all dichorial pairs are monozygotic and about 33% of monozygotic pairs are dichorial.

The general procedures in twin diagnosis cannot be broadly discussed here, but it must be insisted that an investigator desiring to determine the distinctions of dermatoglyphics in monozygotic and dizygotic twins should not include these features among the items in his original diagnoses. Some investigators of twins have fallen into error by not observing this precaution against circular analysis.

According to von Verschuer (252), the hereditary equality of mono-zygotic twins is supported by three lines of evidence. (a) In lieu of direct proof drawn from human twins, which in this relation is unobtainable, he cites the study of Kappert on the flax-plant. One-egg twins, triplets and quadruplets occur in certain stocks of flax. Cultivation by self-pollination demonstrates that the phenotypic differences among the components of these multiples, whether two or more in number, are not hereditary. (b) In a simple and well known hereditary complex (blood groups O, A, B, AB and the M and N agglutinogens) it is definite that gene differences in monozygotic twins do not occur, since the two members of such a pair never differ in blood type. (c) Similarities of monozygotic twins are no greater than those between the right and left halves of the body of one person—and in characteristics which exhibit distinctive unilateral variations the homologous halves of the members of a mono-zygotic twin pair are more nearly alike than the right and left sides of an individual. This last point, elaborated by Komai and confirmed by other investigators, has come to be universally accepted as a law applicable in twin diagnosis. Both von Verschuer (250) and Meyer-Heydenhagen point out that the rule regarding homolateral and bilateral unlikenesses in twins holds only for characters having different statistical trends of varia-tion on right and left sides.

An excellent demonstration of the contrast between monozygotic and dizygotic twins, with respect to degrees of homolateral and heterolateral differences, is provided by the correlations of quantitative value. Monozygotic and dizygotic twins are widely different in these comparisons (Table 41), though equal in their intra-individual, or bilateral, differences.

TABLE 41

COEFFICIENTS OF CORRELATION IN QUANTITATIVE VALUES OF FINGER PRINTS IN TWINS

Combination	Monozygotic twins		Dizygotic twins			Author
	MM	*FF*	*MM*	*MF*	*FF*	
Both hands of twin *A* and both hands of twin *B*	0.97	0.96	0.36	0.24	0.23	Fukuoka
		0.92		0.54		Bonnevie
		0.95		0.46		Newman
Right hand and left hand of the same individual	0.91	0.89	0.91	0.94	0.83	Fukuoka
		0.86				Bonnevie
		0.93		0.93		Newman
Left hand of *A* and left hand of *B*	0.92	0.92	0.37	0.29	0.38	Fukuoka
		0.93		0.50		Newman
Right hand of *A* and right hand of *B*	0.93	0.93	0.41	0.19	0.35	Fukuoka
		0.92		0.34		Newman

The same is true when quantitative value, pattern type and palmar configurations are analyzed by the method of average differences (Table 42).

It will be recalled that among the members of the family studied by Heindl (60), resemblances and differences of finger prints are correlated to some degree with resemblances and differences in other bodily and mental characteristics. In the main this correlation is borne out in observations on twins. Obonai, who examined about 200 pairs of twins, emphasizes that some pairs of monozygotic twins may have finger patterns that are very unlike.

The reliability of dermatoglyphics as a diagnostic aid is illustrated in the experience of several workers. Newman (227) reports that of 42 pairs of twins in his series, 40 were correctly diagnosed by dermatoglyphics alone. Meyer-Heydenhagen asserts that 90% of monozygotic twins may be diagnosed by their similarities in palmar dermatoglyphics. An especially significant test is reported by Rife (237), who had submitted to MacArthur, another experienced student of twins, only the prints of 61 pairs, including both monozygotics and dizygotics. MacArthur correctly diagnosed 58 of the 61 pairs, and it is noteworthy that two of his three diagnoses which disagreed with Rife's judgment based on other traits were tentative.

Lauterbach doubts the usefulness of palmar dermatoglyphics in twin diagnosis. His reservation is made because of the close likenesses of these features occurring in some twins whose dizygosity is certain because they are opposite-sexed. Cummins (180), analyzing the dermatoglyphics in eight pairs of twins, at the time without other information which might give clues to zygosity, makes diagnoses of two pairs inconsistent with the data on fetal membranes. The diagnosis of two pairs as dizygotic, in disagreement with monochorionic membranes, is open to the explanation, since emphasized by von Verschuer, Essen-Moller and others, that fetal membranes may not be reliable indicators of zygosity.

Ford, Brown and McCreary report on a pair of twins presenting every evidence of monozygosity except in dermatoglyphics. In this case the parakinetic mechanism responsible for dermatoglyphic unlikenesses is identified with a functional handicap in intrauterine development, which is shown to be probable in view of demonstrated abnormal relations of the fetal membranes. Of similar significance from the standpoint of para-kinetic factors are observations on joined monozygotic twins, popularly called "Siamese" twins. Their dermatoglyphics are more dissimilar than in monozygotic twins generally (181, 182, 228, 234). The developmental processes of individuals so united obviously are disturbed, and characteristics susceptible to such influence would not be expressed geno-typically. Unlikenesses of patterns in a supernumerary digit and the corresponding digit of the normal series are further illustrations of para-kinetic effects. In the absence of such influences it might be expected that a supernumerary thumb, for example, would bear a pattern closely resembling the pattern of the normal thumb. Actually, major discrepancies, even of pattern type, occur in a large proportion of these cases.

Grüneberg (203) urges that in studies of inheritance the single-born should be compared with twins, and he illustrates how such material may be quantitatively analyzed to secure a measure of paratypic influences.

Specific Methods, with Comparisons of Twin Types

MacArthur regards finger-print traits as more reliable than palmar features in distinguishing the twin varieties, at least as he analyzed them, and considers ridge counts more effective than pattern type. He follows an exacting method in analyzing the dermatoglyphics of twins and in comparing twins with their parents and siblings:

(a) Total ridge counts for the five digits of each hand are compared in the right and left hands of the one individual, between corresponding hands of the members of the pair, and between their opposite hands. The difference obtained in each of these comparisons is expressed as a percent fraction of the average ridge count in the general population (about 66 ridges per hand in the material chosen by MacArthur).

(b) Pattern type and pattern direction are evaluated and the differences are rated by empirical values. A unit difference is assigned to unlikenesses as distinct as those represented by the main pattern types: whorls, ulnar loops, radial loops, simple arches, tented arches. A half-unit difference is assigned when two patterns belong to the same general type, but differ as do minor varieties of whorls. A half-unit difference applies also to two patterns morphologically closely allied to each other, such as an ordinary ulnar loop and one practically reduced to an arch. The total difference in the comparison is the sum of the unit and half-unit differences. Its percent value is expressed in relation to the maximum difference possible for the specific comparison—in five couplets or ten, according to whether the comparison concerns single hands or right and left hands combined. The same procedure is followed in the palmar features, below.

(c) Specific differences in palmar main lines and axial triradii also are rated by empirical values. There are five items in this comparison, four main lines and the axial triradius. Unit values are recorded when corresponding main lines end in zones as widely separated as 11 and 9, 9 and 7, 6 and 5, or when one of the lines is absent. Half-unit values apply to corresponding lines which terminate in adjoining positions such as $5'$ and $5''$, $5'$ and 4, 4 and 3, upper zone of 3 and lower zone of 3, 10 and 9, 10 and 11, X and x, X and 9, X and 8 or 7. An independent termination in one line and a dual termination in the other, with one main number in common, such as 11 and $11/7$, or 9-7 and 7, also is valued as a half-unit. For axial triradii, t is valued as one unit difference from O, t'', or $t't''$; t is a half-unit difference from t' or tt', as are t' from t'', and the presence of an ulnarward t as distinguished from its usual absence.

(d) Each of the five palmar configurational areas is subjected to a similar quantitative analysis. In the hypothenar area, A^u is one unit difference from A^c and from L^r, W, L^r/A^c, or other true patterns. Except as noted below, loops of the thenar and interdigital areas are rated as of one unit difference from W, D, d, V, M or O. Half-unit differences are entered when two compared hypothenars are A^u and A^u/A^c; A^u and O; A^r and L^r (or T^r); L^r and L^{rw}; also for thenar and interdigital configurations L and L/V (or L/O); L and l, D and d, O and V (or M), V and M.[1]

---

[1] The assignment of some of these values should be revised, to obviate duplicated ratings of difference. For example, the half-unit difference between A^u and A^u/A^c is a repetition of the value already assigned to the t and t' which are the associates of these configurations.

MacArthur recommends additionally: indices of pattern form, presence or absence of twisting, ridge counts on toes, pattern types on toes, plantar main lines, plantar patterns. He mentions further that the configurations of the basal phalanges of fingers have proved useful. With this method, MacArthur makes comparisons of bilateral, homolateral and heterolateral differences in twins and in single-born individuals (Table 42).

TABLE 42

AVERAGE NUMBERS OF DIFFERENCES IN QUANTITATIVE VALUE, PATTERN TYPE, PALMAR MAIN-LINE TERMINATIONS AND PALMAR PATTERNS. IN COMPUTING THE AVERAGE PERCENT DIFFERENCE EQUAL WEIGHTS ARE GIVEN THE FOUR TRAITS

(*MacArthur*)

Hand comparison	Ridge counts	Finger patterns	Palm lines	Palm patterns	Average percent difference
Bilateral					
100 identical twins..........	7.16	2.58	4.25	3.00	26.9
100 fraternal twins..........	8.14	2.61	3.64	3.28	26.5
100 single born.............	8.00	3.49	4.24	2.89	29.2
Homolateral					
50 prs. identical twins.......	5.88	1.88	2.84	2.09	19.0
50 prs. fraternal twins.......	22.94	4.38	4.15	3.65	37.9
62 prs. single sibs..........	22.52	4.77	4.54	3.69	39.8
150 prs. random pairs........	28.61	5.60	5.34	4.56	48.1
Heterolateral					
50 prs. identical twins........	6.86	2.51	4.04	2.96	26.0
50 prs. fraternal twins........	22.98	4.40	4.75	4.18	40.8
62 prs. single sibs...........	22.59	5.15	5.40	4.14	44.1

In the monozygotic pairs bilateral differences usually are greater than homolateral differences, this being reversed in dizygotics. In 84% of dizygotic pairs both homolateral and heterolateral differences are greater than bilateral differences; in the same proportion of monozygotics both bilateral and heterolateral differences are greater than the homolateral, though in instances of "asymmetry reversal" the heterolateral difference is reduced. MacArthur formulates this rule: "If a pair has no more than 30 percent homolateral difference in hands, the probability is 84 percent that they are monozygotic; if they have more than 30 percent homolateral difference the probability is 90 percent that they are dizygotic."

Essen-Moller (189) introduces a diagnostic formula for twins (in principle the same as his formula applied in questioned paternity). The formula depends on the relationship of frequency of a character in dizygotic twins (B) as compared to the frequency of the same character in monozygotics (A). The unlike proportions of monozygotics and dizygotics are adjusted by a factor derived from the proportion of mono-zygotics among same-sexed twins (26:63, in the population which he analyzes). The factor is $\dfrac{63 - 26}{26} = 1.423$. The formula (applied to a single character, as it would be in the instance of a selected trait such as the ridge number) is $\dfrac{1}{1 + 1.423 \times \dfrac{B}{A}}$. It may be extended by continued multiplication of B/A for each of the traits observed, thus:

$$\frac{1}{1 + 1.423 \times \dfrac{B_1}{A_1} \times \dfrac{B_2}{A_2} \times \dfrac{B_3}{A_3} \cdots}.$$

The value signifies positive monozygosity when it approaches 100%, and positive dizygosity in approaching 0%. The mean probability in dizygotics is 30.6% and in monozygotics 69.4% (190). Using as finger-print criteria the difference in total ridge count, Essen-Moller compares a group of dizygotic pairs (the diagnoses being unquestionable since the blood groups differ) with a series of monozygotic twins diagnosed by several criteria (Table 43).

TABLE 43
DIFFERENCES IN TOTAL RIDGE COUNT, THEIR FREQUENCIES AND THE PROBABILITY VALUES
(*Essen-Moller*)

Differences in total ridge number	Dizygotics (73 pairs)	Monozygotics (42 pairs)	Probability
40–	41.4%	0.19%	0.5%
30–39	12.6	1.77	12.3
20–29	14.3	10.00	41.2
10–19	15.7	31.70	66.7
0– 9	16.0	56.30	78.1

PATTERN TYPE. Stocks (245) makes homolateral comparisons of corresponding digits in each twin pair. If seven or more couplets have similar patterns the pair is diagnosed as monozygotic. When there are five or less agreements the pair is dizygotic, and if there are six agreements (or a doubt between five and six, or between six and seven), other bodily traits must be used for diagnosis. This author holds that one out of four pairs may be diagnosed by finger prints alone. In an alternative method, heterolateral comparisons are included. In elaborating on the method (246) he adds that seven digital couplets with like pattern type give odds of 50:1 in favor of monozygosity.

In his 1941 publication Geipel refers to a study, in press, on concordance of pattern type. Comparing homologous digits of the two members of a pair, he reports in 583 same-sexed dizygotic pairs, 5.2% of cases in which more than seven digital couplets are discordant. Among 596 monozygotic pairs there is no pair showing more than seven discordant digital couplets. He concludes, therefore, that a twin pair showing discordance of pattern type in more than seven digital couplets is almost certainly dizygotic.

In Danner's series of 85 pairs of twins, Stocks' dictum regarding pattern type fails in 19 pairs. Fourteen of the fraternal pairs have more than six couplets of like patterns and there are 5 pairs classed as monozygotic having less than six couplets of the same type.

TABLE 44
LOTTIG'S VALUES OF DIFFERENCES IN PATTERN TYPE AND DIRECTION

Differences	Difference Values
Loop and whorl.	1.0
Loop and arch.	1.0
Arch and whorl.	2.0
Loop and transitional pattern.	0.5
Whorl and transitional pattern.	0.5
Arch and transitional pattern.	0.5
Ulnar and radial directions of the same pattern type.	0.5
Symmetry reversal of right and left.	0.5
Difference of pattern in digits III and IV.	0.5
Difference of pattern in digits IV and V.	0.5
Difference of pattern in digits I and II.	0.5
Difference of pattern between I and III, IV or V.	1.0
Difference of pattern between II and III, IV, V.	1.0

Volotzkoy uses pattern intensity rather than the descriptive pattern type. He claims that intra-pair differences of six or more triradii indicate dizygosity. In the intra-pair comparisons of monozygotic twins he finds cases, contrary to Stocks, in which five, six or even seven pairs of digits are discordant in pattern type.

Most authors compare pattern type, as well as some other fingerprint traits, in couplets of homologous fingers. Lauer and Poll, however, show that there is a relation not only between corresponding digits, but also among fingers of the same hand. The digits particularly thus associated are III with IV, and IV with V; digits I and II also are associated in an obscure way, but rarely is there an indication of such relation between I or II and any of the other digits.

Lottig applies this principle in a twin analysis, and though his series is small (ten pairs each of monozygotics and dizygotics), the results suggest possibilities of further investigation. Like MacArthur, he constructs a scale of arbitrary numerical values (Table 44) for rating the differences of pattern type and direction, and reports the quantitative differences (Table 45).

TABLE 45
DIFFERENCE VALUES OF PATTERN TYPE AND DIRECTION IN 20 PAIRS OF TWINS
(*Lottig*)

Monozygotics	Dizygotics
0.0	1.0
0.5	2.0
0.5	3.5
1.0	3.5
1.0	4.0
1.0	4.5
1.0	5.0
2.0	5.5
2.5	6.5
2.5	12.0
Average 1.2	4.8

PATTERN FORM. Ennenbach finds that the maximum intra-pair difference in the form index (ten-digit average) of monozygotic twins is 10.3. He agrees with Geipel that a difference of 15 or more points in the index would indicate dizygosity. However, among his dizygotic pairs the majority display differences less than 15 points, showing that the diagnostic value of the form index is limited. Ennenbach regards quantitative value as the most important dermatoglyphic items in twin diagnosis, cushioning as a useful supplement and pattern form as of slight aid.

Fukuoka, judging pattern form mainly on the basis of digit IV, reports that in 125 pairs of monozygotic twins there is no instance of intra-pair discordance, which contrasts with a discordance of 53% in opposite-sexed dizygotics.

QUANTITATIVE VALUE. Geipel concludes that a pair of same-sexed twins presenting a difference of more than 40 ridges in a total count may be considered almost with certainty dizygotic (Table 35). He cautions that in instances presenting a difference of about 40 ridges reliance must be placed on other characteristics. In twins with a difference greater than 60 ridges the diagnosis of dizygosity can be made with certainty.

Fukuoka observes in dizygotic twins an average difference in quantitative value nearly six times as great as in monozygotics when all ten digits are considered, and three to four times as great when the hands are compared separately. In monozygotic twins the average bilateral differences are somewhat higher than homolateral differences. The coefficient of correlation between corresponding hands of monozygotics is slightly higher than that between right and left hands of the same individual; the same trends are reported for ridge counts between palmar digital triradii.

Danner records a range of difference of 0–11 ridges in monozygotics and 0–36 ridges in dizygotics.

Rife (236) analyzes 20 pairs of carefully diagnosed monozygotic twins. The mean intra-pair difference in quantitative value is 4.0, and the mean in 100 sibling pairs is 14.9. The maximum intra-pair difference in the twins is 8, and in the siblings it is 51. In four twin pairs there is no difference in quantitative value, while among the 100 pairs of siblings only two pairs are equivalent.

MINOR CONFIGURATIONAL CHARACTERS. Newman (225) places weight on close resemblances in minor configurational features, believing that resemblances such as those shown in figure 144 are sufficient to indicate monozygosity. The resemblance to which he refers is of course not a correspondence in minutiae, though the disposition of ridge details may be similar in two patterns. (Even this degree of likeness is not an absolutely dependable guide to monozygosity, for even with unusual and complex configurations a striking resemblance may exist in two individuals who are fraternal twins, siblings or parent and child.)

PALMS AND SOLES. Meyer-Heydenhagen provides detailed information relating to the palmar dermatoglyphics in a large series of twins. The unlikenesses of palmar dermatoglyphics in monozygotic and dizygotic twins, already indicated in MacArthur's scheme of diagnosis, are in full agreement with the contrasts in finger prints. One of her general conclusions of particular interest is that reversal of asymmetry is not a characteristic of monozygotic twins, contrary to the claim of Newman and others. The same negative finding is reported by Rife and Cummins. Viewing the palmar characteristics from the standpoint of the developmental mechanism, Meyer-Heydenhagen concludes that most of the dimensional and configurational features, particularly the hypothenar area, are quite environment-labile. The most environment-stable traits are: larger whorls in the thenar and fourth interdigital areas; well expressed loops in the thenar/first interdigital area; loops with accessory triradii in interdigital areas II, III and IV. All triradii appear more stable than the patterns associated with them.

Montgomery analyzes the plantar patterns in 57 pairs of same-sexed and 30 pairs of opposite-sexed twins. Aiming to determine how many pairs are "identical" he sets the following specifications: (a) Either all four soles, or both right and both left soles must have the same pattern formulae (Wilder's formulation); (b) There must be no marked differences in configurational character of patterns having the same formula. Thirteen of the 87 pairs (14.9%) conform to these specifications, and all except one of these pairs are of like sex. The formula in the exceptional case is a frequent one, occurring in about 10% of the general population, hence the concordance here is not significant. If the concordant pairs are accepted as monozygotic, there must remain among the 57 like-sexed pairs a number of monozygotics whose intra-pair differences exclude them from concordance as defined. Montgomery concludes that while conformity to these specifications may point to monozygosity, non-conformity does not necessarily indicate dizygosity.

QUESTIONED PATERNITY

PERSPECTIVES

ADVANCES in development of methods for evaluating the probability of paternity have been made mainly in Germany and in Austria, and especially through the contributions of Joseph Weninger and associates in the Anthropological Institute of the University of Vienna. A group of investigators attached to this Institute has been engaged in a program of studies directed toward the evaluation of a wide variety of structural and physiological traits for proof or exclusion of paternity.

Blood groups can be relied upon in some cases to exclude the possibility of paternity, but never do they serve to establish relationship. Unless the possibility of paternity is eliminated by blood groups, resort must be made to other traits in the attempt to exclude or incriminate the putative father. So far, dermatoglyphics have figured only in a small way in cases of questioned paternity.

Excellent discussions of the field of questioned paternity are available in articles by J. Weninger and by Schrader. Harrasser (205) reviews the statistics on 200 cases investigated by the Institute in Vienna. His digest (including dermatoglyphics but largely concerned with other traits) embraces a total of 236 putative fathers. In 53% of these cases the evidences were of great value, and in 20% they were useful, leaving 27% unsolved. The numbers of instances of proof of paternity and of exclusion of paternity are nearly equal.

A case reported in 1928 by Schläger illustrates the action of a court which at that time was justifiably hesitant to accept finger-print testimony in the issue of questioned paternity. A lower court had granted the claim of a plaintiff that a certain man was his illegitimate father. The defendant then took the case to a higher court, where blood groups and finger prints were presented in evidence. Paternity could not be excluded on the basis of blood groups, but the finger-print expert declared that the accused could be excluded with a "probability bordering on certainty." The higher court did not reverse the earlier decision on this evidence, taking the position that the use of finger prints in this connection was too contested and the methods too recent and untried. Even in the present state of knowledge, dermatoglyphics can claim a place only as a minor accessory in cases of questioned paternity; there are as yet no laws of inheritance so firmly substantiated that they qualify for rule-of-thumb practice.

Specific Methods

Geyer points out that the criteria used in problems of questioned paternity vary in significance, according to several qualitative and quantitative attributes. To meet the demands fully, a characteristic must be clearly definable, its mode of inheritance must be known, and it must be environment-stable and age-stable. Finally, the frequency of a characteristic in the population at large must be considered in relation to its occurrence in the examined individuals, since in general the probative value of a concordance between a child and putative father varies inversely with the frequency of the trait.

In 1937 Essen-Moller published his formula for assessing the chance that a putative father is the true father of a child in question. The formula, embodying a series of anatomical and serological items, resolves the probability in percent. The probability of paternity (P) is determined in terms of: first, the frequency in "true fathers" of occurrence or absence of a particular characteristic in their children (X); second, the frequency of the occurrence or absence of this characteristic among "false fathers" (Y), that is to say, in the general population of the same racial stock, and in males if there is a sexual difference in frequency. Frequencies in the general population (Y) are determined empirically, and values for many dermatoglyphic characteristics are already available in published statistics. Since the genetic process in most dermatoglyphic features is complex and but little known, it is not feasible to calculate frequencies in true fathers (X), hence collections of family material must be examined for obtaining observed frequencies.

The formula, where only one trait is considered, is $P = \dfrac{1}{1 + \dfrac{Y}{X}}$. For a series of traits the formula is expanded to: $P = \dfrac{1}{1 + \dfrac{Y_1}{X_1} \times \dfrac{Y_2}{X_2} \times \dfrac{Y_3}{X_3} \cdots}$.

An example presented by Geyer may be mentioned as an illustration of the formula in use. A certain characteristic of the ear (band-formed helix) occurs in 1.77% (0.018) of the Viennese population; it is age-stable and of like frequency in the sexes. This value is Y. Among true fathers of children who possess this character the frequency is 13.3% (0.133), this being X. With these values inserted in the formula, a probability of 88.3% is obtained, indicating that if there were 100 such cases the putative fathers would be judged as true fathers about 88 times and excluded from paternity about 12 times. When paternity is not excluded by blood groups the Y/X values of a series of traits are determined, selecting traits which are genetically independent. Thus one would not include both hair color and eye color, because of their genetic association. So far as finger prints are concerned, the independence of epidermal thickness (V), radial cushioning (R) and ulnar cushioning (U) seems to be established. For the same reason some palmar and plantar dermatoglyphic features would justify inclusion in the diagnostic formula. To continue with Geyer's example: The child and putative father both have the band-formed helix; both have blood group O; epidermal thickness in the child is VV, and in the putative father it is Vv. The respective Y/X values for these traits (as determined in the Viennese population) are 0.133, 0.592 and 0.638—which when inserted in the formula give a probability of paternity of 95.2%.

Bonnevie is cautious with regard to the use of her analyses of the genetic process in proving or excluding paternity, though she predicts that with further investigation finger prints may take their place with other characters which have a simpler mechanism of inheritance. She states, however, that paternity might be determined in cases having rare patterns or rare combinations. It may be added that minor pattern characteristics would be of service in instances of close resemblance between child and putative father. Other authors also urge caution, especially when the observations can not be supplemented by examination of relatives of those immediately concerned in the case. Hahne, in a very limited material of seven families and with rather inexact methods of pattern comparison, is unable to point to a single instance in which resemblance between father and child would aid in establishing paternity. (He alludes, however, to instances of resemblance between mother and child.)

PATTERN TYPE. Böhmer and Harren state that in cases presenting conspicuous similarity of infrequent patterns, pattern type may be valuable as an indication of paternity. It is their opinion that the configurational expression is too variable to admit classification under a few set types or values, and they consider that the evidence must be evaluated in each case individually. In at least one-third of their cases they note a distinct resemblance to one of the parents.

DOUBLE-CORED PATTERNS. On the basis of his rules regarding the inheritance of double loops (Chap. 13), Nürnberger formulates the following principles: (a) When the child and one putative father have double loops, which are lacking both in mother and other putative father, the man bearing double loops is the more probable father. (b) When mother and child bear double loops this pattern character is not applicable in the question of paternity. (c) When a child lacks double loops, and they are present in both the mother and assumed father, this is no evidence against the paternity of the man in question.

Bonnevie, with whom Müller and Ting agree, considers that the genetic process of double loops and other double-cored patterns is too uncertain to allow for application in paternity cases.

PATTERN FORM. Mueller suggests that his rules on the inheritance of pattern form (Chap. 13) may be occasionally useful in determination or exclusion of paternity, though he makes the reservation that age changes of pattern form may disqualify this trait when young children are involved. He formulates three rules: (a) If a mother has in each hand at least one elliptical pattern, and the child only circular patterns, the presence of elliptical patterns in both hands of the putative father would speak against his paternity. (b) If a child has in each hand at least one elliptical pattern and if the mother has all circular patterns, the true father is expected to have at least one elliptical pattern in at least one hand. (c) Paternity is improbable when the mother has only circular patterns, the putative father only circular patterns and the child has in either hand at least one intermediate pattern.

Nürnberger formulates these general rules: (a) If one of two putative fathers has elliptical patterns and the other does not, the latter is excluded when the child has elliptical patterns and the mother none. (b) If the child and one putative father have circular patterns, while the mother and other putative father have elliptical patterns, it is highly improbable that the man with elliptical patterns is the father. (c) When the child and mother both have elliptical or circular patterns it is impossible to make any determination of paternity.

Müller and Ting regard Nürnberger's rules as invalid. Though these critics offer no real evidence against the method, Geipel points out that the extreme infrequency of elliptical patterns (e.g., 1.9% on digit IV) would render the rules largely inapplicable in practice.

Geipel uses the average index of the ten fingers, and while warning against over-confidence in any rules he presents the following: (a) When mother and child both have a low ten-digit index it is improbable, theoretically impossible, that the child's father would be one with a large average index. The reverse situation is equally true. (b) If mother and child both have an intermediate average index, probability of paternity usually cannot be established. (c) If the mother has a high index and the child a low one, the establishment of paternity is theoretically impossible. He adds that instances with intermediate form indices involve special difficulty.

Geipel (198) reports a case in which the accused man had a small index, below 80, the mother an intermediate index, below 110, and the child a high one, over 120. The accused, according to this, could not be the father, a conclusion which agreed with the collateral evidence.

QUANTITATIVE VALUE. Von Wehren, in a large family material, estimates the efficiency of quantitative value for the exclusion of paternity. Transposing fathers from one family unit to another in the comparison of prints, he finds that in ten different combinations paternity may be excluded on an average of 1.9% of the children and 2.1% of the "families." By the same exchange method Mueller (221) finds that paternity can be excluded in 5.3% of children and 7.8% of "families." Bonnevie's earlier method (44) is considered by von Wehren superior to the newer one since it yields fewer exceptions to the rule that quantitative values of the children lie within the variational limits of the parents.

RACIAL VARIATION

CONCEPTS UNDERLYING RACIAL COMPARISONS

CLASSIFICATIONS of peoples may be founded on physical characters, culture, language or geographic distribution. Consideration of structural and physiological characters lies in the field of physical anthropology. Many physical characters (e.g., stature, head form, nose form, skin color, eye color, hair color, hair form, blood groups) have been used in defining races. The classification obtained with one character or set of characters may conflict with that resolved from others. Dermatoglyphics, it will be shown, display racial variations which in general are in accord with classifications based upon other traits.

A troublesome but apparently unavoidable complication is use of the word "race," a term so variously applied and so ill-reputed that its sense in this discussion of racial variation must be explained. In our sense, "race" is equivalent to "breed," with the same biological connotation as that applying in breeds of dogs, cattle or other domesticated animals. Just as reference is sometimes made to "the human race," designating a group of beings distinct from all other forms, there may be set apart in accord with biological qualities differing from those of other chief groups, a broad division of mankind, e.g., "White race." Again, the "White race" might be divided into "races," each having distinctive physical characters. The sense of "race" in these examples applies to a group, whether comprehensive or limited, marked by common characteristics traceable to inheritance. One shortcoming in such use of the word is lack of indication of major or subordinate rank. Fortunately, we are not attempting to establish a specific classification and have no need of a scaled nomenclature for races. Our naming of racial samples is not planned to conform to any consistent classification of races. At one moment it may be convenient to refer to Whites as a major race, and the next mention of a racial difference may contrast Norwegians and Italians, the designations being based upon nations. National populations are not on a par with groups separated on the basis of biological characters, the races of customary anthropological usage. The distribution of biological qualities does not conform to political boundaries. In Italy, for example, two races are represented—Alpines in the north, and Mediterraneans in the south.

It is necessary, however, to construct a working classification, so that related racial samples may be combined. In terming any group a race there is no intent to conflict with established classifications. Since many writers on anthropology adopt a classification comprising three main races—White, Yellow-brown and Black—this grouping is followed here.

Included in the group of *Whites* are the populations of Europe and of sections of Asia and Africa bordering the Mediterranean Sea. In the usage of most authors three or more races of Whites are distinguished. The *Mediterraneans* comprise European and extra-European populations of regions neighboring the Mediterranean Sea; the *Alpines* are typified by inhabitants of Switzerland, northern Italy, southern France and southern Germany, while *Nordics* are typified by peoples of the Scandinavian countries and northern Germany. Among Whites also are the Hindus and, closely related in many characters though of doubtful position, some other groups such as the Aino. The *Yellow-brown* peoples, *Mongolians*, include not only Japanese, Chinese and related Asiatics, but also Indians of the Americas. The third main racial group, the *Blacks*, embraces the Negroes of Africa, both typical and dwarf types, Philippine Negritos and Melanesians.

Two landmarks in the history of knowledge of racial variation in dermatoglyphics are Galton's *Finger Prints* and Wilder's *Racial differences in palm and sole configuration.* In his Chapter 12, Galton compares four racial series (English, Welsh, Jews and Negroes) with regard to frequencies of arches on index fingers. The only outstanding contrast in the four groups is between the English and Jews, where the respective frequencies of arches are 13.6% and 7.9%. In Jews the lower frequency of arches, and to some extent of loops also, is compensated by increase in whorls. Galton states emphatically that there is no peculiar pattern which is characteristic of any of these groups and that the only differences observed are unlike frequencies of the same pattern types.

In a general article on palms and soles, Wilder remarked in 1902 that "it would be of much interest to compare the sculpture of the palms and soles in the various races of men, as it is at least possible that there may be sufficient difference to constitute important racial characteristics." His paper of 1904 concerns an investigation of palms and soles in Maya Indians, Whites, Negroes and a few Chinese. Among other contrasts, he observes in the Maya a high frequency of palmar thenar/first interdigital patterns and infrequent hypothenar patterns. His observations on the distinctions of Maya Indians, Whites and Negroes have been repeatedly confirmed. Like Galton, Wilder stresses the absence of morphological peculiarities diagnostic of race in the individual. The distinctions observed are therefore unlikenesses in the frequencies of characters that occur in all races.

With the accumulation of records for many racial series, it is now assured that racial differences in dermatoglyphics are real. The misunderstanding of a distinguished British anatomist, writing as late as 1939, may be typical of an erroneous view held possibly by others. This anatomist states, without indicating in context whether the remark applies to morphological characters or to statistical trends: "Attempts to establish racial differences in the papillary ridge pattern of the fingers and of the palm of the hand have led to negative results." Heindl, an outstanding authority in his own field of finger-print identification and criminology, published in 1935 a pointed denial of the reality of statistical expressions of racial difference. Noting that the frequencies of finger-print types in European peoples are fairly uniform, he claims that all the reported departures therefrom in other racial series are due solely to the use of samples too small to yield reliable frequencies. His argument ignores the fact that reliability of racial differences is demonstrated both by accepted tests for statistical significance and by the repeated finding of the same distinctive trends in different collections from the same racial stock, even when the series are small.

The status of racial variation in dermatoglyphics may be better appreciated in the light of differences in other traits. Some racial characteristics are so deeply ingrained genetically that they appear in all individuals of a race. It would not be difficult to recognize as a Mongollan an individual with straight black hair, yellowish-tinged skin and epicanthic folds of the upper eye-lids. If, however, one confined examination to some isolated feature—e.g., head form, stature or blood group—an individual would not be assignable to his race because each of these traits varies inter-racially only with respect to frequencies. A race might be predominatingly short-statured, round-headed or of blood group O. Similarly, a race might be distinguished by relatively many arches and few whorls among finger patterns. An individual who has many arches and few whorls can not be diagnosed as to race any more readily, on the basis of this characteristic alone, than an individual about whom we know only that he is short in stature, round-headed or of blood group O. All such traits enter into the racial character of a mass sample. Their more frequent occurrence in individuals of some races determines the trend which makes the group distinctive.

DERMATOGLYPHICS AS CRITERIA FOR RACIAL COMPARISONS

BIOLOGICAL AND TECHNOLOGICAL QUALIFICATIONS. In a valuable critique of methods of classifying mankind, Boyd[1] enumerates certain requirements which should be satisfied by criteria chosen for human classifications. These requirements are here listed, and under each the degree of qualification of dermatoglyphics is briefly indicated.

(a) The criteria must be objective, so that individuals will be classified consistently by different observers. The methodology of dermatoglyphics is now so standardized that constancy in determinations is sufficiently assured. As a result of intensive interest in finger prints. descriptive methods for these features progressed rapidly to the point of stability, and abundant data from different races are on record. In the case of palms and soles less material has been accumulated; additionally, some of the early records, based upon methods now superseded, admit at best only tentative translation into terms of current methods.

(b) The traits used in racial classification must not be subject to extensive environmental modification. This requirement is met by dermatoglyphics, which are not modifiable post-natally.

(c) Ideally a criterion chosen for racial comparison should be one controlled by a simple and known genetic process. Dermatoglyphic features, unfortunately, are like most other traits which figure in racial classifications, being regulated by a complex and incompletely understood genetic mechanism.

(d) The traits should be non-adaptive, thus eliminating effects of natural selection. Dermatoglyphics satisfy this condition probably as well as any physical characteristic, and better than many. The superiority of patterns over patternless configurations, both in heightening frictional resistance and in increasing tactile acuity is recognized (Chap. 2), but it is extremely doubtful that the difference between a pattern and a patternless configuration or between two pattern types has any selective value whatsoever. Grüneberg (202) concedes the improbability of a direct selection of qualities of dermatoglyphics, but he holds that selection may still have been indirectly responsible for effecting racial differences in these features. He asserts, without offering evidence, that there may be genetic linkage with traits which do have a selective value. Actually, dermatoglyphics are not thus correlated with characteristics that have been tested (Chap. 16), and their genetic independence (from head form, nasal form, general body build and blood groups) adds a distinct advantage for use in racial comparison.

---

[1] Am. J. Phys. Anthropol., vol. 27, pp. 337–364, 1940.

(e) To be fully qualified, the criterion should not be subject to a high rate of mutation. No investigations have been made on mutation rate in dermatoglyphics, but the character of dermatoglyphic variation suggests that mutation is a negligible factor in the production of racial differences.

CHOICE OF TRAITS. Dermatoglyphic characters are heritable, hence dependent upon the action of genes, and since races vary statistically in frequencies of particular features, it follows that they vary also in frequencies of genes. Characterization of a race would be stated ideally in terms of gene frequencies, because the actual expression of features in the individual (phenotype) may differ from the genetic prospect (genotype). These matters are discussed in Chapter 12, where all the available calculations of gene frequencies are brought together in table 38. Few racial samples are represented, and the only genes thus far investigated are determined from ridge counts in finger patterns (epidermal thickness, V; radial cushioning, R; ulnar cushioning, U). Pending confirmation of the genetic process in dermatoglyphics and accumulation of proved data on gene frequencies in many representative racial samples, it will be necessary, as in the case of most bodily traits, to compare races only on the basis of phenotypes.

Having limited the comparison to phenotypes, the first question involves the selection of regions and specific dermatoglyphic characters which meet the needs for racial comparison. Shall it be fingers, palms, soles or toes—or shall all regions be considered? This question is in part already answered by limitations of available records. Frequencies of pattern types in toes are known only in four racial samples (Table 17). Racial distinctions are evident, but this material is too meager for comprehensive comparisons. The situation is more satisfactory with regard to data on plantar configurations, and still larger material is available for palms. Finger prints have been studied most extensively and are thus favorable as the principal foundation for racial comparisons. Two points are significant in connection with this emphasis on finger prints. Twin studies indicate that finger patterns may be more rigidly controlled genetically than dermatoglyphics of other regions (Chaps. 12 and 13). There is a degree of correlation in pattern expressions of different regions—fingers and palms, fingers and toes, palms and soles (Chap. 11); to that degree, therefore, trends of palmar, plantar and toe configurations would only reinforce conclusions drawn from analysis of finger patterns.

A rough measure of interracial variability in different dermatoglyphic regions is obtained from the following analysis. Finger patterns, palmar main lines, palmar patterns, and patterns of the distal sole (but not toe patterns) are all available from sufficiently diverse populations to provide for the desired calculation: European-Americans, Germans (or Italians in the instance of finger patterns and plantar patterns), New Mexicans of Spanish descent (available in two samples, one of which shows signs of Indian admixture), Jews, Eskimos, North American Indians, Indians of Mexico and Middle America, Chinese, Japanese, Gilyaks, Oroks, Siamese (for soles alone), Negroes (East African Negroes for fingers and Liberian Negroes for other features). Values for finger and plantar patterns are calculated from indices of pattern intensity, palmar patterns from percent frequencies, and palmar main lines from main-line indices. In the case of palmar patterns calculations are made not only for all configurational areas collectively (average of the percent frequencies of patterns in the five areas) but also for the individual configurational areas; the same procedure is followed for patterns of the distal sole, where four configurational areas are analyzed. In each determination, e.g., pattern intensities of finger prints or main-line indices, the eleven values are averaged. Deviations from this mean are then averaged, and the result stated as the average deviation: finger prints, 6.4%; palmar main lines, 7.8%; palmar patterns (collectively), 10.5%; plantar patterns (collectively), 18.6%. Higher deviations indicate greater variability among these racial groups.

It is to be noted that unlike technical methods are applied in different dermatoglyphic regions. Such technical unlikeness, for example between the statement of total pattern intensity for finger prints and the evaluation of palmar patterns in terms of percent frequency, might introduce discrepancies in the weights of the different regions. The fact remains, however, that the technical methods applied in obtaining these results are the same methods which are to be relied upon in racial comparisons.

Two factors must be considered in interpretation of the data just presented: (a) It is impossible in this material to discriminate between phenotypic variation and genetic variation. Twin studies disclose a similar order of increasing phenotypic variation in the several regions, and interracial variation is in all likelihood equally subject to phenotypic influences. (b) Whether the variants are genetic or phenotypic in origin, massing of the five palmar, or the four plantar, configurational areas obviously obscures the distinctions of individual areas. The numerical values for average deviations (Table 46) must inevitably be lower for the several configurational areas collectively than for any single area. In general, variations of these values are related, inversely to some degree, with pattern frequencies in the individual areas.

Not all the analytic methods applicable in any one region are used in the various samples. Pattern-type determinations in finger prints are uniformly available, but ridge counts, measurements of pattern form and similarly specialized analyses are made so infrequently that attention is here almost confined to total frequencies of pattern type. Consideration of even these data in detail would require an inordinate amount of tabular or graphic records.

TABLE 46

AVERAGE DEVIATIONS AMONG RACES OF PATTERN OCCURRENCES IN THE PALM AND SOLE

Area	Palm	Sole
Hypothenar..	39.5%	
Thenar/Interdigital I*..	49.7	13.3%
Interdigital II...	58.3	45.8
Interdigital III..	33.2	22.5
Interdigital IV...	17.6	54.3

* Hallucal, in sole.

All dermatoglyphic traits embodied in racial comparisons are determined by objective methods. Standard definitions prescribe that a finger print is to be interpreted as a loop, a whorl or an arch, that a palmar or plantar configurational area is of a specific configurational type, and that a palmar main line courses in a particular manner. There is common understanding in the use of such methods because both the methods and the features to which they are applied can be precisely described.

It is possible that racial differences occur also in features for which a descriptive technique has not been devised. This possibility was recognized by Galton, though with his characteristic caution he makes no final pronouncement on the question. After pointing out that finger-print patterns of Negroes are not definably different from those of the other races examined, he continues:

> Still, whether it be from pure fancy on my part, or from the way in which they were printed, or from some real peculiarity, the general aspect of the Negro print strikes me as characteristic. The width of the ridges seems more uniform, their intervals more regular, and their courses more parallel than with us. In short, they give an idea of greater simplicity, due to causes that I have not yet succeeded in submitting to the test of measurement.

The same experience is indicated in a comment by Bridges (46):

> There is little doubt that skin patterns do display some general race characteristics, especially in pure-blooded groups of little intermingling. This is notably true of Negroes and Orientals, whose patterns are commonly distinctive enough to be recognized in any accumulation of miscellaneous prints. With familiarity, the skilled technician finds it

possible to discriminate, although the aptitude is more easily acquired than described.

In our own contacts with comparative racial material we have sensed at times that there are some trends of variation which elude objective treatment. For instance, while examining the dermatoglyphics of a series of Eskimos we were impressed by peculiarities of the hallucal area of the sole:

> Open fields present a singular high frequency [23%]. . . . A further point, which can be appreciated only by examination of the prints themselves and comparison with other series, is the frequent weak and irregular expression of the type forms of patterns, especially the form known as $A[L^d]$. One who is accustomed to the usual expanse and contour of $A[L^d]$ patterns cannot fail to be impressed by the occurrence in this collection of many configurations which are distinctly atypical, often appearing as if they were about to be effaced as true patterns, to be superseded by open fields. This irregularity suggests that the same factors conditioning the high frequency of open fields have operated to suppress the full development of true patterns. (Am. J. Phys. Anthropol., vol. 16, pp. 41–49, 1931.)

MATERIAL AND METHOD OF STUDY

RACIAL SAMPLES. A racial sample is composed of a number of persons so chosen from a population as to represent fairly the character of the population as a whole. The composition of the sample by ages of the subjects is unimportant inasmuch as dermatoglyphics are age stable. To be representative, a sample for analysis of dermatoglyphics must satisfy certain requirements.

The sample must be selected at random. It is obvious that dermatoglyphic traits can not be permitted to influence the selection. In view of known differences among some constitutional types (Chap. 16) and the possibility of distinctive trends in others which have not been investigated, samples should not be obtained from sources likely to have concentrations of particular constitutional types (such as hospitals for the insane and penal institutions).

Sexual composition is important, since the sexes differ in trends of variation. The most satisfactory sample would contain both sexes, each adequately represented in number. (Many samples on record represent males alone, or males and females combined in widely unequal numbers.)

Exclusion of related individuals is particularly important in small samples, since introduction of familial peculiarities would produce deviations from trends characteristic of the population at large. Abel's series of 68 Eskimos of eastern Greenland (265) may be mentioned as an example of possibly distorted statistics attributable to familial composition. In the finger prints of this series there is a remarkable incidence of 72.2% whorls and 0.8% arches. This result is to be compared with respective whorl and arch frequencies of 43.8% and 3.4% in 273 Eskimos from other localities. (The latter values are obtained from three independent samples, collected in western Greenland, St. Lawrence Island and Point Barrow. The three samples differ insignificantly among themselves, the values cited being weighted averages of their separately reported frequencies.) Abel's material comprises several families, with as many as six, seven or eight siblings. It seems quite possible, therefore, that this series is not a representative racial sample. A high whorl frequency (with attendant reduction of arches) in one or more of these families may have vitiated the characteristic racial trend. Accordingly, Abel's sample of Eskimos as well as the Cummins and Steggerda sample of Dutch (the latter, 113 individuals, assembled designedly as a family series), are here omitted from racial comparisons.

Many of the recorded samples are from criminal populations. Such records consist of relatively enormous numbers, but it is questionable that the advantage of numbers in these instances compensates for the lack of specific information concerning racial origins (as well as the possibility of statistical distortion by concentration of constitutional types). Some reported racial samples, especially those collected among generally inaccessible peoples, are relatively small. Dankmeijer (280) excludes from his comparative tables all samples containing less than 200 persons. Such exclusion is not always advisable, for there may be available a small sample, say only 25-100 individuals, from a population important for racial comparison. Use of small samples calls for caution in evaluating trends of variation. The standard methods of statistics may be used to test the significance of results in small series. Small collections may reveal characteristic racial trends, as illustrated by several samples of Middle American Indians, where time after time the same directions of variation are repeated. This is not intended to indicate that a report of the dermatoglyphics in several individuals (e.g., Hill on three Veddahs, or Abel on six natives of Tierra del Fuego) would be a significant contribution to racial dermatoglyphics. The case might be different if races varied in morphological characters, but a series of several persons is patently useless for revealing statistical trends.

RACIAL COMPARISONS

Figures 145-148 are records of data gathered from published sources and adapted for graphic presentation. These records, for the features

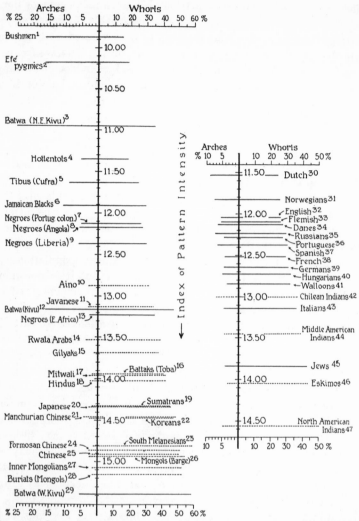

FIG. 145.—Comparison of racial samples with regard to percent frequencies of arches and whorls, arranged in the order of increasing pattern intensity. Peoples of Asia and Africa are grouped in the section at the left; peoples of Europe and the Americas are included in the section at the right.

Sources of the material are here identified by the reference numbers in the graph, the authors and the number of subjects being indicated. In instances in which two or more samples are combined, the values shown in the graph are weighted averages. In most cases the samples include both males and females. 1—M. Weninger, 32. 2—Valsik, 143; Dankmeijer, 207. 3—M. Weninger, 84. 4—Fleischhacker, 50. 5—Sabatini, 104. 6—Davenport and Steggerda, 124. 7—de Pina, 275. 8—Sarmento, 174. 9—Dankmeijer, 343; Cummins, 58. 10—Hasebe, 55. 11—Dankmeijer, 2000. 12—M. Weninger, 174. 13—de Zwaan, 1300. 14—Shanklin and Cummins, 200. 15—Suda, 28. 16—Maasland, 1000. 17—Cummins and Shanklin, 138. 18—Biswas, 50. 19—de Zwaan, 500. 20—Iseki, 359; Hasebe, 276; Shute, 5064; Furuse, 1528;

selected, form an essentially complete survey of known racial samples. A few reports, mostly Japanese publications, remain inaccessible to us.

WHITES. European populations exhibit in their finger prints (Fig. 145) a fairly definite ordering which conforms to the division into Mediterraneans, Alpines and Nordics. Unfortunately the precise geographic origins of the individuals composing many reported samples are not known. However, it is evident that Nordics are distinguished by low pattern intensity and Mediterraneans by higher intensity, Alpines being probably

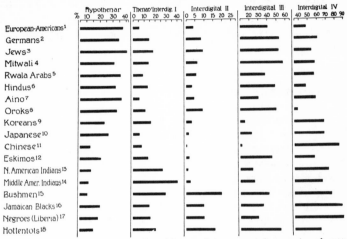

FIG. 146.—Comparison of racial samples with regard to percent frequencies of patterns in the several palmar configurational areas.

Sources are listed as in the legend of figure 145: 1—Cummins, Leche and McClure, 300. 2—Tables 7-10. 3—Cummins and Midlo, 200. 4—Cummins and Shanklin, 138. 5—Shanklin and Cummins, 230. 6—Biswas, 50. 7—Hasebe, 50. 8—Suda, 50. 9—Miyake, 134. 10—Hasebe, Wilder, 461. 11—Wilder, 100. 12—Midlo and Cummins, Cummins, 86. 13—Cummins, Cummins and Goldstein, 350. 14—Cummins, Leche, Steggerda, Steggerda and Lane, Wilder, 848. 15—M. Weninger, 25. 16—Davenport and Steggerda, 67. 17—Cummins, 75. 18—Fleischhacker, 50.

intermediate. It is noteworthy that Hindus, Arabs, Syrians (Mitwali) and Jews show pattern intensities somewhat higher than those of European Mediterraneans. Perhaps significant is the level of pattern intensity in the Aino, a people of problematic relationship; in pattern intensity, as in some other physical traits, this population closely resembles White stocks.

Kubo, 1000; Shima, 380; Kanaseki et al., 1386; Kutsuna et al., 215. 21—Furuse, 3350. 22—Kubo, 700; Takeya, 3191. 23—Hesch, 35. 24—Kutsuna et al., 475; Matuyama et al., 550. 25—Kubo, 500. 26—Yokoh, 138. 27—Yokoh, 191. 28—Yokoh, 55. 29—M. Weninger, 76. 30—Piebenga, 400; Dankmeijer, 2500. 31—Bonnevie, 24,518. 32—Waite, 2000; Scotland Yard series, 5000. 33—Piebenga, 200. 34—Bugge, 101,511. 35—Semenovsky, 22,000. 36—de Pina, 2000; Lopez, 1000; Valladares, 2000. 37—Oloriz, 10,000. 38—Bayle, 15,000. 39—Steiner, 4542; Karl, 556; Heindl, 99,400 and 200,000. 40—Bonnevie, 833. 41—Piebenga, 200. 42—Henckel, 246. 43—Sabatini, 550; Falco, 1579. 44—Cummins, Leche, Cummins and Steggerda, 633. 45—Cummins and Midlo, 200. 46—Cummins, Hansen, Midlo and Cummins. 273. 47—Cummins, Downey, Cummins and Goldstein, 400.

In palmar patterns (Fig. 146) there is no opportunity, for want of material, to examine the possibility of distinctions among Nordics, Alpines and Mediterraneans. It is suggested, however, that European-Americans and Germans, the only representatives of European Whites, differ only slightly from Hindus, Arabs, Syrians (Mitwali), Jews and Aino.

With regard to plantar patterns (Fig. 147) the material is inadequate for broad comparisons, only European-Americans, Italians and Jews being represented. Jews tend to have higher pattern intensity than other Whites; this applies to finger prints, most palmar areas and all plantar areas.

Palmar main lines (Fig. 148) in Whites, both European and extra-European, agree in presenting marked transversality, as indicated in the

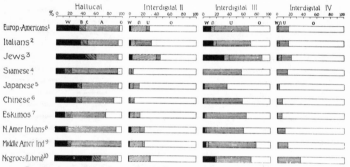

FIG. 147.—Comparison of racial samples with regard to percent frequencies of configurational types in the four areas of the distal sole.
Sources are listed as in the legend of figure 145: 1—Cummins and Midlo, Montgomery, Wilder, 2400. 2—Sabatini, 552. 3—Cummins and Midlo, 100. 4—Cummins, 76. 5—Kanaseki et al., 796. 6—Takeya, 1000. 7—Midlo and Cummins, Cummins, 95. 8—Cummins, 311. 9—Cummins and Steggerda, 124. 10—Cummins, 96.

main-line index and in the high proportion of type *11* of line *D*. In this item the Aino show a less close relationship to the characteristics of Whites, the frequencies of types *11* and *7* being more allied to Yellow-browns and Blacks.

YELLOW-BROWNS. The general characteristics of Yellow-brown, or Mongolian, peoples (as contrasted with Whites) are: high pattern intensity in fingers (Fig. 145); reduction of patterns in palmar hypothenar, second interdigital and third interdigital areas, and, in Indians of Middle America, a spectacular rise of thenar/first interdigital patterns (Fig. 146); reduced pattern intensity in all four plantar configurational areas of the distal sole (Fig. 147); tendency of palmar main lines toward longitudinal alignment, the Eskimo being an exception (Fig. 148).

BLACKS. Blacks are distinguished by great dispersion with respect to pattern intensity of finger prints (Fig. 145). The samples of typical

Negroes present intensities within the range of European Whites. Bushmen have the lowest pattern intensity yet reported (9.87), and the Efé pygmies are but little higher. At the other extreme are the South Mela-

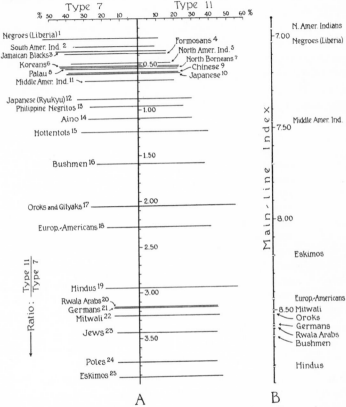

FIG. 148.—A. Frequencies of modal types of palmar main lines. Percent frequencies of types 7 and 11 are indicated, type 9 being implied in the remainders. The racial samples are arranged in the order of increase of the ratio Type 11 ÷ Type 7. B. A comparison based upon the main-line index.

Sources are listed as in the legend of figure 145. Japanese sources are identified by serial numbers in the list of Kanaseki and Shima. 1—Cummins, 75. 2—Keith, 64. 3—Davenport and Steggerda, 67. 4—Nos. 69-71, 79. 5—Cummins, and Cummins and Goldstein, 350. 6—Nos. 63-64, 281. 7—Ride, 133. 8—No. 75, 170. 9—Nos. 66-68, 608. 10—Nos. 38-61, 6315. 11—Steggerda and Steggerda, Leche, Cummins, 749. 12—Nos. 30-35, 1482. 13—No. 72, 47. 14—Nos. 28-29, 171. 15—Fleischhacker, 50. 16—M. Weninger, 25. 17—No. 27, 36. 18—Cummins and Midlo, Cummins, Leche and McClure, 700. 19—Biswas, 50. 20—Shanklin and Cummins, 229. 21—Table 5. 22—Cummins and Shanklin, 138. 23—Cummins and Midlo, 200. 24—Loth, 107. 25—Midlo and Cummins, Cummins, 86.

nesians and the Batwa of West Kivu with extremely high pattern intensities. Palmar hypothenar patterns, though less rare than in Yellow-brown peoples generally, are less frequent than in Whites, while second and fourth interdigital patterns tend to be especially abundant (Fig. 146). In the plantar configurational areas, especially hallucal and interdigital IV, pattern intensity is high (Fig. 147). Palmar main lines tend toward longitudinal alignment, a character shared with the Yellow-browns (Fig. 148).

INTERPRETATION OF RACIAL DIFFERENCES. The ultimate objective of racial comparisons is the tracing of lines of racial descent. Questions at once arise as to whether the resemblances here catalogued indicate relationship, and whether differences may be relied upon in tracing racial derivation. The solution of these questions must await more extensive investigation, but in the meantime it is profitable to review the prospects of such applications.

A crucial problem is to determine the signs which suggest that one stock is more generalized, or "primitive," than another. Clues to "primitiveness" of dermatoglyphics among races are furnished by comparative anatomy (Chap. 9). With regard to finger prints it may be concluded that the sequence *whorl-loop-arch* represents successive departures from the primitive. A race presenting a high frequency of whorls thus would be more primitive (disregarding bodily traits generally, culture, or any other criterion that might be used in human classifications) than a stock presenting a low frequency of whorls. Some human populations are more primitive, with regard to finger prints, than apes (e.g., chimpanzee). Indeed, other dermatoglyphic regions in man also indicate a degree of primitiveness suggesting that man stemmed from an ancestral stock more primitive than any recent ape, having dermatoglyphic traits more closely allied to those of monkeys (Chap. 9). Even granting the assumption that abundance of whorls is a sign of primitiveness, it may not be justified to conclude that two races having equally high pattern intensity are on a par with regard to racial genealogy, or that a race presenting lower pattern intensity is farther removed in the genealogical tree. The factors underlying racial divergence are complex, and it is impossible to assign shares to ancientness, degree of isolation and other factors which render the history of races so involved. The student of dermatoglyphics will not fall into the error of presuming that dermatoglyphic features now provide ready answers for refractory questions in the history of races, particularly when he sees that attacks from many quarters have failed to yield a completely knit scheme of the affinities of races.

Difficulties in tracing racial affinities are multiplied when dermatoglyphic regions other than fingers are considered. It is not unwarranted to assume that, as an indication of primitiveness, high pattern intensity in palmar and plantar configurational areas has the same significance as high pattern intensity in fingers. The dilemma arising from this view is that a population presenting high pattern intensity in fingers may present relatively low intensity in palmar and plantar configurations, as in the Chinese for example. It seems, therefore, that different dermatoglyphic regions may have independent courses of specialization in racial evolution. The situation becomes even more complicated when the courses of palmar main lines are introduced in racial comparisons. There is reason to think that the trend toward longitudinal alignment (indicated in reduced frequency of type *II* and reduced values of the main-line index) is a derived condition, the tendency to transverse alignment being more primitive. As a rule, races having high pattern intensity in fingers exhibit the longitudinal or specialized trend in palmar main lines.

For reasons already stated it is possible that greater reliance in tracing racial affinities may be placed upon finger prints. Accepting this, the Yellow-browns embrace the most primitive stocks, and the most specialized are certain components of the Blacks and, among Whites, the Nordics. Whites, in general, and typical Negroes may be regarded as representing a fulcrum of pattern intensity. They show intermediate degrees of intensity, being thus neither much specialized nor near the primitive.

Gross geographic trends of pattern intensity are recognizable. In Africa, Asia and the Americas there is a tendency toward progressive reduction of pattern intensity from north to south, while in Europe the line of reducing pattern intensity is from south to north.

The possibility that ancient lines of dispersion might be reflected in dermatoglyphics is suggested by these distributions of finger-print types. Early human migrations have been traced by numerous investigators. Taylor[2] emphasizes that early migrations must be considered with the idea that the continents are three "peninsular" offshoots from central Asia. The three peninsulas are Europe-Africa, southeast Asia with Australasia, and northeast Asia with the Americas. Taylor suggests that early migrations into the three peninsulas were mainly in the order of accessibility: Europe-Africa, Australasia and the Americas. Significantly, the postulated center of distribution in Asia coincides with recent populations characterized by high pattern intensity. In passing northward in Europe, southward in Africa and southward in the Americas the populations exhibit progressively reduced pattern intensity. This reduction reaches its maximum in Africa, in the southern extremity (Bushmen) and in the central area (pygmies). Next in order of reduction of pattern intensity are populations of northern Europe, especially the Scandinavian countries.

---

[2] Human Biol., vol. 13, pp. 390–397, 1941.

Though in the Americas there is a progression of diminishing pattern intensity from north to south, the level of intensity is relatively high; this is suggestive in the light of the supposition that migrations to the Americas were relatively late.

INTRARACIAL VARIABILITY. Expressions of variability within a single race, a race in the most comprehensive sense, are conspicuous. Whites, for example, are divisible into races showing distinctive differences in dermatoglyphics as well as other traits. Within a single nation, say Italy or Germany, unlike trends of variation in dermatoglyphics are indications of the heterogeneous biological composition of a political region. Only in Germany and Japan have local variations been extensively investigated. The German studies are cited to illustrate such local differences.

Abel (267) reports variations in finger prints in individuals from 40 localities in Germany, though his results are presented in incomplete form since the account is only preliminary. Poll (302) makes an exhaustive study of populations from 19 arbitrarily divided regions covering all Germany (as of 1937) and Germanic Poland. The material comprises 8041 persons, each of whom is classified according to his birthplace (ignoring birthplaces of forebears). The data are analyzed by an elaborate method, and to present the full results would require a lengthy description of his procedure. The populations of major geographic divisions of Germany may be characterized, however, in the simple terms of the descriptive method adopted here. Populations of the north and west have relatively many arches and few whorls, while in the south and east there are fewer arches and increased whorls. Populations of the middle sections present intermediate frequencies of these pattern types. The described distribution conforms to the generalization that whorls are found to diminish in passing northward in Europe. It agrees also with the separation of the German population into two races, the Nordic and the Alpine, on the score of other physical traits.

Steiner surveys finger-prints in 3582 school children born and residing in the Tettnang district. He analyzes the native material, using the whorl/arch index, in correlation with archeological and judiciary history. The local series which yield an index above 2.00 are from communities where there are pre-Roman relics and where the judicial system is distinctive (lower courts being independent of the upper). The series having indices smaller than 2.00 originate from communities which were settled later, communities lacking pre-Roman relics and having the ordinary court system. It is Steiner's opinion that the localities having independent lower courts probably preserve the influence in this respect of pre-Germanic populations. These populations, he believes, were distinguished by a higher whorl/arch index than that of the Germans who later occupied the section. As a supplement, Steiner studied a few populations in Ravensburg, a locality having an historical background not much different from that of Tettnang. Here he found that series originating from towns with old names yield high indices while those from towns with recent names yield lower indices. Though Steiner's results are in need of verification, they are suggestive that dermatoglyphics may have promise for correlation with the history of peoples.

RACIAL HYBRIDS

It is doubtful that any racial sample, of the sort here considered in treating racial variation, is strictly homogeneous, or pure. Admixtures of unknown kind and degree enter into the makeup of a race. There are, however, some recent admixtures which involve groups having contrasting characteristics and in which there is opportunity to test the behavior of the trends present in the two original races. Observations in two hybrid groups are here presented, White $\times$ Black, and White (Spanish) $\times$ North American Indians.

The study on Blacks, Browns and Whites in Jamaica is by Davenport and Steggerda. The results warrant attention, though the numbers of individuals are too small to provide stable values. Finger prints, palmar patterns, and palmar main lines are investigated. For finger prints there are 124 Blacks, 213 Browns and 47 Whites; the numbers of subjects available for the study of palms are even smaller. Frequencies of whorl and arch patterns of fingers form a graded series, Browns being intermediate between Blacks and Whites; the frequencies of whorls are 30%, 25% and 22% for Blacks, Browns and Whites respectively. The corresponding figures for arches are 11%, 10% and 7%. Calculations of pattern intensities have been made from the data of these authors and are here given separately for the sexes. For males: Blacks 12.01, Browns 11.63, Whites 11.69; for females: Blacks 11.76, Browns 11.39; Whites 11.16. These data would suggest that there is a blending in the hybrid Browns of the trends of Blacks and Whites. Such intermediate values in Browns occur also in pattern frequencies of two palmar areas, the hypothenar and fourth interdigital, but the other three configurational areas show a different relationship. In Browns there are more thenar/first interdigital and second interdigital patterns than in Blacks, while third interdigital patterns are even less frequent than in the Blacks. The frequencies in these last three areas may indicate that in the Browns there is an accentuation rather than a leveling of the traits distinctive of the Blacks.

The same accentuation may be present in the palmar main lines where, it will be recalled, typical Negroes differ from Whites in having more longitudinal alignments. Main-line indices calculated from the original data are: Blacks 8.43, Browns 8.38, Whites 8.52.

The results are not very illuminating, and in evaluating them two factors must be kept in mind. First, the samples are too small to yield statistically reliable frequencies; second, the Blacks as well as the Browns may carry admixture, present in such degree as to vitiate the comparison. This might be illustrated by reference to the main-line index, which in Liberian Negroes drops to 7.03, a value in keeping with the typical longitudinality in the Negro, while in neither Jamaican Browns nor Blacks is this figure approximated.

Two series of New Mexicans of Spanish descent, and three groups of American Indians from the same locality, are reported by Cummins (274). The New Mexican samples are 110 persons from Chamita and 97 from Bernalillo. The finger prints of the Bernalillo series are representative of other series of Spanish, but in the Chamita sample the high frequency of whorls approaches that of the Indians. Even the symmetry relations, as expressed in the dactylodiagrams, agree with the indication that there is Indian admixture in the Chamita series. In the Chamita sample of Spanish, as in Indians, arches and whorls conform to the rule of all pairs rather than the pair-group rule. With regard to frequencies of palmar hypothenar and thenar/first interdigital patterns, the Chamita sample is intermediate between the Bernalillo-Spanish and Indians. The third interdigital area, repeating the trend noted in connection with Negro-White hybrids, shows a higher pattern frequency than either of the two original stocks. Palmar main lines, approaching the trait distinctive of Indians, are slightly more longitudinal in the Chamita sample than in the Bernalillo sample. Curiously, and again recalling a situation noted in the Jamaican Negro-White material, the Bernalillo series does not reach the expected high value—perhaps suggesting that there is Indian admixture even here. There is no question that the signs of Indian traits in the Chamita series are significant, and it may be of interest to add that the locality furnishing this sample is one figuring in the early Spanish domination when, according to historians, interbreeding was frequent.

CONSTITUTION

CONSTITUTION comprises all the structural, physiological and psychological traits of an individual. Constitution is determined in part by inherited factors and in part by environment. Different traits vary in susceptibility to environmental influences. Certain ones, blood groups for example, are immune to the action of environment. For most traits the genetic mechanism is not so rigid, and modifications are introduced in the phenotype. The effective environment, it must be understood, embraces not only agencies external to the individual but also complexes within the body which constitute an intrinsic environment. Further, the effective environment is not limited to the period after birth. For some traits it extends into the prenatal period as far back as the union of the spermatozoön and the egg cell which produce the individual, and even includes action on these sex cells in the parent bodies.

Dermatoglyphics represent a part of the structural constitution. They are heritable, though prenatal environmental influences may mask or modify the genetically prospective traits (Chap. 12). It is highly improbable that environmental influences can introduce any departures from the dermatoglyphic genotype after about the middle of intra-uterine existence (Chap. 10). Investigation of constitution in dermatoglyphics necessarily confines itself to a consideration of *phenotypes*—the traits as expressed in individuals—without discriminating the determinations of the traits by inheritance and their modification by environment.

One aspect of constitution is represented by the racial characteristics treated in Chapter 15, set apart because of the special nature and bulk of the material. Indeed, all phases of morphology, asymmetry and the like concern constitution. The present chapter is devoted to certain more special aspects of constitution, including sex differences, the unlike trends of variation in right-handed and left-handed persons, and the distinctive trends associated with certain diseases.

Constitutional trends are revealed only by statistical analysis of mass samples, as already illustrated by racial variation. It is impossible to recognize the race of an individual in the dermatoglyphics, and as a parallel, dermatoglyphics in the individual do not indicate handedness, sex, criminality or predisposition to disease. It would be unexpected if any of these non-dermatoglyphic constitutional traits were invariably registered in the dermatoglyphics. This would depend on a much more consistent correlation in individuals than any yet demonstrated. In principle, all constitutional trends are comparable to the racial distinctions discussed in the previous chapter. Even if it is true that a relatively small proportion of individuals conform to the direction of variation revealed in the mass sample, the existence of this proportion denotes a significant deviation. Once a correlation between dermatoglyphics and some other aspect of constitution is substantiated, it becomes clear that the constitutional bond is one dating to the prenatal period. In itself this finding does not indicate whether the correlation has a genetic or a non-genetic basis.

Correlations between dermatoglyphics and certain diseases are to be presented. The dermatoglyphic traits concerned are morphological variants, which are in existence from the very first differentiation of ridged skin in the fetus. There is to be distinguished a quite different aspect of disease in its relation to dermatoglyphics, which will receive only this passing mention. We refer to conditions in which the dermatoglyphics are directly altered by the disease process. The skin of the ridged surfaces may show damage resulting from leprosy (36), from increased deposition of cornified elements (318), from fungus infection, excessive sweating (328) and from cutting of nerves to the part (329, 330, 331). Such structural damage to dermatoglyphics, like scarring of the ridged skin, involves pathological alteration of features already formed, and is unrelated to the constitutional aspect of dermatoglyphic morphology.

CORRELATIONS WITH BODY MEASUREMENTS AND BLOOD GROUPS

BODY MEASUREMENTS. Collins suggests that there may be a correlation between head form (as measured by cephalic index) and occurrences of finger-print types. His material includes 5000 Chinese, 2000 Hindus and 5000 Englishmen. The Chinese (generally brachycephalic) have total frequencies of whorls and arches (38.7% and 4.2% respectively) distinct from those of his English (dolichocephalic) sample (frequencies 20.2% and 5%). This suggested to Collins that narrowing of the head is associated with reduction of whorls and increase of arches, a conclusion apparently supported by his comparisons of brachycephalic and dolichocephalic Hindus. The brachycephalic Hindus show 36% whorls and 3% arches, and the dolichocephalic group 30.5% and 4.5% respectively.

It is probable, however, that these mass comparisons fail to differentiate all the factors concerned, because exacting statistical analysis does not indicate a significant correlation between head form and pattern types, i.e., between cephalic index and the index of pattern intensity. Cummins and Steggerda (337) calculate the coefficient of correlation in 72 Maya Indians as 0.059, and in 61 Netherlanders as 0.042—coefficients so small that correlation is lacking or insignificant. (In the same material there are no significant correlations of pattern intensity with nose form and general body build.) Karl likewise finds no correlation between pattern types and cephalic index.

Pattern size, in the Maya and Dutch material, also is apparently independent of head form, nose form and general body build. Pattern form, as related to the same anthropometric indices, yields in this small material statistically insignificant correlations, but with a suggestive indication that there may be a slight inverse relationship, i.e., that the broader patterns tend to be associated with narrow head, narrow nose and slender body (Table 47). To substantiate this suggestion would require a material large enough to give reliability to the low correlations.

TABLE 47
CORRELATIONS OF PATTERN FORM AND CERTAIN ANTHROPOMETRIC INDICES
(*Cummins and Steggerda*)

	Maya	Dutch
Average pattern form—Cephalic index...............	.124 ± .08	−.159 ± .08
Average pattern form—Nasal index..................	−.113 ± .08	−.205 ± .08
Average pattern form—Index of body build..........	−.089 ± .08	−.198 ± .08

BLOOD GROUPS. There is no convincingly demonstrated correlation between dermatoglyphics and blood groups. Hesch announced such a correlation (between whorls and group *B*, and possibly between loops and group *A*), which he claimed to be the first report of correlation of blood groups with any physical character. Actually he was preceded by Hahne, who asserts (from a study of 100 persons) that blood group *O* is associated with more loops and less whorls than blood group *A*. The Blotevogels also suggest that there may be correlations, but neither their evidence nor that of Hesch and Hahne is conclusive. Geipel shows, in a series of 381 Germans, the absence of significant correlation:

Group *B*—Whorls .047 ± .02
Group *A*—Loops −.015 ± .016.

These findings are in agreement with Karl's failure to demonstrate a correlation between group B and whorls, or between group A and loops.

SEXUAL VARIATION

RIDGE BREADTH. The first trait likely to suggest itself for comparison in the sexes is ridge breadth. Inasmuch as females generally have smaller bodies than males, it might be expected that their ridges would be narrower—and they are. In young adult males (24) the mean number of ridges per centimeter (considering all apical patterns and palmar areas together) is 20.7, a value to be compared with 23.4 in young adult females (30). Ridges in the female are significantly finer, since on the average

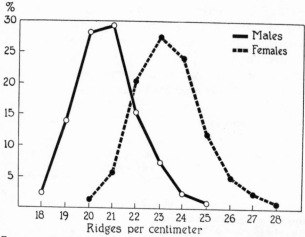

FIG. 149.—Frequency distributions of ridge counts per centimeter (average of all fingers and palmar areas) compared in the sexes.

there are 2.7 ± .09 more ridges to the centimeter than in the male. This sexual difference, of course, expresses itself only in the general trend, with which individual cases may or may not agree (Fig. 149). The distinction is correlated with the tendency toward smaller hand size in the female, but it is also partly independent of hand size, since ridges tend to be narrower in females even when under comparison with males having the same hand lengths. It may be concluded, therefore, that the conditioning of differential ridge breadth in the sexes involves both a direct genetic mechanism and an indirect one, through loose correlation of ridge breadth and body size.

FINGER-PRINT TYPES. Among various racial samples (Table 48) females almost universally differ from males in having more arches, and usually they differ also in bearing fewer whorls. The arch/whorl index of Dankmeijer is almost without exception higher in females. Radial loops are fewer in females. According to Geipel's observations (197) on 315 males and 287 females, there are no sexual distinctions in pattern form.

TABLE 48

PATTERN-TYPE FREQUENCIES AND ARCH/WHORL INDICES COMPARED IN THE SEXES

	Males					Females				
	A	R	U	W	A/W Index	A	R	U	W	A/W Index
Tobabataks (Maasland)	1.6 %	3.1 %	52.2 %	43.0 %	3.7	1.9 %	2.7 %	55.8 %	39.6 %	4.8
Koreans (Kubo)	2.3	3.7	52.5	44.7	5.1	2.8	2.6	51.2	45.7	6.1
Portuguese (Valadares)	2.4	65.1		32.4	7.4	2.8	68.1		29.0	9.7
Javanese (Dankmeijer)	2.7	2.8	58.5	35.9	7.5	3.3	2.1	61.9	32.7	10.1
Jews (Cummins-Midlo)	4.6	2.7	50.6	42.1	10.9	3.9	3.3	49.4	43.4	9.0
Chilean-Spanish (Henckel)	4.8	4.4	54.5	36.3	13.2	7.8	3.7	56.4	32.1	24.3
Portuguese (de Pina)	4.2	68.6		26.9	15.6	5.9	72.4		21.5	27.4
Danes (Bugge)	5.4	5.5	59.3	29.8	18.1	7.5	4.4	61.9	26.2	28.6
Negroes (Dankmeijer)	5.5	3.3	62.2	28.8	19.1	8.5	2.2	61.4	27.9	30.5
Russians (Semenowsky)	6.2	61.7		32.1	19.3	8.4	64.3		27.3	30.8
Portuguese (Lopes)	6.1	67.0		26.9	22.7	6.7	66.0		27.2	24.6
Germans (Karl)	6.7	67.1		26.3	25.5	8.1	64.9		27.0	30.0
Dutch and Belgians (Piebenga)	6.8	5.9	61.5	26.5	25.7	4.6	63.2		24.2	33.1
Angola Negroes (Sarmento)	6.7	67.5		25.7	26.1	5.1	64.9		29.9	17.1
Dutch (Dankmeijer)	7.7	5.4	60.7	26.2	29.4	9.6	3.7	63.5	23.2	41.4
Efé pygmies (Dankmeijer)	15.9	2.8	61.6	19.6	81.1	17.0	2.0	60.7	19.6	86.7

There are indications in some races that the usual sexual distinction may be leveled or even inverted. However, these exceptions to rule noted in some racial samples may be due to inadequacy of numbers, differences of method in classifying pattern types or lack of homogeneity of race in the compared samples. Since sex is but one aspect of constitution, a fully dependable comparison of the sexes can be achieved only if the samples are homogeneous in all respects except sex. This would require racial purity and consistence in all other phases of constitution, an ideal which may not be attainable.

The crude result obtained by dealing with total pattern-type frequencies and arch/whorl indices is substantiated by more refined methods of analysis, including the manuar, ambimanuar (348) and dactylodiagram (356). Analysis of individual fingers is of further interest in sexual comparison, since the contrasts are more discriminative.

Pattern-type frequencies in toes differ in the sexes in the same directions as those of fingers (119). As in fingers, whorls are more abundant and arches less frequent in toes of males than in toes of females.

Females generally present less bimanual difference than males. The level of this difference may be first exemplified by the values in Piebenga's comparison of 400 males and 400 females (299). In that series the sum of the differences of frequencies on right and left hands of the four pattern types (arches, radial loops, ulnar loops and whorls) is 5.3% in females, 15.3% in males. The corresponding values in Henckel's (288) much larger series are 7.0% and 15.0%. Another manifestation of symmetry which may differ in the sexes is conformity and non-conformity to the pair-group rule.

PALMAR CONFIGURATIONS. The frequencies of patterns in the five configurational areas of the palm are unequal in the sexes, like frequencies of whorls and arches on fingers and toes. In White stocks (four series: 86, 333 and two unpublished series, Germans and German Jews) females present consistently larger frequencies of hypothenar and fourth interdigital patterns and lesser frequencies in the remaining palmar areas (thenar/interdigital I, interdigitals II and III). In the palmar features, as in finger prints, females present a lessened degree of bimanual asymmetry. This distinction extends to pattern frequencies and to such dimensions as distances between palmar triradii (86) and bimanual inequality in alignment of palmar main lines (336).

HANDEDNESS

Investigations which attempt to correlate dermatoglyphics with right-handedness and left-handedness face many difficulties. As in other constitutional studies, samples would be ideal only if they were uniform in all respects except the trait which is to be studied in correlation with dermatoglyphics. It is fortunate, since there are sex differences in dermatoglyphics, that the sexual composition of the samples can be absolutely controlled. Racial composition is not so readily standardized. The racial differences detailed in Chapter 15 indicate that a study of handedness might be seriously vitiated if the samples of right-handed and left-handed subjects were not from a common racial source.

Classifying the subjects as to handedness presents a major difficulty. Handedness is expressed variably in its degree of fixation, and the classification must be founded on adequate tests. These tests should be reliable indicators of handedness and should differentiate the degrees of fixation. The compared samples should be composed of individuals old enough to exhibit definitive functional handedness. If a correlation between dermatoglyphics and handedness is demonstrable at all, subjects with most extreme left-handedness and right-handedness would be presumably the most promising.

No investigator has worked with material selected as rigorously as the ideal demands, and it is not surprising that the distinctions between handedness groups reported by several authors are at some points inconsistent.

With the appearance of the studies by Rife (357) and by Cromwell and Rife, unlike trends in the dermatoglyphics of left-handed and right-handed persons may be accepted as established. These authors report on the largest material yet assembled by any investigator. The material for the latter study includes 300 right-handed males, 300 right-handed females, 430 left-handed males and 323 left-handed females. Handedness was diagnosed by the following unimanual operations: writing, throwing, sewing, hammering, sawing, shooting marbles, use of knife, bowling, use of scissors and spoon. When all these acts were performed with the right hand the subject was classed as right-handed, and if the left hand was used in one or more of them, the subject was assigned to the left-handed group. The findings of particular interest are: (a) Increase of patterns in the third interdigital area in left hands of left-handed subjects of both sexes; this conforms to the results of all other investigators of the problem; (b) Increased frequency of thenar/first interdigital patterns in both hands of left-handed females; (c) Lessened frequency of patterns in the fourth interdigital area of left hands of left-handed females. Cromwell and Rife restate the comparisons in another form, this time in the light of bimanual differences of pattern frequency (or, in fingers, in the frequency of whorls as compared with other patterns). There are five areas characterized by large bimanual difference. The ring finger, with its large excess of whorls on the right hand, is like the second and third interdigital areas in the palm, where patterns occur more frequently in right hands. Left hands have greater pattern frequencies in the thenar/first interdigital and fourth interdigital areas. For each of these five configurational areas, Cromwell and Rife refer to the hand which carries the larger frequency as "superior" and to the hand having the smaller pattern frequency as "inferior." In each of the five areas the inferior hands of left-handed females present increase of pattern frequency. Also, in left-handed males the inferior hands show increase of pattern frequency, except in the fourth interdigital area where the value remains as in right-handers. In the left-handed groups there is a slight lessening of bimanual difference in pattern frequencies. Cummins (335) demonstrates such a decrease in bilateral asymmetry of fingers in left-handed males, and an increase in bilateral asymmetry in left-handed females, the net effect being, as in the palmar features, a leveling of the "normal" sex distinction in bilateral asymmetry.

CONSTITUTION AND DISEASE

Constitutional groups separated by race, by sex and by handedness are defined in accord with what may be termed normal variants of human beings. This section is concerned with subjects who are afflicted with certain diseases. The central question here is whether persons so afflicted are distinguished from the non-diseased by characteristics of the dermatoglyphics. If such distinctions exist they are of the utmost moment in analysis of the constitution of disease, because they demonstrate that susceptibility to the disease, like the distinctions in dermatoglyphics with which it is correlated, is inborn.

This aspect of investigation attracted early attention. Some studies were made in the latter part of the nineteenth and beginning of the twentieth centuries, at the time when finger prints received wide notice through their introduction for personal identification. D'Abundo describes the finger prints of imbeciles and idiots as being similar to those of monkeys, pointing out that monomorphic hands are frequent. Forgeot, de Sanctis and Toscano, Féré, and Cevidalli examined finger prints in idiots, imbeciles and psychopaths of various types, claiming distinctive statistical trends. As pointed out by Møller, these pioneer workers were handicapped by inadequate methods. Furthermore, peculiarities of classification and lack of proper control make it difficult to evaluate some of the reported findings. This account is accordingly limited to the more recent investigations.

NEUROFIBROMATOSIS. This is a heritable disease characterized by the formation of multiple tumors of nerves. Blotevogel examines finger prints (as well as blood groups and body dimensions) in 30 cases, 15 of each sex. The bimanuars show no departure from distribution of patterns in the normal population. It is curious that the author, having only 30 subjects, considers it probable that a larger material would not disclose distinctive trends. The finding of interest is the frequent occurrence of central pockets. Thirteen of the 27 patients finger-printed present one or more central pockets, which are confined to the little fingers of both hands and the left ring finger. With 48% of individuals bearing such patterns, as contrasted with 6% in his normal series, and with the surprising frequency on digit V (compare Table 1), it is evident that an aberrant fingerprint trend distinguishes this group.

PSORIASIS. One hundred patients presenting this heritable skin disease are investigated by Krieger, and compared with normals from the same racial stock. Palmar patterns as well as finger prints are considered. The following distinctions are reported in the psoriasis group: more frequent whorls on digit IV (50% and 41% for right and left, respectively, as compared with 46% and 38.5% in the control material); more frequent patterns in the fourth interdigital area of the left palm (38% and 47% for right and left as compared with 38% and 39% in the control). Other distinctions, especially in symmetry relations, are noted, but it is doubtful whether any of the claimed distinctions are significant; the material is small and there is no separation of data for the sexes.

SCHIZOPHRENIA. This is a mental disease in which manifestations of split personality are prominent. The first comprehensive study of dermatoglyphics in patients presenting this condition is by Poll, who analyzes finger prints of 232 males and 545 females, comparing them with normals of the same racial stock (Germans, Berlin). The analytical method mainly utilized is the dactylodiagram, though even the total frequencies of whorls and arches indicate a tendency to leveling of the normal sex difference, each sex showing either decrease or increase toward the value of the other (Table 49). The dactylodiagram for males exhibits a shifting to the left and above, brought about by the decrease of whorls and increase of arches.

TABLE 49

FREQUENCIES OF WHORLS AND ARCHES IN THREE INDEPENDENT SERIES OF SCHIZOPHRENICS, COMPARED WITH CONTROLS FROM THE GENERAL POPULATIONS

Germans (Poll)				East Prussians* (Duis)		Danes (Møller)			
Control		Schizophrenics		Schizophrenics		Control		Schizophrenics	
(845) Male	(776) Female	(232) Male	(545) Female	(416) Male	(356) Female	(86654) Male	(14857) Female	(450) Male	(583) Female
Whorls....... 33.6%	26.8%	28.5%	28.1%	30.2%	29.6%	29.8%	25.3%	27.0%	26.2%
Arches....... 4.3	7.6	5.7	6.6	5.2	7.8	5.4	7.5	7.7	8.2

* The geneaology of all these subjects was traced at least as far as through their grandparents, and East Prussian origin of each generation was established. In the absence of a control, it should be explained that the higher whorl frequencies, as compared with Poll's material, are the expected associate of more frequent whorls in the general population of this territory.

These results are anticipated in the earlier study by Blümel and Poll. Here the bimanuar serves as the chief analytical method, and the material differs in that various psychoses, including schizophrenia, are combined.

Møller (353) confirms Poll's observations. His findings in schizophrenic Danes (Table 49) are closely parallel to the findings by Poll in schizophrenic Germans. Møller observes that the schizophrenic Danes and Germans retain the racial contrasts which distinguish normal Danes and normal Germans. There is accordingly no universal schizophrenic type, but rather a schizophrenic type confined within the limits of the racial variants.

Duis investigates a schizophrenic material numbering 416 males and 356 females (East Prussians). He claims that the sex difference is the same as in the normal population, an assertion hardly reconcilable with his own record (Table 49) of practically equal frequencies of whorls in males and females, 30.2% and 29.6% respectively (with arches, 5.2% in males and 7.8% in females). Inconsistently, he regards the schizophrenics as showing no special distinction in total frequencies of patterns in the face of data which agree with Poll and Møller.

EPILEPSY. Brown and Paskind compare the finger prints in 146 mentally deteriorated epileptic patients with 115 non-deteriorated epileptics. Earlier studies by the same authors reveal anthropometric and other evidences of a constitutional distinction between these two epileptic types. Arches are increased in the deteriorated group, and the sex difference is lessened (deteriorated: males, 9.7%, females 10.9%; non-deteriorated: 2.3% and 7.2%). The deteriorated patients show fewer whorls than the non-deteriorated. The deteriorated group shows a significantly smaller quantitative value than the non-deteriorated. This reduction is not merely the associate of increased frequency of arches, since the separately compared values of loops and whorls indicate an actual difference of pattern size in the two groups. The deteriorated group presents a larger frequency of anomalies of ridge construction, including defects similar to those shown in figure 129.

FEEBLE-MINDEDNESS. Bonnevie (322) compares the finger prints in a series of 535 feeble-minded children with 300 mentally normal children. The intelligence quotients of all these subjects had been determined by the Stanford revision of the Binet-Simon test. The quotients of the feeble-minded group are mainly clustered in the range 55-70, and the normals in the range 80-100.

There is no correlation (0.01 ± .05) between intelligence quotients and quantitative values, though when the quantitative values are arranged in curves of distribution it appears that the feeble-minded may have a greater number of large patterns. The feeble-minded show more variability of quantitative values among the ten digits in individuals. Composites appear in larger numbers in the feeble-minded and they are more evenly distributed among the digits than in normals. Poll also investigates the feeble-minded, comparing 124 such subjects with 972 normal persons, reporting that the number of individuals lacking whorls is greater in the feeble-minded.

IMBECILITY AND IDIOCY. Møller (354) makes a study of 282 male imbeciles, excluding from his material cases with inferior mentality acquired through birth injury or other extrinsic causes. A normal series of 2000 males of the same racial stock is his control. Few dermatoglyphic differences are found and they are not statistically significant. In imbeciles the greatest difference is reduction of whorls on the right index and ring fingers. In the two groups the unimanuars of the left hands are nearly identical, though in right hands the unimanuars indicate a reduction of whorls.

Mongoloid idiots present outstanding distinctions in finger prints and palmar configurations. Studies on two independent series, by Cummins (334) and by Workman, agree in all essential respects. Palmar hypothenar patterns are nearly twice as abundant as in the normal and they are distinctive in the large representation of expanded patterns (such as L^u and L^c) and arches (A^c) associated with an axial triradius located centrally in the palm (t''). Thenar/first interdigital patterns are reduced in number, size and complexity. Second and third interdigital patterns are more frequent than in normals, and fourth interdigital patterns are less frequent. Transverse coursing of palmar main lines is accentuated (the main-line index being unprecedentedly high, 11.11) and bimanual asymmetry of ridge direction much reduced. In finger prints, whorl frequency is reduced (19.8% in the Cummins series of 54 cases), the compensation for this reduction being limited to increase of ulnar loops. Radial loops shift their maximum frequency from the normal position on digit II to digits IV and V.

The peculiar conformation of the hand in mongoloid idiots is certainly a developmental associate of variants in the dermatoglyphics. Perhaps some of the distinctions in the palmar dermatoglyphics are correlated specifically with the presence of the simian line, a modified distal transverse flexion crease coursing continuously from radial to ulnar margins of the palm. The simian line, occasional in normal persons, occurs quite frequently in mongoloid idiots (316).

POLIOMYELITIS. Poliomyelitis, or infantile paralysis, is produced by a virus which affects nerve cells in the spinal cord and brain. The series of 282 cases studied by the Blotevogels consists only of patients presenting serious crippling as a result of this disease. It may be assumed that the series represents an extreme accentuation of predisposition and that, if structural constitutional signs of this predisposition occur, the signs would appear in a series so selected. The normal control, from the same racial stock, is mainly the material of Kirchmair. In diseased males whorls are increased and arches diminished. Diseased females also show an increase of whorls, and at the same time there is an increase of arches, so that loops are reduced in frequency. The number of males having ten-loop combinations is 5% greater than in the normal. The normal difference in pattern-type distribution in right and left hands is absent. Kirchmair (349), working with 288 cases of infantile paralysis and using his ambimanuar method, confirms this finding of lessened asymmetry. The sex difference in quantities of whorls and arches persists, though deviated from the normal. There are no distinctive frequencies of rare patterns (such as the central pockets noted in neurofibromatosis).

CRIMINALITY AND DEGENERACY

Ascarelli analyzes the finger prints of 100 prostitutes, whom he classes as a type of degenerates. Radial loops are increased, especially in the little finger. There is a higher frequency of what he terms primitive patterns, forms similar to patterns of some non-human primates (10.7% vs. 6.2% in 200 women not classed as prostitutes). Mutrux-Bornoz insists that increased occurrence of such "primitive" patterns, of the palm as well as fingers, characterizes criminals also.

The most extensive and recent study is that of Bugge and Poll, devoted to an examination of 2056 Danish criminals (offenses: rape, immoral conduct, homosexuality) and 4000 German criminals (murderers, burglars, thieves, etc.). The Danish sex offenders present fewer whorls than non-criminal Danes, though this difference is not statistically significant. The Germans present the same contrast between criminals and non-criminals, and the difference is here significant. Shifting of the dactylo-diagram to the left (as a result of decreased whorls) is evident both in Danes and in Germans as compared with the non-criminal controls. The bimanuars display significant differences, showing concentrations of frequencies in the fields of O-whorls. There are no distinctions of symmetry between criminal and non-criminal groups in either Danes or Germans.

It will be recalled (Chap. 10) that Abel observes defects of ridge formation (Figs. 129–130) in some criminals, and in the non-criminal population only in association with imbecility, insanity and the like.

CHARACTER AND TEMPERAMENT

In its broadest scope, dactylomancy (Chap. 1) extends to the reading of past, present and future, as in the similar pseudo-science of palmistry. To the extent that dactylomancy concerns itself with a search for signs of constitutional makeup it merits attention as genuine scientific inquiry. As an object of investigation, this is not so far-fetched as it may seem to be at first thought. Since flexion creases (341) and dermato-glyphics vary in other constitutional expressions, a correlation between dermatoglyphics and the character-temperament constitution may be ultimately demonstrated.

Takashima (quoted from Kubo, 296) gives an account of Japanese folk dactylomancy, claiming the following attributes of pattern types:

> The whorl signifies dexterity in handicrafts and is also a sign of stubbornness.
> The composite is a sign of a liar, a faithless and unreliable character.
> The loop indicates lack of perseverance.
> The arch denotes a merciless, crude character.

In making the reading of a male the fingers of the left hand are chosen, and of a female, the fingers of the right hand. Attention is paid to the finger or fingers bearing whorls, and the combinations are made into a code for reading character and temperament and for prediction of the future.

Kojima (quoted from Kubo) claims to have examined the finger prints of 200,000 criminals and to have evaluated character and temperament for correlation with the prints. His general conclusions are:

> A person with ulnar loops on all fingers is clear-spirited, mild-mannered, strong-willed, perhaps melancholy, and is likely to be cool in judgment and ruthless in business dealings.
> A person having whorls on all fingers is restless, vacillating, doubting, sensitive, clever, eager for action and inclined to crime.
> A mixture of loops and whorls signifies a neutral character, a person who is kind, obedient, truthful, but often undecided and impatient.
> Arches or radial loops occur on persons who are ambitious, cold-blooded, stubborn, disobedient, defiant and rebellious.

Present information on the association of dermatoglyphics with character and temperament is a mixture of folk-lore and questionable deductions lacking scientific control. It is difficult enough to evaluate character and temperament with the aid of truly scientific methods. This phase of constitution is mentioned primarily to indicate that an interesting field of investigation remains to be explored.

SUPPLEMENT

IDENTIFICATION IN ACTION

THE term "personal identification" applies to all the various means of establishing the identity of an individual, showing either that he is or is not the person in question. In everyday life, this is a simple matter of sight recognition (or nonrecognition). Sight recognition is notoriously fallible, and everyone has had the experience of mistaking one person for another. In some situations such a mistake is of little consequence, but there are many circumstances in which an error cannot be tolerated; even a human life may depend upon the identification.

Difficulties are compounded when the person to be identified and the necessary records are in different places. Though a description and photographs of the individual are helpful, there is a degree of possible error. What is desired is a foolproof and mechanically simple procedure that provides for identification on a scale involving hundreds, or thousands, or millions of individuals wherever they may be. *Fingerprint identification,* which meets these requirements, is now in virtual world-wide use.

An example contrasting the results of three different approaches in personal identification may serve to show the shortcomings of sight recognition and of the Bertillon method (based principally on body measurements) which was superseded long ago by fingerprint identification. The example goes back to 1903, a time when fingerprint identification was first gaining its merited acceptance as a positive method. The scene was the federal prison at Leavenworth, Kansas, and the principals were two Negroes, William West and Will West. William had been confined, two years before, on a life sentence for murder. Will, a new prisoner, was brought to the record office for photographs and Bertillon measurements. The clerk "recognized" Will and remarked that he had been there before. When Will stoutly denied this, the clerk proceeded with the regulation Bertillon measurements, then went to the file and secured the card indicated by the collective measurements. The photograph pasted on the card was shown to Will, who "recognized" it as his own picture and was puzzled as to how it could have been obtained. But the card, despite the correspondence in features and in body measurements, was that of William, whose presence in the institution was enough to prove that Will was not he. Both sight recognition and body measurements had failed to distinguish these two men, who by strange coincidence had virtually the same name and careers that led to imprisonment. But the coincidence ended at once with examination of their fingerprints. Their finger patterns differed materially and even a small part of one print was sufficient to show distinctiveness.

Fingerprints Never Lie is the title of the autobiography of Fred Cherrill, long-time member of the Fingerprint Bureau of New Scotland Yard and its chief superintendent for many years preceding his retirement in 1953. Mr. Cherrill is right: fingerprints tell the truth. But they can do so only in their own language, and one cannot hope to understand how they reveal truth without having some acquaintance with this unique language.

Fingerprints have special virtues as means of personal identification. (1) Their features are permanent, unchanged through the lifetime of the individual, and persisting after death until the skin disintegrates. (2) The finer characteristics (minutiae of single ridges) are so highly variable that one print or even a portion of it is unique. Each person, and each finger, therefore has an absolute individuality, an assemblage of characteristics that has no match. (3) The major features lend themselves to classification. Classification, which may be extended to progressively subordinate ranks in accord with the demands of a large file, provides for ready searching. When a fingerprint card has been classified, the prints filed under its class must be inspected to determine whether the person in question is represented; if he is, the earlier card provides information concerning the person and establishes his identification even if the name is falsified. (4) Although suitable precautions must be taken in fingerprinting to ensure that the prints are complete and clearly registered, the process of recording is simple. Furthermore, the prints are actual impressions of the fingers themselves, hence they are not liable to the human errors that may be introduced in various other forms of record. (5) Finally, fingers come into contact with objects and leave their impressions; in criminal investigation these chance prints supply evidence.

Some of the principles of fingerprint variation are explained in Chapter 4, and Chapter 8 presents an elementary outline of how fingerprints are used in identification. However, it is desirable to review some of this material for emphasis on working principles.

FINGERPRINTS DEFINED

Even without magnification, one can see fine, closely spaced ridges on the skin of the grasping surface of the fingers (including the thumbs, which are "fingers" in the sense of fingerprint identification). These ridges are aligned in systems of patterning. The terminal segments of the fingers bear the patterns that are routinely used, when registered as prints, in individual identification. However, any area characterized by similarly corrugated skin would be adequate for establishing an identification—the other segments of the fingers, the palms, toes and soles. Although this chapter is mainly concerned with fingerprints, it should be understood that with the exception of descriptions of specific pattern types the principles apply to all areas of ridged skin.

A fingerprint is an impression made by contact of the ridged skin. Such an impression might be a solid smudge useless for identification, but under optimum conditions (as when prints are made for purposes of record or when a chance contact is favorable) the print is comparable to printing from metal type or a rubber stamp. Like the elevated type faces, the summits of the ridges come into contact with the ink and all their details are faithfully registered in prints. From the standpoint of their common use in identification, fingerprints are of two classes: record prints and chance prints.

Record prints are those made for an identification file, or for a search to determine whether the person has a previously filed fingerprint record, or for comparison with chance prints discovered at the scene of crime. Record prints, as distinguished from chance prints, are recorded with purpose and with attention to their clear decipherability. These prints, registered on white cards, are made with an ink similar to ordinary printer's ink.

The usual form of fingerprint card (Fig. 41) has assigned spaces for the two sets of prints, and space for various entries including the classification of the fingerprint characteristics that denotes the place of the card in the file. The first set of ten prints (upper part of the card) consists of "rolled" impressions, which extend part way along the sides of the digits and thus ensure registration of the complete patterns. The other set contains "plain" or "dab" impressions, made by contact of the inked digits without any rolling.

The basic types of patterns are whorls, loops and arches (Fig. 29,) but intergrading forms occur (Fig. 48), and there are occasional extreme deviations from these types. In Caucasian peoples, about two-thirds of all patterns are loops, of which the large majority (ulnar loops) have their open ends directed toward the little finger, while the others (radial loops) open thumbward. Identification practice makes use of two variables within the same pattern type, namely counts of ridges and ridge tracing. Counting the number of ridges included in a pattern affords a convenient means of subclassifying the one pattern type; this is especially useful for loops. If one examines a large series of ulnar loops he will see that they vary widely in size, size being determined by the number of ridges composing the pattern. The count of ridges along a prescribed line (Fig. 53) thus makes it possible to describe an ulnar loop more specifically. In whorls, tracings of ridges originating from prescribed points (as illustrated in Fig. 48, examples 2–8) are of similar value in providing for subclassification of patterns belonging to this type. Classification is a prime essential because fingerprint cards must be filed in a systematic manner providing for the ready location of cards that are to be compared with the card of the individual whose identity is under search (see pp. 145–147). The magnitude of the search and the needed refinement of classification vary with the size of the identification file, which might range from perhaps a few hundreds of cards up to enormous proportions. The active files of the Federal Bureau of Investigation contained (as of July 1, 1960) 36,333,153 fingerprint cards of criminals and 119,785,546 cards of non-criminals. (These figures are available through the courtesy of J. Edgar Hoover.) The files of certain agencies, notably the Federal Bureau of Investigation and the Department of Correction of the State of New York, are so enormous that machine searching has been adopted. With this method, of course, the pertinent data must be punched on IBM cards and handled in the sorting machine for the initial phase of the search. Regardless of the size of the file, the search for a record corresponding to that of a card at hand involves direct visual comparison with the several or many cards falling under the same classification. In such inspection, differing general characters of pattern configuration are clearly recognizable to the expert, though an untrained person might regard two or more compared patterns as identical. More detailed examination, with a magnification of several times, reveals many fine details of individual ridges (minutiae, or ridge characteristics—see Figs. 28 and 98). Two patterns of the same type, ulnar loops for example, may agree exactly in their over-all configuration and in ridge count; but comparison of even small corresponding areas in the prints immediately discloses striking differences in these details.

Up to this point, references to identification files concern fingerprint cards carrying impressions of all ten fingers of individuals (with special provisions for classifying cases in which digits are missing or unprintable or in which malformations occur). Some identification offices have files of single finger prints, in addition to the ten-finger cards. In this situation the ten prints of an individual might be widely separated in the file because each is separately classified, using features common to the ten-finger system supplemented by coding of such details as the minutiae of single ridges. A file of this sort is designed to expedite the search for identification of single prints discovered at the scene of crime.

Thousands upon thousands of fingerprint identifications are made daily over the world. The cases at issue, each originating with a fingerprint card referred for searching, involve varied elements of the population: criminals and noncriminals, employees in certain occupations where national security must be safeguarded, personnel of the armed forces, the unidentified dead, etc. A few abbreviated histories of actual cases will be presented to illustrate this variety and the procedure of the identification.

IDENTIFICATION FROM TEN-FINGER RECORDS

One G.C. was under a four-year sentence for obtaining money under false pretenses. He was confined, in 1916, in the Oklahoma State Penitentiary, but was soon transferred to a reformatory where he was assigned work at a farm camp. One night he walked away and was not apprehended. He first went to Missouri and then, after three years, moved to Texas and assumed a new name. Here he led a respectable life as a farmer and family man. Little did he realize that his fingerprints would eventually reveal his criminal history and escape from prison authority; thirty-nine years passed before this disclosure. In 1955 he suffered an illness and was admitted to a Texas state hospital, where fingerprinting is a regular part of the admittance procedure. On learning that fingerprinting was to be done, he freely told about his escape and expressed relief that this history had come to light. The hospital prints, checked against the original record, proved that he was G.C. though under another name. This story has a happy ending. The authorities, in view of his long record of upright life, decided against returning him for completion of his sentence.

An assault to kill resulted in a five-year sentence for W.M., and he was confined in the Oklahoma State Penitentiary. About a year later he was transferred to the State Reformatory, from which he escaped with less than half of his sentence completed. Twenty-five years after the escape he was arrested in Kansas on a charge of theft. He was fingerprinted, the record was sent to the FBI, and there he was identified as the escapee who had enjoyed a quarter-century of freedom. W.M. did not fare as well as G.C. of the preceding account, because he was returned to complete his sentence.

Sometimes arrest on a petty offense leads to the disclosure of prior major crime, as in the instance of E.C. (alias) who was arrested in Phoenix, Arizona, on suspicion of stealing a watch. His fingerprints were recorded as a part of the ordinary routine and referred for identification. He proved to be H.C., wanted in California for the murder of a woman and her teen-age daughter.

The next example concerns a man who was picked up in the railroad yards in Pueblo, Colorado. Railroad officers took him to jail after discovering that he had suffered loss of memory (amnesia.) He was held in jail for a week on suspicion that he was F.C., an escaped convict from another state. F.C.'s brother, brought to Pueblo for the purpose, saw the amnesic man and found him to be of the same size and general appearance as F.C. but did not make a positive identification. Fingerprints of the amnesic were made and sent to the FBI, which promptly reported the identification as T.M.H., of Lawrence, Kansas, who had served in the Navy. Had it not been for the routine of fingerprinting personnel in the armed forces, T.M.H. would not have been thus identified for return to his family.

A binge resulted in trouble for W.C.B., a Californian. After an attack on a night watchman he was jailed and brought to court on charges of intoxication and assault. The judge sentenced him to 30 days on the first charge and 150 days on the assault. When W.C.B. started to remonstrate the judge halted him and declared that the sentence was severe because of his record. W.C.B. insisted that he had no record, but the judge retorted that the long record included an arrest in Colorado for seduction and another in California for violation of the Dyer Act. W.C.B. again denied having a police record. Though the judge pointed out that the description from the cited record fitted exactly, his confidence was weakened and he postponed sentence until fingerprints could be taken and compared with those of the record. They did not match and W.C.B. was relieved of the onus of another man's police record.

Mrs. E.T. of Beaumont, Texas, was murdered by two hitchhikers. Her automobile, when found at a roadside, contained pieces of woman's apparel. Several days after this a woman's body was discovered in a thicket, 100 miles from the location of the abandoned car. The body was tentatively identified by shreds of clothing that fitted the description of garments worn by Mrs. E.T. when she left Beaumont. Although the body had been extensively mutilated, the right hand and left little finger were intact; prints adequate for identification were obtained from the left little finger. The police secured a lead indicating that Mrs. E.T. had worked at a shipyard in Beaumont during World War II and that she had been fingerprinted as an applicant for employment. Prints from the left little finger were sent to the FBI for comparison with the fingerprints that had been filed there nine years before. The identification, which up to this time had been only tentative, was thus conclusively established. Both hitchhikers were convicted, one being sentenced to life imprisonment and the other to death in the electric chair.

Another gruesome story is that of Miss B.J., a twenty-one-year-old waitress of Dallas, Texas. Her murderer decapitated the body and amputated the hands. The headless body was found in a dry creek bed in Oklahoma; the head and hands were recovered from a river six miles away. There were no significant clues to the identification, and when the identification officers printed the fingers of the amputated hands it was considered unlikely that so young a woman would have been printed previously. However, her description and the fingerprint record were circulated to local and state police in Texas, Oklahoma, and neighboring states. Her identity was quickly discovered because she had a criminal record in Texas and Oklahoma; her fingerprints were on file, and the post-mortem prints matched them.

P.B., a West Virginian twice convicted of murder, had been jailed for a year. Developments showed that he was innocent of the crime for which he was charged and convicted. Seven years previously, C.B. (the same surname) was arrested. On his way to the jail, accompanied by a Justice of the Peace and a constable, he requested and was granted permission to stop at his home for a change of shoes. He emerged from the house with a gun, fired, and killed the Justice. The unarmed constable fled from the scene and the killer escaped. Later, in Norfolk, Virginia, P.B. was arrested as the claimed murderer. P.B. denied knowledge of the crime and declared that he was not C.B., but he was tried twice and found guilty. A third trial was imminent, but at long last he was freed after proof that he was P.B., not C.B. The proof came through P.B.'s fingerprints, that had been recorded when he entered military service. This case of mistaken identity had serious enough consequences for its victim, and they would have been grave indeed in the lack of the positive identification furnished by his wartime fingerprint record.

M.R.R., a mining engineer, was arrested under the impression that he was M.D., a Chicago murderer who was being sought all over the United States. There was a physical resemblance between the two men and both drove the same type of car. M.R.R.'s car was followed through three California counties by deputy sheriffs who had orders to "shoot first and arrest afterwards." He was taken into custody in Los Angeles, luckily without being harmed. Here his fingerprints were recorded and they immediately eliminated his identification with the wanted criminal whose prints were already on record.

A veteran of World War I, P.W.K. spent his final period of hand-to-mouth existence in the Bowery area of New York City. An illness required that he be sent to Bellevue Hospital, and there he died. His body, unclaimed by relatives or friends, was buried in the city cemetery on Hart's Island. Fourteen months after the death, P.W.K.'s brother John went to the Missing Persons Bureau in the attempt to trace P.W.K., from whom there had been no word for two years. He found P.W.K.'s photograph among the pictures of persons who had been given pauper burial or whose bodies were in the city morgue awaiting identification. The body of P.W.K. was exhumed and fingerprints were taken. These prints were identified in Washington as those of P.W.K., who had enlisted eighteen years earlier. P.W.K.'s body was given a military funeral and his mother received the insurance and bonus money which only this positive identification could have released.

A baby born to an unmarried girl was left in a truck that was unattended while the driver stopped for coffee in Rockville, Connecticut. The state police were called and the infant was placed in Rockville Hospital. Footprints of the infant were taken and within a week matching prints were located in a local hospital where the child had been born. The name and address, as given by the mother, were fictitious but her thumb print was on the footprint card. No matching thumb print was found in the file and none came through the identification office. But hospitals had been alerted to report any woman admitted under circumstances out of the ordinary. Finally, seven years after the baby was abandoned, one such call turned up the elusive mother; her thumb matched the print recorded at the birth of her baby.

IDENTIFICATION BY CHANCE FINGERPRINTS

All the foregoing cases involve comparison of a previously filed ten-finger set of prints with the prints of an individual, living or dead, recorded for this purpose. The next group of examples involves chance prints, prints left without intention by contact of the fingers. A common form of chance print is demonstrated if one grasps a drinking glass or a polished metal object. The resulting fingerprints are visible if the surface is examined at a suitable angle and with favorable illumination. They represent an impression of the thin, oily film that adheres to the fingers from their contact with the face and scalp. Such a print is "latent" in the strict sense of the word, for it can be "developed" into a clearly visible impression by one or another method—for example, dusting with fine powder selected for dark-and-light or color contrast with the background. The skin surface also carries a deposit from sweat which, like the oily film, can be developed by chemical means. Chance prints may be impressed in a clearly visible medium, such as blood or paint, and they may be literally sculptured as in wax.

Mention has been made of files of single fingerprints. When a file of this type is available the search for a matching print is expedited, but usually the search must be made otherwise as in the following examples.

Most commonly, latent prints figure in the hunt for lawbreakers, but occasionally they serve other purposes. The police of Marysville, California, picked up on suspicion a man who was carrying an electric flatiron. Several fingerprints on the iron were developed. Some of the prints were those of the suspect and others did not match any of his fingers. A search of the civilian fingerprint file led to the identification of the remaining prints with a local housewife, who farsightedly had been fingerprinted as a safeguard. The safeguard on this occasion resulted only in the recovery of her flatiron, but prints on file may some day prove far more useful to the housewife or her family.

The notorious Jake Fleagle was in a four-man gang that held up a bank in Colorado, killed the bank president and his son, kidnapped a physician to have him attend a wounded bandit and then murdered him. When the physician's body was found, in his abandoned car, a usable print was developed on a window glass. This print was forwarded to the FBI, where Director J. Edgar Hoover requested the identification workers to memorize its characteristics and to be watchful for the pattern on incoming cards. Some twenty months passed; a card received from Stockton, California, bore the telltale print. Jake Fleagle was soon under arrest. Four men who had been falsely convicted were freed.

A fourteen-year-old girl was alone in her home one night, sitting in the music room with a book, when someone outside shot through the French window, wounding her. The intruder ripped the wire of the back screen door, broke a pane of glass, and then reached through to remove a large piece of the glass which he threw down. After criminally assaulting the dying girl, he fled. Only two bits of evidence were available, a print on the piece of glass and the recovered bullet. A matching print was not found in the files and a call went out, asking that all males in the community over thirteen years of age appear for fingerprinting. Over three thousand were printed and eliminated as suspects. There remained a half-dozen who had not been fingerprinted, and among them E.S., who was thought to be an ex-convict. When his prints were examined, the right thumb was identical to the print on the piece of glass. He confessed to the crime.

Palms and Soles

The ridge patternings of palms and soles, and toes as well, conform in all fundamental principles of identification to those of fingers. They are highly variable in their major features and may be classified, though few identification offices maintain classified files of such prints. Ordinarily, therefore, identifications are approached as in the examples to be related.

A series of safe-blowings, described as the most extensive in the history of crime in Norway, was solved when one of the culprits was identified by palm prints. In investigating one of the cases, in Oslo, the search for chance fingerprints was fruitless. Imprints of gloves, on a glass-topped desk, explained the absence of fingerprints. But the criminal had neglected the fact that a section of the palm exposed at the glove opening provides for an identification no less positive than that afforded by fingerprints. He had so placed both hands on the desk as to leave imprints of this exposed area. The palm-print files, which were started in Oslo in 1947, were searched without success and the identification was not made until three years after the incident reported above. Three men were arrested on charges of safe-blowing in communities outside Oslo. When their palm prints were recorded, one of the men was shown to be the glove-wearer who had impressed a patch of each palm on the desk glass in Oslo.

A killer in a London suburb left a palm print at the scene of his crime. A large-scale project was undertaken in the community, the palmprinting of every male over sixteen years of age. Scotland Yard experts were assigned the task of comparing the chance print with each of some 9,000 palms that had been recorded. Success came with the 4,605th comparison. The seventeen-year-old youth whose record print matched the chance print confessed.

Burglars may make their entries in bare feet, as did this criminal in Florida. He entered a house after removal of a plate glass panel from the kitchen door, which he placed flat on the floor. The investigators of the burglary considered it likely that fingerprints would be present on the glass. However, dusting of the marginal area, where prints would be expected from the handling, did not reveal any impressions. Though no fingerprints appeared as the dusting proceeded centrally, a clear right footprint developed. Within a few days, a man was arrested for breaking and entering a store in the same town. His footprints were made; the right one was identical to the latent print on the glass in the home that had been burglarized.

Dismembered parts of a woman's body had been found in Boston Harbor over a span of nearly a month. The police were informed by a concerned friend that Mrs. G.M.A. had been missing from her summer cottage in a Boston suburb. The police entered the cottage and found a shambles. On the bathroom floor, which had been carelessly mopped, there was a naked footprint in blood. Two men were suspects, of whom one was apprehended. His footprints were recorded in prison. One foot was identical to the bathroom print; he was found guilty of murder in the first degree, sentenced and executed.

UNIVERSAL FINGERPRINT REGISTRATION

Step by step, there has been progress through the years in the fingerprint registration of law-abiding citizens. Millions of persons, realizing the benefits of such registration, have been fingerprinted voluntarily. Others have accepted in good spirit the necessity of recording their prints: men and women in the armed forces, applicants for positions of trust that require this safeguard. Mothers of newborn infants are grateful for the protection afforded in the record of their own fingerprints and the prints (usually soles) of their infants. All this, and more examples which might be mentioned, is gratifying because the potential benefits of the fingerprint record are being extended to a rapidly increasing number of people. Furthermore, it is a good sign of decreasing prejudice against fingerprints through their association with the criminal element of the population. The existence of such prejudice is difficult to explain, when the person has no cause to fear that his prints would lead to disclosure of a blemished past. The prejudice is on a par with objection to being photographed, if anyone ever so objected, on grounds that criminals are routinely photographed.

Consider some of the registrations of our modern living: marriage license, birth, death, census, voting, Selective Service, Social Security. The day will come when fingerprinting will be likewise a commonplace, when every person will take for granted that his fingerprints must be recorded in the interest of himself, his family, and the population at large. So far, efforts toward securing legislation in the direction of nation-wide fingerprinting have failed but the legislation will come eventually. Perhaps it will be modeled along the principle of an unsuccessful bill introduced in 1943 by Senator William Langer of North Dakota, which provided for the initial fingerprinting of persons twelve years of age or older and, thereafter, the printing of those reaching the age of twelve. It is obvious that any bill would set an age at which registration is compulsory and that differences of opinion on the appropriate age are inevitable. But whatever the age proposed, parents may still take advantage of earlier registration of their children on a voluntary basis, just as many have done and are doing now. Protests may be voiced by some on the basic issue of compulsion, the argument being that fingerprinting is a violation of personal rights and liberties. Such an argument loses force in the face of the obvious fact that fingerprinting is for the benefit of good people, both in its use in combatting crime and in its civil applications.

The case histories recorded in this chapter illustrate .benefits received through identification by fingerprints. Some of the cases involve protection to society by criminal identifications. Others are direct personal advantages. T.M.H., suffering from loss of memory, was restored to his family. W.C.B. was absolved from blame for another man's police record. The confusion between C.B. the killer and the innocent P.B. was cleared. M.R.R. was mistaken for the murderer M.D., and his prints proved the mistake. The family of P.W.K. was assured of his death; the mother received his service benefits. Such cases are typical of thousands that occur every year. And many other varieties could be added, drawn from records of floods, storms, fires, explosions, and wrecks of automobiles, trains, and ships. Fingerprint identifications of checks and documents and pocket identification cards already are gaining headway. An article published in 1937 is headed: "Finger Print Everybody? Yes—says John Edgar Hoover." He and many others are still saying "Yes."

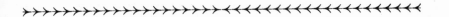

BIBLIOGRAPHY

THE following is a representative working bibliography of dermatoglyphics, though of necessity it is an incomplete list of the literature available. The articles and books are grouped under headings of the chapters to which they have primary reference. The individual publications are numbered in a sequence carried continuously through the bibliography. These reference numbers are cited in the text when the bibliography for the particular chapter contains more than one work by the same author, and when a book or article is included in the bibliography of a chapter other than that in which the reference is made. Often, for the sake of brevity, the reference number alone is cited.

CHAPTER I. HISTORY

1. Bidloo, G. *Anatomia Humani Corporis*. Amsterdam, 1685. (Utrecht edition, 1728. Cited by Dankmeijer, 280.)
2. Bridges, B. C. *Personal identification through the ages*. Finger Print and Ident. Mag., vol. 19, no. 5, 1937.
3. Copits, L. W. *Sir [William] Herschel's historic contract*. Finger Print and Ident. Mag., vol. 19, no. 8, 1938.
4. Cummins, H. *The "finger-print" carvings of Stone-Age men in Brittany*. Sci. Monthly, vol. 31, pp. 273–279, 1930.
5. ———. *Ancient finger prints in clay*. Sci. Monthly, vol. 52, pp. 389–402, 1941.
6. Dilnot, G. *The Story of Scotland Yard*. Boston, Houghton Mifflin & Co., 1927.
7. de Forest, H. P. *The evolution of dactyloscopy in the United States, with an historical note on the first finger print bureau in the United States and a bibliography of personal identification*. Reprinted from Proc. Internat. Assoc. for Ident., 1930 and 1931, pp. 33 (of privately issued reprint).
8. Heindl, R. *Die erste deutsche Arbeit über das Fingerabdruckverfahren als polizeiliches Identifizierungsmittel*. Arch. f. Kriminol., vol. 85, pp. 30–69, 1929.
9. Herschel, W. J. *The Origin of Finger Printing*. London, Oxford Univ. Press, 1916.
10. Laufer, B. *History of the finger-print system*. Ann. Report, Smithsonian Inst., pp. 631–652, 1912.
11. Malpighi, M. *De Externo Tactus Organo*. London, 1686.
12. Mayer, J. C. A. *Anatomische Kupfertafeln nebst dazu gehörigen Erklärungen*. 1783–88 (Finger prints described in the last section, 1788).
13. Myers, H. J., II. *History of identification in the United States*. Finger Print and Ident. Mag., vol. 20, no. 4, 1938. Ibid., vol. 24, no. 6, 1942. (See also: *Supplementary note on early American identification procedures*, ibid., vol. 20, no. 10, 1939.)
14. de Pina, L. *Dactiloscopia*. Lisbon, Bertrand, 1938.

15. *Heinrich Poll Papers*. Owing to the circumstances of the latter years (1934–1939) of his life in Germany, Poll was apprehensive about the safety of his collection of prints and notes on research. To ensure safe-keeping he placed all this material in the custody of the present authors.

16. Purkinje, J. E. *Commentatio de Examine Physiologico Organi Visus et Systematis Cutanei.* Breslau, 1823. (Translated into English by Cummins, H., and R. W. Kennedy, Am. J. Crim. Law and Criminol., vol. 31, pp. 343–356, 1940.)

17. Schröter, J. F. *Das menschliche Gefühl oder Organ des Getastes.* Leipzig, 1814.

18. Wilton, G. W. *Fingerprints: History, Law and Romance.* London, William Hodge & Co., Ltd., 1938.

CHAPTER 2. GENERAL CONSIDERATIONS

19. Anonymous. *"Live" palm prints, 50 years apart, revealed.* Finger Print and Ident. Mag., vol. 20, no. 10, 1939.

20. ———. The Illinois Policeman, vol. 8, p. 15, 1942. (Abstracted in J. Crim. Law and Criminol., vol. 32, 1942.) See also on this subject: Finger Print and Ident. Mag., vol. 23, no. 8, 1942.

21. Bettmann, S. *Zur Oberflächenmikroskopie der Haut am lebenden Menschen.* Arch. f. Dermat. u. Syph., vol. 161, pp. 444–455, 1930.

22. Bridges, B. C. *Biological aspects of dermatoglyphics.* Finger Print and Ident. Mag., vol. 18, no. 5, 1936.

23. Cummins, H. *Attempts to alter and obliterate finger prints.* J. Crim. Law and Criminol., vol. 25, pp. 982–991, 1935.

24. Cummins, H., W. J. Waits and J. T. McQuitty. *The breadths of epidermal ridges on the finger tips and palms: a study of variation.* Am. J. Anat., vol. 68, pp. 127–150, 1941.

25. Galton, F. *Prints of scars.* Nature, vol. 53, p. 295, 1896.

26. Hecht, A. F. *Über das Hand- und Fussflächenrelief von Kindern.* Ztschr. f. d. ges. exper. Med., vol. 39, pp. 56–66, 1924.

27. Küstermann, W. *Über die anatomische Beziehung zwischen Schweissdrüsen-Ausführungsgang und Papillarsystem.* Dissertation, Hamburg, 1932.

28. Locard, E. *Les pores et l'identification des criminels.* Biologica, vol. 2, pp. 357–365, 1912.

29. Macaggi, D. *Sulle "linee bianche" delle impronte digitali.* Atti Soc. cult. sci. med. natur. Cagliari, vol. 37, pp. 316–324, 1935.

30. Ohler, E. A., and H. Cummins. *Sexual differences in breadths of epidermal ridges on the finger tips and palms.* Am. J. Phys. Anthropol., vol. 29, pp. 341–362, 1942.

31. O'Neill, M. E. *Bacterial fingerprints.* J. Crim. Law and Criminol., vol. 32, p. 482, 1941.

32. Pessoa, A. *O que é um delta.* Arq. de med. leg. e ident., vol. 11, pp. 20–25, 1933.

33. de Pina, L. *A propósito de alterações das figuras papilares digitais.* Arq. rep. antrop. crim. psicol. Porto, vol. 3, pp. 49–75, 1935.

34. ———. *Traumatologia dermopapilar em operários portugueses.* Proc. I Congresso médico nacional dos desastres do Trabalho, Lisbon, 1938.

35. Pinkus, F. *Die normale Anatomie der Haut.* In *Handbuch der Haut- und Geschlechtskrankheiten,* vol. 1, part 1, pp. 1–378. Berlin, Julius Springer, 1927.

36. Ribeiro, L. *Dáctilo-diagnose: Contribuição da Medicina Legal para a Propêdeutica Médica.* Rio de Janeiro, Imprensa Nacional, 1939.

37. Updegraff, H. L. *Changing of fingerprints.* Am. J. Surg., vol. 26, pp. 533–534, 1934.

38. Welcker, H. *Die Dauerhaftigkeit des Desseins der Riefchen und Fältchen der Hände.* Arch. f. Anthropol., vol. 25, pp. 29–32, 1898.

CHAPTER 3. METHODS OF PRINTING

39. Cummins, H. *Dermatoglyphic prints: neglected records in racial anthropology.* Am. J. Phys. Anthropol., vol. 16, pp. 31–40, 1941.

40. Federal Bureau of Investigation. *Fingerprints.* Washington, Government Printing Office, 1934.
41. Schlaginhaufen, O. *Beobachtungsblatt und Anleitung zur Aufnahme von Hand- und Fussabdrücken.* Korrespondenzbl. d. Deutsch. anthrop. Gesells., vol. 43, pp. 33–36, 1912.
42. Schött, E. D. *En ny, enkel, för den undersökte behaglig metod för tagning av finger-och handavtryck.* . . . Upsala Läk. Förhand., New Series, vol. 33, pp. 347–353, 1928.

CHAPTER 4. FINGERS

43. Battley, H. *Single Finger Prints.* London, H. M. Stationery Office, 1930.
44. Bonnevie, K. *Studies on papillary patterns of human fingers.* J. Genetics, vol. 15, pp. 1–111, 1924.
45. Brayley, F. A. *Arrangement of Finger Prints.* . . . Boston, Worcester Press, 1910.
46. Bridges, B. C. *Practical Fingerprinting.* New York and London, Funk & Wagnalls Co., 1942.
47. Bridges, B. C., and F. M. Boolsen. *Fifty-one Fingerprint Systems.* Privately printed, 1935.
48. Chapel, C. E. *Fingerprinting.* New York, Coward McCann, Inc., 1941.
49. Crosskey, W. C. S. *The Single Finger Print Identification System.* San Francisco, Privately printed, 1923.
50. Cummins, H. *Finger prints and the "Margery" mediumship: The strange case of Dr. X. and Mr. Y.* Boston Soc. for Psychic Research, Bull. 22, pp. 1–26, 1934.
51. Falco, G. *Sulla evoluzione delle figure papillari dei polpastrelli delle dita nell'uomo.* Riv. di antropol., vol. 22, pp. 175–192, 1917–18.
52. Faulds, H. *Guide to Finger-print Identification.* Hanley, Wood, Mitchell & Co., Ltd., 1905.
53. ———. *A Manual of Practical Dactylography.* London, Police Review Pub. Co., 1923.
54. Federal Bureau of Investigation. *Classification of Fingerprints.* Washington, Government Printing Office, 1941.
55. Furuhata, T. *The difference of the index of finger prints according to race.* Japan Med. World, vol. 7, pp. 162–164, 1927.
56. Galton, F. *Method of indexing finger-marks.* Proc. Roy. Soc. London, vol. 49, pp. 540–548, 1891.
57. ———. *Finger Prints.* London, Macmillan & Co., 1892.
58. ———. *Fingerprint Directories.* London, Macmillan & Co., 1895.
59. Geipel, G. *Anleitung zur erbbiologischen Beurteilung der Finger- und Handleisten.* München, J. F. Lehmann, 1935.
60. Heindl, R. *System und Praxis der Daktyloskopie.* Third edition. Berlin and Leipzig, de Gruyter & Co., 1927.
61. Henry, E. R. *Classification and Uses of Finger Prints.* Eighth edition. London, H. M. Stationery Office, 1937.
62. Holt, J. *Finger Prints Simplified.* Chicago, F. J. Drake & Co., 1941.
63. King, W. W. *Die Hautleisten am Mittel- und Grundgliede von Chinesenhänden und deren übriges Leistensystem.* Ztschr. f. Morphol. u. Anthropol., vol. 38, pp. 309–342, 1939.
64. Kirchmair, H., and H. Poll. *Zur Charakteristik des Rassenunterschiedes des Daktylogramms. Deltie, Strobotoxie und Brochie.* Biol. generalis, vol. 12, pp. 202–216, 1936.
65. Kuhne, F. *The Finger Print Instructor.* Third edition. New York, Munn & Co., 1942.
66. Larson, J. A. *Single Fingerprint System.* New York, D. Appleton & Co., 1924.
67. Locard, E. *Traité de Criminalistique.* Lyon, Desvigne, 1931.
68. ———. *Manuel de Technique Policière.* Paris, Payot, 1939.
69. Mairs, G. T. *Finger prints indexed numerically.* Finger Print and Ident. Mag., vol. 15, nos. 4 and 5, 1933.
70. ———. *Fingerprint Study Data.* New York, The Delehanty Institute, 1938.
71. ———. *A study of the Henry accidentals.* Finger Print and Ident. Mag., vol. 25, no. 2, 1943.
72. Ploetz-Radmann, M. *Die Hautleistenmuster der unteren beiden Fingerglieder der menschlichen Hand.* Ztschr. f. Morphol. u. Anthropol., vol. 36, pp. 281–310, 1937.

73. Poll, H. *Seltene Menschen.* Anat. Anz., vol. 66, pp. 18–30, 1928.
74. ———. *Das Manuar oder die Verteilung der Fingerleistenmuster bei verschiedenen Rassen.* Verhandl. d. Ges. f. phys. Anthrop., vol. 5, pp. 49–59, 1931. [This paper is sometimes erroneously credited to H. Virchow, who had merely presented it for Poll before a meeting of the German Association of Physical Anthropology.]
75. Roscher, G. *Handbuch der Daktyloskopie.* Leipzig, C. L. Hirschfeld, 1905.
76. Seymour, L. *Finger Print Classification.* Los Angeles, Privately printed, 1913.
77. Stephens, E. O., G. T. Mairs, et al. *Report of Science and Practice Committee.* Proc. Internat. Assoc. Ident., 1925.
78. Vucetich, J. *Dactiloscopia Comparada.* La Plata, Peuser, 1904.
79. Wentworth, B., and H. H. Wilder. *Personal Identification.* Second edition. Chicago, T. G. Cooke, 1932.

CHAPTER 5. PALMS

80. Beletti, F. M. G. *Identificando a Impressão Palmar.* Rio de Janeiro, Inst. de Ident., 1934.
81. Bettmann, S. *Über Papillarleistenzeichnungen am menschlichen Daumenballen.* Ztschr. f. Anat. u. Entwicklungsgesch., vol. 96, pp. 427–452, 1931.
82. Cummins, H. *Morphology of the palmar hypothenar dermatoglyphics in man.* Human Biol., vol. 7, pp. 1–23, 1935.
83. ———. *Methodology in palmar dermatoglyphics.* Middle American Research Series, Tulane Univ., pub. 7, pp. 23–81, 1936.
84. Cummins, H., H. H. Keith, C. Midlo, R. B. Montgomery, H. H. Wilder and I. W. Wilder. *Study of error in interpretation and formulation of palmar dermatoglyphics.* Am. J. Phys. Anthropol., vol. 11, pp. 501–521, 1928.
85. ———. *Revised methods of interpreting and formulating palmar dermatoglyphics.* Am. J. Phys. Anthropol., vol. 12, pp. 415–473, 1929.
86. Cummins, H., S. Leche and K. McClure. *Bimanual variation in palmar dermatoglyphics.* Am. J. Anat., vol. 48, pp. 199–230, 1931.
87. Ferrer, R. *Manual de Identification Judicial.* Madrid, Reus, 1921.
88. Lecha-Marzo, A. *Las impresiones palmares; contribución al estudio de los bucles.* Rev. Ibero-Am. de cien. med., vol. 27, pp. 336–344, 1912.
89. ———. *Las impresiones palmares; contribución al estudio de los deltas.* Rev. de med. y cirurg. pract., vol. 96, pp. 361–369, 1912.
90. ———. *Los dibujos papilares de la palma de la mano como medio de identificacion.* Rev. d. Ident., vol. 2, pp. 570–608, 1934.
91. Pond, G. P. *Positive and permanent identification of the new born.* Ill. Med. J., vol. 69, pp. 327–377, 1936. (Reprinted in Finger Print and Ident. Mag., vol. 18, no. 2, 1936.)
92. Ride, L. *An improved formula for expressing the distribution of papillary ridges on the hand and its possible use as a basis for racial distribution.* Proc. Fifth Pacific Science Congress, p. 2743, 1933.
93. ———. *Statistical studies of palmar formulae.* The Caduceus (Univ. of Hongkong), vol. 14, no. 2, 1935.
94. Sharp, V. *Palm Prints.* Cape Town, Mercantile-Atlas Printing Co., 1937.
95. Steggerda, I. D., M. Steggerda and M. S. Lane. *A racial study of palmar dermatoglyphics with special reference to the Maya Indians of Yucatan.* Middle American Research Series, Tulane Univ., pub. 7, pp. 129–194, 1936.
96. Stockis, E. *Les empreintes palmaires.* Arch. de med. leg., 1910.
97. Valsik, J. A. *An essay on a new expression of the epidermic formulas of the human palm.* Časopisu lékařů českých, vol. 67, pp. 281–283, 1928. [In Czech, with summary in English.]
98. ———. *The papillar number in dermatoglyphics.* Časopisu lékařů českých., vol. 37, 1932. [In Czech, with summary in English.]

99. ———. *X-ray skeletotopics of palmar dermatoglyphics with reference to some actual problems.* Biologicke Listy, vol. 18, pp. 21–62, 1933. [In Czech, with summary in English.]
100. Wilder, H. H. *Scientific palmistry.* Pop. Sci. Monthly, vol. 61, pp. 41–54, 1902.
101. ———. *Palm and sole studies.* Biol. Bull., vol. 30, pp. 135–172 and 211–252, 1916.
102. Wood Jones, F. *The Principles of Anatomy as Seen in the Hand.* London, J. & A. Churchill, 1920.

CHAPTER 6. SOLES

103. Féré, C. *Les lignes papillaires de la plante du pied.* J. de l'anat. et de la physiol., vol. 36, pp. 602–618, 1900.
104. ———. *Note sur les lignes papillaires du talon.* C. R. Soc. Biol., vol. 61, pp. 44–46, 1906.
105. Harkness-Miller, F. *Application of a new method of formulating plantar dermatoglyphics with a statistical study of the palm and sole prints of a hundred women.* Thesis, Univ. of Toronto. [Microfilm by courtesy of Dr. Norma Ford.]
106. Hozyo, H. *Über die Einteilung der Hautleistenfiguren der Fusssohle.* Hanzai Z., vol. 10, pp. 1–18, 1936.
107. Montgomery, R. B. *Sole prints of newborn babies.* Am. J. Med. Sci., vol. 169, pp. 830–837, 1925.
108. ———. *Sole patterns. A study of the footprints of two thousand individuals.* Anat. Rec., vol. 33, pp. 107–114, 1926.
109. ———. *Classification of foot-prints.* J. Crim. Law and Criminol., vol. 18, pp. 105–110, 1927.
110. Sabatini, A. *Le figure ad ansa della regione plantare del calcagno.* Riv. di antropol., vol. 28, 1928–29.
111. ———. *I rilievi cutanei della regione plantare.* Riv. di antropol., vol. 29, pp. 257–315, 1930–32 (1933).
112. ———. *Valori morfometrici e figure tattili della regione plantare.* Riv. di antropol., vol. 29, pp. 375–384, 1930–32 (1933).
113. Takeya, S. *Ueber die Hautleistenfigur der Planta der Chinesen.* J. Orient. Med., vol. 20, pp. 54–58 and 495–523, 1934.
114. Wilder, H. H. *Palm and sole impressions and their use for purposes of personal identification.* Pop. Sci. Monthly, vol. 63, pp. 385–410, 1903.
115. ———. *The phylogeny of the human foot; the testimony presented by the configuration of the friction ridges.* Ztschr. f. Morphol. u. Anthropol., vol. 24, pp. 111–124, 1924.

CHAPTER 7. TOES

116. Féré, C. *Les empreintes des doigts et des orteils.* J. de l'anat. et de la physiol., vol. 29, pp. 223–237, 1893.
117. Féré, C., and P. Batigne. *Note sur les empreintes de la pulpe des doigts et des orteils.* C. R. Soc. Biol., vol. 44, pp. 802–806, 1892.
118. Newman, M. T. *A comparative study of finger prints and toe prints.* Human Biol., vol. 8, pp. 531–552, 1936.
119. Steffens, C. *Über Zehenleisten bei Zwillingen.* Ztschr. f. Morphol. u. Anthropol., vol. 37, pp. 218–258, 1938.
120. Takeya, S. *Ueber die Hautleistenfigur der Zehen der Chinesen.* J. Orient. Med., vol. 19, pp. 36–56, 1933.

CHAPTER 8. PERSONAL IDENTIFICATION

121. Balthazard, V. *De la certitude dans l'identification par les empreintes digitales.* Bull. Soc. de méd. lég. de France, An. 43, 2nd series, vol. 8, pp. 106–115, 1911.
122. Castellanos, I. *Identification Problems, Criminal and Civil.* Brooklyn, R. V. Basuino, 1939.

123. Hoover, J. E. *Criminal Identification and the Functions of the Identification Division.* Washington, U. S. Dept. of Justice, 1938.

124. Inbau, F. E. *Scientific evidence in criminal cases. III. Finger-prints and palm-prints.* J. Crim. Law and Criminol., vol. 25, pp. 500–516, 1934.

125. Locard, E. *La Preuve Judiciaire par les Empreintes Digitales.* Lyons, A. Rey, 1914.

126. O'Neill, M. E. *Fingerprints in criminal investigation.* J. Crim. Law and Criminol., vol. 30, pp. 929–940, 1940.

CHAPTER 9. COMPARATIVE DERMATOGLYPHICS

127. Bychowska, M. *The courses of palmar papillary lines in primates.* Folia morphol., vol. 2, pp. 69–121, 1930. [In Polish, with French summary.]

128. Cummins, H. *Dermatoglyphics* [of Macaca mulatta]. In *The Anatomy of the Rhesus Monkey.* Baltimore, The Williams & Wilkins Company, 1933.

129. Cummins, H., and S. D. S. Spragg. *Dermatoglyphics in the chimpanzee: description and comparison with man.* Human Biol., vol. 10, pp. 457–510, 1938.

130. Dankmeijer, J. *Zur biologischen Anatomie der Hautleisten bei den Beuteltieren.* Morphol. Jahrb., vol. 82, pp. 293–312, 1938.

131. Féré, C. *Notes sur les mains et les empreintes digitales de quelque singes.* J. de l'anat. et de la physiol., vol. 36, pp. 255–267, 1900.

132. Hepburn, D. *The papillary ridges on the hands and feet of monkeys and men.* Sci. Trans. Roy. Dublin Soc., vol. 5, ser. 2, pp. 525–538, 1895.

133. Kidd, W. *The Sense of Touch in Mammals and Birds.* London, Adam and Charles Black, 1907.

134. ———. *Initiative in Evolution.* London, H. F. & G. Witherby, 1920.

135. Klaatsch, H. *Zur Morphologie der Tastballen der Säugetiere.* Morphol. Jahrb., vol. 14, pp. 407–435, 1888.

136. Kollmann, A. *Der Tastapparat der Hand der menschlichen Rassen und der Affen.* Hamburg and Leipzig, Leopold Voss, 1883.

137. ———. *Der Tastapparat des Fusses von Affe und Mensch.* Arch. f. Anat. u. Entwick., pp. 56–103, 1885.

138. Midlo, C. *Dermatoglyphics in primates with special reference to man.* (Abstract) Anat. Rec., vol. 45, p. 232, 1930.

139. ———. *Dermatoglyphics in Tupaia lacernata lacernata.* J. Mammal., vol. 16, pp. 35–37, 1935.

140. ———. *A comparative study of volar epidermal ridge configurations in primates.* Proc. La. Acad. Sci., vol. 4, pp. 136–141, 1938.

141. Midlo, C., and H. Cummins. *Palmar and Plantar Dermatoglyphics in Primates.* American Anatomical Memoirs, No. 20. Philadelphia, Wistar Institute of Anatomy and Biology, 1942.

142. Miranda Pinto, O. *Les crêtes papillaires dans la série animale.* Rev. internat. Criminalist., vol. 2, pp. 406–431, 1930.

143. Mutrux-Bornoz, H. *Les Troublantes Révélations de l'Empreinte Digitale et Palmaire.* Lausanne, F. Roth & Cie., 1937.

144. Schlaginhaufen, O. *Das Hautleistensystem der Primatenplanta unter Mitberücksichtigung der Palma.* Morphol. Jahrb., vol. 33, pp. 577–671; vol. 34, pp. 1–125, 1905.

145. ———. *Über das Leistenrelief der Hohlhand- und Fusssohlen-Fläche der Halbaffen, Affen und Menschenrassen.* Ergebn. Anat. u. Entwick,. vol. 15, pp. 628–662, 1905.

146. Schultz, A. H. *Fetal growth and development of the rhesus monkey.* Contrib. to Embryol., Carnegie Inst. of Wash., vol. 26, pp. 71–97, 1937.

147. Whipple, I. L. [Mrs. Inez Whipple Wilder]. *The ventral surface of the mammalian chiridium.* Ztschr. f. Morphol. u. Anthropol., vol. 7, pp. 261–368, 1904.

148. Wilder, H. H. *On the disposition of the epidermic folds upon the palms and soles of primates.* Anat. Anz., vol. 13, pp. 250–256, 1897.

149. Wolff, C. *The form and dermatoglyphs of the hands and feet of certain anthropoid apes.* Proc. Zool. Soc. London, Ser. A, vol. 107, pp. 347–350, 1937.

150. ———. *A comparative study of the form and dermatoglyphs of the extremities of primates.* Proc. Zool. Soc. London, Ser. A, vol. 108, pp. 143–161, 1938.

CHAPTER 10. EMBRYOLOGY

151. Abel, W. *Kritische Studien über die Entwicklung der Papillarmuster auf den Fingerbeeren.* Ztschr. f. menschl. Vererb.-u. Konstitutionslehre, vol. 21, pp. 497–529, 1938.

152. Bellelli, F. *Le linee papillari nelle sindattilie.* Arch. ital. di anat. e di embriol., vol. 42, pp. 423–438, 1939.

153. Bonnevie, K. *Die ersten Entwicklungsstadien der Papillarmuster der menschlichen Fingerballen.* Nyt Mag. f. Naturv., vol. 65, pp. 19–56, 1927.

154. ———. *Was lehrt die Embryologie der Papillarmuster über ihre Bedeutung als Rassen- und Familiencharakter?* Ztschr. f. indukt. Abst.- u. Vererbungslehre, vol, 50, pp. 219–274, 1929.

155. ———. *Zur Mechanik der Papillarmusterbildung. I. Die Epidermis als formativer Faktor in der Entwicklung der Fingerbeeren und der Papillarmuster.* Arch. f. Entwicklungs-mechn. d. Organ., vol. 117, pp. 384–420, 1929.

156. ———. *Zur Mechanik der Papillarmusterbildung. II. Anomalien der menschlichen Finger- und Zehenbeeren, nebst Diskussion über die Natur der hier wirksamen Epidermispolster.* Arch. f. Entwicklungsmechn. d. Organ., vol. 126, pp. 348–372, 1932.

157. Cummins, H. *Epidermal-ridge configurations in developmental defects, with particular reference to the ontogenetic factors which condition ridge direction.* Am. J. Anat., vol. 38, pp. 89–151, 1926.

158. ———. *Evidence limiting the time of inception of intrauterine digital amputations.* Proc. Soc. Exper. Biol. & Med., vol. 23, pp. 847–848, 1926.

159. ———. *The topographic history of the volar pads (walking pads; Tastballen) in the human embryo.* Contrib. to Embryol., Carnegie Inst. of Wash., vol. 20, pp. 103–126, 1929.

160. ———. *Spontaneous amputation of human supernumerary digits: pedunculated postminimi.* Am. J. Anat., vol. 51, pp. 381–416, 1932. (See also: Anat. Rec., vol. 60, pp. 273–277, 1934.)

161. Evatt, E. J. *The development and evolution of the "papillary" ridges and patterns of the volar surface of the hand.* J. Anat., vol. 41, pp. 66–70, 1906.

162. MacArthur, J. W., and E. McCullough. *Apical dystrophy—an inherited defect of hands and feet.* Human Biol., vol. 4, pp. 179–207, 1932.

163. de Pina, L. *Les anomalies de la main et la morphologie des crêtes papillaires.* L'Anthrop., vol. 49, pp. 55–71, 1939.

164. Pinkus, F. *The development of the integument.* In Keibel and Mall, *Manual of Human Embryology,* vol. 1. Philadelphia and London, J. B. Lippincott Co., 1910.

165. Schaeuble, J. *Die Entstehung der palmaren digitalen Triradien.* Ztschr. f. Morphol. u. Anthropol., vol. 31, pp. 403–438, 1933.

CHAPTER 11. SYMMETRY AND OTHER ASPECTS OF SPECIAL MORPHOLOGY

166. Cummins, H., and J. Sicomo. *Plantar epidermal configurations in low-grade syndactylism (zygodactyly) of the second and third toes.* Anat. Rec., vol. 25, pp. 355–389, 1923.

167. Dankmeijer, J., and R. C. Renes. *General rules in the symmetrical occurrence of papillary patterns.* Am. J. Phys. Anthropol., vol. 24, pp. 67–79, 1938.

168. Poll, H. *Two unlike expressions of symmetry of finger-tip patterns.* Human Biol., vol. 10, pp. 77–92, 1938.

169. Waite, H. *Association of finger-prints.* Biometrika, vol. 10, pp. 421–478, 1915.

170. Wilder, H. H. *The morphology of the hypothenar of the hand: a study in the variation and degeneration of a typical pattern.* Biol. Bull., vol. 50, pp. 393–405, 1926.

171. Wilder, I. W. *The morphology of the palmar digital triradii and main lines.* J Morphol. vol. 49, pp. 153–208, 1930.

CHAPTER 12. INHERITANCE

CHAPTER 13. TWIN DIAGNOSIS

CHAPTER 14. QUESTIONED PATERNITY

172. Boas, K. *Vaterschaft und Fingerabdruck.* Arch. f. Kriminol., vol. 53, pp. 326–327, 1913.
173. Böhmer, K., and F. Harren. *Die Vererbung der Papillarlinien und ihre Bedeutung für den Nachweis der Vaterschaft.* Deutsche Ztschr. f. d. ges. gerichtl. Med., vol. 32, pp. 73–82, 1939.
174. Bonnevie, K. *Lassen sich die Papillarmuster der Fingerbeere für Vaterschaftsfragen praktisch verwerten?* Zentralbl. f. Gynäk., vol. 51, pp. 539–543, 1927.
175. ———. *Was lehrt die Embryologie der Papillarmuster über ihre Bedeutung als Rassen- und Familiencharakter?* III. *Zur Genetik des quantitativen Wertes der Papillarmuster.* Ztschr. f. indukt. Abst.- u. Vererbungslehre, vol. 59, pp. 1–60, 1931.
176. Carrière, R. *Über Erblichkeit und Rasseneigentümlichkeit der Finger- und Handlinienmuster.* Arch. f. Rassenbiol., vol. 15, pp. 151–155, 1923.
177. Cevidalli, A. *Contributo allo studio delle linee papillari in rapporto alla ereditarietà.* Bol. Soc. med. chir. di Modena, vol. 13, pp. 547–551, 1911.
178. Clarke, A. E., and D. G. Revell. *Monozygotic triplets in man.* J. Hered., vol. 21, pp. 147–156, 1930.
179. Csik, L., and M. Malan. *Zur Erblichkeit der Hauptlinien und Muster der menschlichen Hand.* Ztschr. f. menschl. Vererb.- u. Konstitutionslehre, vol. 21, pp. 186–205, 1937.
180. Cummins, H. *Dermatoglyphics in twins of known chorionic history, with reference to diagnosis of the twin varieties.* Anat. Rec., vol. 46, pp. 179–198, 1930.
181. ———. *Finger prints in "Siamese" twins.* Eugenical News, vol. 21, pp. 89–95, 1936.
182. Cummins, H., and G. T. Mairs. *Finger prints of conjoined twins.* J. Hered., vol. 25, pp. 237–243, 1934.
183. Dalla Volta, A. *Le figure digitali in rapporto all' eredita.* Arch. per l'antropol., vol. 43, pp. 187–230, 1913.
184. Dankmeijer, J. *De Erfelijkheid van het Vingerpatroon.* Nederl. tijdschr. v. geneesk., vol. 84, pp. 4785–4792, 1940.
185. Danner, M. R. W. *A comparative study of human twins.* Thesis, Univ. of Illinois, 1934.
186. Elderton, E. M. *On the inheritance of the finger-print.* Biometrika, vol. 12, pp. 57–91, 1920.
187. Ennenbach, S. *Fingerabdrücke bei ein- und zweieiigen Zwillingen.* Ztschr. f. menschl. Vererb.- u. Konstitutionslehre, vol. 23, pp. 555–586, 1939.
188. Essen-Moller, E. *Die Beweiskraft der Ähnlichkeit im Vaterschaftsnachweis. Theoretische Grundlagen.* Mitt. anthrop. Ges. Wien, vol. 67, pp. 9–53, 1937.
189. ———. *Zur Theorie der Ähnlichkeitsdiagnose von Zwillingen.* Arch. f. Rassenbiol., vol. 32, pp. 1–10, 1938.
190. ———. *Empirische Ähnlichkeitsdiagnose bei Zwillingen.* Hereditas, vol. 27, pp. 1–50, 1941.
191. Essen-Moller, E., and C. E. Quensel. *Zur Theorie des Vaterschaftsnachweises auf Grund von Ähnlichkeitsbefunden.* Deutsche Ztschr. f. d. ges. gerichtl. Med., vol. 31, pp. 70–96, 1939.
192. Fischer, E. *Versuch einer Phänogenetik der normalen körperlichen Eigenschaften des Menschen.* Ztschr. f. indukt. Abst.- u. Vererbungslehre, vol. 76, pp. 47–115, 1939.
193. Ford, N. *Evidence of monozygosity and disturbance of growth in twins with pyloric stenosis.* Am. J. Dis. Child., vol. 61, pp. 41–53, 1941.
194. Fukuoka, G. *Anthropometric and psychometric studies on Japanese twins.* In *Contributions to the Genetics of the Japanese Race*, Kyoto, 1937.
195. Ganther, R., and E. Rominger. *Über die Bedeutung des Handleistenbildes für die Zwillingsforschung.* Ztschr. f. Kinderh., vol. 36, pp. 212–220, 1923.

196. Gardner, I. C., and D. C. Rife. *The diagnosis of five sets of triplets.* J. Hered., vol. 32, pp. 27–32, 1941.
197. Geipel, G. *Der Formindex der Fingerleistenmuster.* Ztschr. f. Morphol. u. Anthropol., vol. 36, pp. 330–361, 1937.
198. ———. *Fingerabdrücke bei ein- und zweieiigen Zwillingen.* Ztschr. f. menschl. Vererb.- u. Konstitutionslehre, vol. 24, pp. 113–115, 1939.
199. ———. *Die Gesamtanzahl der Fingerleisten als neues Merkmal zur Zwillingsdiagnose.* Der Erbarzt, vol. 9, pp. 16–19, 1941.
200. Geyer, E. *Die Beweiskraft der Ähnlichkeit im Vaterschaftsnachweis. Praktische Anwendung.* Mitt. anthrop. Ges. Wien, vol. 68, pp. 54–87, 1938.
201. ———. *Zwillinge mit verschiedenen Vätern.* Volk und Rasse, no. 9, pp. 135–136, 1940.
202. Grüneberg, H. *Die Vererbung der menschlichen Tastfiguren.* Ztschr. f. indukt. Abst.- u. Vererbungslehre, vol. 46, pp. 285–310, 1928.
203. ———. *Idiotyp und Paratyp in der menschlichen Erbforschung.* Ztschr. f. indukt. Abst.- u. Vererbungslehre, vol. 50, pp. 76–96, 1929.
204. Harrasser, A. *Die anthropologisch-erbbiologische Vaterschaftsprobe und ihre Anwendung in der Rechtspflege.* Med. Welt, no. 38, 1934.
205. ———. *Ergebnisse der anthropologisch-erbbiologischen Vaterschaftsprobe in der österreichischen Justiz.* Mitt. anthrop. Ges. Wien, vol. 65, pp. 204–232, 1935.
206. Harster, T. *Vaterschaft und Fingerabdruck.* Arch f. Krim.-anthrop., vol. 56, pp. 1–4, 1913.
207. Hellwig, A. *Kriminalistische Abhandlungen. I. Daktyloskopie und Vaterschaft.* Arch. f. Kriminol., vol. 50, pp. 1–2, 1912.
208. Jordan, H. E. *Studies in human heredity.* Bull. Philosoph. Soc. Univ. of Va., vol. 1, pp. 293–317, 1912.
209. Komai, T. *Review of literature on twin studies in Japan.* In *Contributions to the Genetics of the Japanese Race,* Kyoto, 1937.
210. Lauer, A., and H. Poll. *Tracing paternity by finger prints.* Am. J. Police Sci., vol. 1, pp. 92–99, 1930. (Translated from Krim. Monatsh., vol. 10, pp. 217–221.)
211. Leven, L. *Erblichkeit des Papillarliniensystems.* Klin. Wchnschr., vol. 3, pp. 1817–1818, 1924.
212. ———. *Erblichkeit der Tastfiguren und Erbverschiedenheit der Eineier.* Dermat. Wchnschr., vol. 85, pp. 1229–1233, 1927.
213. Lottig, H. *Hamburger Zwillingsstudien.* Ztschr. f. angew. Psychol., Suppl. no. 61, 1931.
214. Lund, S. E. T. *A psycho-biological study of a set of identical girl triplets.* Human Biol., vol. 5, pp. 1–34, 1933.
215. MacArthur, J. W. *Reliability of dermatoglyphics in twin diagnosis.* Human Biol., vol. 10, pp. 12–35, 1938.
216. MacArthur, J. W., and N. H. C. Ford. *A biological study of the Dionne quintuplets—an identical set.* In *Collected studies on the Dionne quintuplets.* Toronto, Univ. of Toronto Press, 1937.
217. MacArthur, J. W., and O. T. MacArthur. *Finger, palm and sole prints of monozygotic quadruplets.* J. Hered., vol. 28, pp. 147–153, 1937.
218. Metzner, I. *Ueber die Häufigkeit des Vorkommens unstimmiger Genformeln für quantitative Werte der Fingerleisten bei Eltern und Kindern.* Ztschr. f. menschl. Vererb.- u. Konstitutionslehre, vol. 22, pp. 669–698, 1939.
219. Meyer Heydenhagen, G. *Die palmaren Hautleisten bei Zwillingen.* Ztschr. f. Morphol. u. Anthropol., vol. 33, pp. 1–42, 1934.
220. Montgomery, R.B. *Sole patterns of twins.* Biol. Bull., vol. 50, pp. 293–300, 1926.
221. Mueller, B. *Untersuchungen über die Erblichkeit von Fingerbeerenmustern unter besonderer Berücksichtigung rechtlicher Fragestellungen.* Ztschr. f. indukt. Abst.- u. Vererbungslehre, vol. 56, pp. 302–382, 1930.
222. ———. *Die Lehre von der Erblichkeit des Reliefs der Hohland und der Fingerbeeren vom gerichtlich-medizinischen Standpunkt aus.* Deutsche Ztschr. f. d. ges. gerichtl. Med., vol. 17, pp. 407–425, 1931.

223. Mueller, B., and W. G. Ting. *Ist die daktyloskopische Untersuchung als Hilfsmittel zum gerichtlich-medizinischen Ausschluss der Vaterschaft brauchbar?* Deutsche Ztschr. f. d. ges. gerichtl. Med., vol. 11, pp. 347–, 1928. (Cited by Geipel, 197.)

224. Newman, H. H. *Studies of human twins. I. Methods of diagnosing monozygotic and dizygotic twins.* Biol. Bull., vol. 55, pp. 283–297, 1928.

225. ———. *The finger prints of twins.* J. Genetics, vol. 23, pp. 415–446, 1930.

226. ———. *Palmar dermatoglyphics of twins.* Am. J. Phys. Anthropol., vol. 14, pp. 331–378, 1930.

227. ———. *Palm-print patterns in twins.* J. Hered., vol. 22, pp. 41–49, 1931.

228. ———. *Differences between conjoined twins.* J. Hered., vol. 22, pp. 201–215, 1931.

229. Nürnberger, L. *Wahrscheinlichkeitsrechnung und Erbanalyse bei gerichtlichen Vaterschaftsgutachten.* Zentralbl. f. Gynäk., vol. 49, pp. 1409–1431, 1925.

230. Obonai, T. *Studies on mental inheritance of twins.* Sinrigaku-Kenkyu, vol. 1, pp. 577–638, 1926. (In Japanese; cited by Komai, 209.)

231. Okuma, Y. *Ueber die Papillarlinien-Faktoren (V, R, U) der Formosonanern.* Taiwan Igakkai Zassi, vol. 40, pp. 482–489, 1941.

232. Poll, H. *Über Zwillingsforschung als Hilfsmittel menschlicher Erbkunde.* Ztschr. f. Ethnol., vol. 46, pp. 87–105, 1914.

233. Raitzin, A. *La hereditariedad dactyloscópica.* Semana méd., vol. 44, pp. 201–211, 1937.

234. Reichle, H. S. *The diagnosis of the type of twinning.* Biol. Bull., vol. 56, pp. 164–176, 1929.

235. Rife, D. C. *Genetic studies of monozygotic twins. I. A. diagnostic formula.* J. Hered., vol. 24, pp. 339–345, 1933.

236. ———. *Genetic studies of monozygotic twins. II. Finger-patterns and eye-color as criteria of monozygosity.* J. Hered., vol. 24, pp. 406–414, 1933.

237. ———. *Contributions of the 1937 national twins' convention to research.* J. Hered., vol. 29, pp. 83–90, 1938.

238. Rife, D. C., and H. Cummins. *Dermatoglyphics and "mirror imaging."* Human Biol., vol. 15, pp. 55–64, 1943.

239. Saller, K. *Einführung in die menschliche Erblichkeitslehre und Eugenik.* Berlin, Julius Springer, 1932.

240. Scheffer, R. *Daktyloskopie und Vaterschaftsfrage.* Zentralbl. f. Gynäk., vol. 50, pp. 2559–2563, 1926.

241. Schläger. *Untersuchung des Blutes und der Papillarlinien im Alimentationsprozess.* München. med. Wchnschr., vol. 175, p. 1969, 1928.

242. Schrader, G. *Gerichtsärztliche Untersuchungen zum Nachweis der Vaterschaft.* Handb. d. biol. meth. Abderhalden, Sect. IV, part 12, second half, pp. 1–36, 1934.

243. Siemens, H. W. *The diagnosis of identity in twins.* J. Hered., vol. 18, pp. 201–209, 1927.

244. Sommer. *Zur forensischen Beurteilung der Erblichkeit von morphologischen Abnormitäten und der Papillarlinien der Finger.* Arch. f. Kriminol., vol. 67, pp. 161–174, 1916.

245. Stocks, P. *A biometric study of twins and their brothers and sisters.* Ann. Eugenics, vol. 4, pp. 49–108, 1930.

246. ———. *A biometric investigation of twins and their brothers and sisters. Part II.* Ann. Eugenics, vol. 5, pp. 1–55, 1933.

247. Tirelli, V. *Contributo allo studio del problema della transmissibilita famigliare dei disegni papillari digitali.* Gior. R. Accad. di med. Torino, vol. 98, 1935.

248. von Verschuer, O. *Die Ähnlichkeitsdiagnose der Eineiigkeit von Zwillingen.* Anthrop. Anz., vol. 5, pp. 244–248, 1928.

249. ———. *Die biologischen Grundlagen der menschlichen Mehrlingsforschung.* Ztschr. f. indukt. Abst.- u. Vererbungslehre, vol. 61, pp. 147–207, 1932.

250. ———. *Neue Ergebnisse der Zwillingsforschung.* Arch. f. Gynäk., vol. 156, pp. 362–375, 1933.

251. ———. Forsch. u. Fortschr., vol. 9, pp. 477–478, 1933. (Cited by Weninger, 260.)

252. ———. *Twin research from the time of Francis Galton to the present day.* Proc. Roy. Soc. London, ser. B., vol. 128, pp. 62–81, 1940.

253. Volotzkoy, M. V. *On the genetics of finger prints.* Proc. Maxim Gorky Medico-Genetical Research Inst., vol. 4, pp. 404–439, 1936. [In Russian, with English summary.]

254. Walker, J. F. *A sex linked recessive fingerprint pattern.* J. Hered., vol. 32, pp. 279–280, 1941.

255. von Wehren, J. *Untersuchungen über die Vererblichkeit des quantitativen Wertes der Fingerbeerenmuster und ihre Verwertbarkeit in gerichtlich-medizinischer Hinsicht.* Dissertation, Göttingen, 1937.

256. Weinand, H. *Familienuntersuchungen über den Hautleistenverlauf der Handfläche.* Ztschr. f. Morphol. u. Anthropol., vol. 36, pp. 418–442, 1937.

257. Weninger, J. *Der naturwissenschaftliche Vaterschaftsbeweis.* Wien. klin. Wchnschr., no. 1, 1935.

258. ———. *Menschliche Erblehre und Anthropologie.* Wien. klin. Wchnschr., no. 26, 1936.

259. Weninger, M. *Familienuntersuchungen über den Hautleistenverlauf am Thenar und am ersten Interdigitalballen der Palma.* Mitt. anthrop. Ges. Wien., vol. 55, pp. 182–193, 1935.

260. ———. *Zur Anwendung der Erbformeln der quantitativen Werte der Fingerbeeren im naturwissenschaftlichen Vaterschaftsnachweis.* Ztschr. f. menschl. Vererb.-u. Konstitutionslehre, vol. 21, pp. 206–219, 1937.

261. Wilder, H. H. *Palms and soles.* Am. J. Anat., vol. 1, pp. 423–441, 1902.

262. ———. *Duplicate twins and double monsters.* Am. J. Anat., vol. 3, pp. 387–472, 1904.

263. ———. *Zur körperlichen Identität bei Zwillingen.* Anat. Anz., vol. 32, pp. 193–200, 1908.

264. ———. *Physical correspondences in two sets of duplicate twins.* J. Hered., vol. 10, pp. 410–420, 1919.

CHAPTER 15. RACIAL DIFFERENCES

265. Abel, W. *Finger- und Handlinienmuster.* Wiss. Ergeb. d. Deutsch. Grönland-Expedition Alfred Wegener 1929 und 1930/1931, vol. 6, pp. 1–23, 1933.

266. ———. *Über die Frage der Symmetrie der menschlichen Fingerbeere und der Rassenunterschiede der Papillarmuster.* Biol. generalis, vol. 9, pp. 13–32, 1933.

267. ———. *Über die Verteilung der Genotypen der Hand- und Fingerbeerenmuster bei europäischen Rassen.* Ztschr. f. indukt. Abst.- u. Verebungslehre, vol. 70, pp. 458–460, 1935.

268. Biswas, P. C. *Über Hand- und Fingerleisten von Indern.* Ztschr. f. Morphol. u. Anthropol., vol. 35, pp. 519–550, 1936.

269. Bugge, J. N. *Til Papillaermonstrenes Statistik.* Meddel. om Danmarks Antrop., vol. 3, pp. 387–392, 1932.

270. Cummins, H. *Dermatoglyphics in Negroes of West Africa.* Am. J. Phys. Anthropol., vol. 14, pp. 9–21, 1930.

271. ———. *Dermatoglyphics in Indians of southern Mexico and Central America.* Am. J. Phys. Anthropol., vol. 15, pp. 123–136, 1930.

272. ———. *Plantar dermatoglyphics and tread area in Siamese.* Am. J. Phys. Anthropol., vol. 19, pp. 321–325, 1934.

273. ———. *Dermatoglyphics in Eskimos from Point Barrow.* Am. J. Phys. Anthropol., vol. 20, pp. 13–17, 1935.

274. ———. *Dermatoglyphics in North American Indians and Spanish-Americans.* Human Biol., vol. 13, pp. 177–188, 1941.

275. Cummins, H., and M. S. Goldstein. *Dermatoglyphics in Comanche Indians.* Am. J. Phys. Anthropol., vol. 17, pp. 229–235, 1932.

276. Cummins, H., and C. Midlo. *Palmar and plantar epidermal ridge configurations (dermatoglyphics) in European-Americans.* Am. J. Phys. Anthropol., vol. 9, pp. 471–502, 1926.

277. ———. *Dermatoglyphics in Jews.* Am. J. Phys. Anthropol., vol. 10, pp. 91–113, 1927.

278. Cummins, H., and W. M. Shanklin. *Dermatoglyphics in peoples of the Near East. I.
Mitwali.* Am. J. Phys. Anthropol., vol. 22, pp. 263–265, 1937.

279. Cummins, H., and M. Steggerda. *Finger prints in a Dutch family series.* Am. J. Phys.
Anthropol., vol. 20, pp. 19–41, 1935.

280. Dankmeijer, J. *De Beteekenis van Vingerafdrukken voor het anthropologisch Onderzoek.*
Dissertation, University of Utrecht. Utrecht, L. E. Bosch & Zoon, 1934.

281. ———. *Some anthropological data on finger prints.* Am. J. Phys. Anthropol., vol. 23, pp.
377–388, 1938.

282. Davenport, C. B., and M. Steggerda. *Race crossing in Jamaica.* Carnegie Inst. of Wash.,
pub. 395, 1929.

283. Falco, G. *Sulle figure papillare dei polpastrelli delle dita nei libici.* Riv. di antropol., vol. 22,
pp. 91–148, 1917–18.

284. Fleischhacker, H. *Untersuchungen über das Hautleistensystem der Hottentotten-Palma.*
Anthrop. Anz., vol. 11, pp. 111–148, 1934.

285. Hansen, V. F. *Fingerabdrücke von Westgrönländern.* Acta path. et microbiol. Scandinav.,
vol. 17, pp. 104–108, 1940.

286. Hasebe, K. *Über das Hautleistensystem der Vola und Planta der Japaner und Aino.* Arb.
a. d. anat. Inst. kaiserlich-japan. Univ. Sendai, no. 1, pp. 13–88, 1918.

287. Heindl, R. *Rassenunterschiede in den Papillarlinienbildern der Fingerhaut?* Arch. f.
Kriminol., vol. 96, pp. 247–248, 1935.

288. Henckel, K. O. *Beiträge zur Anthropologie Chiles. I. Über die Papillarlinienmuster der Fingerbeeren bei der Bevölkerung der Provinz Concepcion.* Ztschr. f. Morphol. u. Anthropol.,
vol. 31, pp. 299–309, 1933.

289. ———. *Beiträge zur Anthropologie Chiles. III. Über die Papillarlinienmuster der Fingerbeeren bei Indianern der Provinz Cautin.* Ztschr. f. Morphol. u. Anthropol., vol. 34, pp.
113–119, 1934.

290. Kanaseki, T. (editor). A series of reports in two volumes, mainly on Japanese material, by
various authors. Arb. a. d. Anthrop. Abt. d. anat. Inst. d. Taihoku kaiserlich-japan.
Univ., 1939.

291. Kanaseki, T., E. Miyauchi and I. Wada. *Palmar dermatoglyphics of Yonaguni-Islanders,
Riukiu.* Taiwan Igakkai Zassi, vol. 38, pp. 989–1018, 1939. [In Japanese, with German
summary.]

292. Kanaseki, T., and Y. Shima. *Palmar main lines, based upon Ride's study of the natives of
north Borneo.* J. Anthrop. Soc. Tokyo, vol. 53, pp. 383–411, 1939. [In Japanese.]

293. Keith, H. H. *Racial differences in the papillary lines.* Am. J. Phys. Anthropol., vol. 7, pp.
165–206, 1924.

294. Kirchmair, H. *Daktylographische Rassenmerkmale im Ambimanuar.* Ztschr. f. Morphol. u.
Anthropol., vol. 33, pp. 49–70, 1934.

295. ———. *Der Fingerabdruck im Dienste der Rassen- und Konstitutionsforschung.* München.
med. Wchnschr., vol. 82, pt. 1, pp. 529–531, 1935.

296. Kubo, T. *Beiträge zur Daktyloskopie der Koreaner.* Mitt. med. Fachschule Keijo, pp. 117–
223, 1918; pp. 1–63, 1919; pp. 1–150, 1921.

297. Leche, S. M. [Four studies on Mexican Indians.] Middle American Research Series,
Tulane Univ., pub. 7, 1936.

298. Miyake, H. *Über das Hautleistensystem der Vola der Koreaner.* Ztschr. f. Morphol. u.
Anthropol., vol. 25, pp. 419–434 1926.

299. Piebenga, H. T. *Systematische und erbbiologische Untersuchungen über das Hautleistensystem der Friesen, Flamen und Wallonen.* Ztschr. f. Morphol. u. Anthropol., vol. 37,
pp. 140–165, 1938.

300. de Pina, L. *Variedades na distribuïção das cristas papillares da mão nos Portugueses de
Norte.* Arq. rep. antrop. crimin. psicol. Porto., vol. 4, pp. 56–76, 1936.

301. Poll, H. *Das Manuar oder die Verteilung der Fingerleistenmuster bei verschiedenen Rassen.*
Verhandl. d. Ges. f. phys. Anthrop., vol. 5, pp. 49–59, 1931.

302. ——. *Beiträge zu einer anthropologischen Daktylographie.* Biol. generalis, vol. 12, pp. 437-454, 1937; vol. 13, pp. 175-218, 1937.

303. Poll, H., and J. N. Bugge. *Studio comparitivo delle impronte digitali Danesi e Tedesche.* Arch. di antropol. crim., vol. 16, pp. 785-813, 1938.

304. Sabatini, A. *Il valore dei rilieve cutanei digito-palmari quale carattere distintivo delle razze.* Atti d. soc. Italiana per il Progresso delle Scienze, XXIII Riunione, vol. 3, 1934.

305. Sarmento, A. *Dactiloscopia Angolana.* Trab. Soc. Portuguesa de antropol. e etnol., vol. 9, 1941.

306. Shanklin, W. M., and H. Cummins. *Dermatoglyphics in Rwala Bedouins.* Human Biol., vol. 9, pp. 357-365, 1937.

307. Shima, Y. *Anthropologische Untersuchungen über die Eingeborenen in Formosa. I. Ueber das Hautleistensystem der Vola bei den Rassen der pazifischen Küste in Formosa.* J. Med. Assoc. Formosa, vol. 38, Suppl., 1939.

308. Steiner, O. *Die Verteilung der Fingerabdruckmuster im Kreis Tettnang Württemberg (Bodenseegebiet), und ihre Beziehungen zur Siedlungsgeschichte.* Anthrop. Anz., vol. 13, pp. 271-281, 1936-37.

309. Weninger, M. *Untersuchungen über das Hautleistensystem der Buschmänner. Ein Beitrag zur Stellung der Buschmannrasse.* Mitt. anthrop. Ges. Wien, vol. 66, pp. 30-46, 1936.

310. ——. *Fingerabdrücke von zentralafrikanischen Batwa-Pygmoiden des Kivu-Gebietes.* Mitt. anthrop. Ges. Wien, vol. 67, pp. 162-168, 1937.

311. Wilder, H. H. *Racial differences in palm and sole configuration.* Am. Anthrop., vol. 6, pp. 244-292, 1904.

312. ——. *Racial differences in palm and sole configuration. Palm and sole prints of Japanese and Chinese.* Am. J. Phys. Anthropol., vol. 5, pp. 143-206, 1922.

CHAPTER 16. CONSTITUTION

313. Abel, W. *Über Störungen der Papillarmuster. I. Gestörte Papillarmuster in Verbindung mit einigen körperlichen und geistigen Anomalien.* Ztschr. f. Morphol. u. Anthropol., vol. 36, pp. 1-37, 1936.

314. D'Abundo. *Contributo allo studio delle impronte digitali.* Arch. di. Psichiat., 1891; Riforma med., 1894.

315. Ascarelli, A. *Le impronte digitali nelle prostitute.* Arch. di Psichiat., vol. 27, pp. 812-821, 1906.

316. Bettmann, S. *Über die Vierfingerfurche.* Ztschr. f. Anat. u. Entwicklungsgesch., vol. 98, pp. 487-503, 1932.

317. ——. *Die Papillarleistenzeichnung der Handfläche in ihrer Beziehung zur Händigkeit.* Ztschr. f. Anat. u. Entwicklungsgesch., vol. 98, pp. 649-674, 1932.

318. ——. *Haut und Konstitution.* Ztschr. f. Konstitutionslehre, vol. 16, pp. 484-501, 1932.

319. Blotevogel, H. *Das Charakterbild der Neurofibromatose (Recklinghausen).* Dermat. Wchnschr., vol. 96, pp. 361-368, 1933.

320. Blotevogel, H., and W. Blotevogel. *Blutgruppe und Daktylogramm als Konstitutionsmerkmale der Poliomyelitiskranken.* Ztschr. f. Kinderh., vol. 56, pp. 143-169, 1934.

321. Blümel, P., and H. Poll. *Fingerlinienmuster und geistige Norm.* Med. Klin., vol. 24, pp. 1424-1430, 1928.

322. Bonnevie, K. *Papillarmuster und psychische Eigenschaften.* Hereditas, vol. 9, pp. 180-192, 1927.

323. ——. *Papillarmuster bei Linkshändigen.* Hereditas, vol. 18, pp. 129-139, 1933.

324. Brown, M., and H. A. Paskind. *Constitutional differences between deteriorated and nondeteriorated patients with epilepsy: dactylographic studies.* J. Nerv. & Mental Dis., vol. 92, pp. 579-604, 1940.

325. Bugge, J. N., and H. Poll. *Esistono differenze dattiloscopiche fra criminali e normali?* Arch. di antropol. crim., vol. 16, pp. 815-843, 1938.

326. Castellanos, I. *The biological examination of finger prints.* Finger Print and Ident. Mag., vol. 11, no. 6, 1929.

327. ———. *Acerca del estudio de los dactilogramas.* Arch. de med. leg., vol. 4, 1934.

328. ———. *Dactiloscopia clinica.* Biblioteca de la Revista Vida Neuva, vol. 4, Havana, 1935.

329. Cestan, R., P. Descomps and J. Euzière. *Les altérations des empreintes digitales dans les lésions des nerfs périphérique du membre supérieur.* Bull. et mém. Soc. de méd. de hôp. d : Paris, pp. 652–674, 1916.

330. ———. *Les empreintes digitales dans les lésions nerveuses du membre supérieur.* Presse méd., vol. 24, pp. 258–262, 1916.

331. Claude, H., and S. Chauvet. *Sémiologie Reelle des Sections Totalis des Nerfs Mixtes Périphériques.* Maloine, Paris, 1911.

332. Collins, W. *Permanence of Geographical Control over Men.* London, 1913. (Quoted from Stockis by Bonnevie, 44.)

333. Cromwell, H., and D. C. Rife. *Dermatoglyphics in relation to functional handedness.* Human Biol., vol. 14, pp. 516–526, 1942.

334. Cummins, H. *Dermatoglyphic stigmata in mongoloid imbeciles.* Anat. Rec., vol. 73, pp. 407–415, 1939.

335. ———. *Finger prints correlated with handedness.* Am. J. Phys. Anthropol., vol. 26, pp. 151–166, 1940.

336. ———. *Bimanual asymmetry of the palmar main lines.* Quart. Phi Beta Pi, C. M. Jackson issue, vol. 39, pp. 4–10, 1942.

337. Cummins, H., and M. Steggerda. *Finger prints in Maya Indians.* Middle American Research Series, Tulane Univ., pub. 7, pp. 103–126, 1936.

338. Downey, J. E. *Types of dextrality and their implications.* Am. J. Psychol., vol. 38, pp. 317–367, 1927.

339. Duis, B. T. *Fingerleisten bei Schizophrenen.* Ztschr. f. Morphol. u. Anthropol., vol. 36, pp. 391–417, 1937.

340. Féré, C. *Les empreintes digitales dans plusieurs croupes de psychopathes.* J. de l'anat. et de la physiol., vol. 41, pp. 394–410, 1905.

341. Friedemann, A. *Handbau und Psychose.* Arch. f. Psychiat., vol. 82, pp. 439–499, 1928.

342. Gasti, G. *Sui disegni papillari in normali e delinquenti.* Atti d. Soc. Rom. di antropol., vol. 13, pp. 187–194, 1907.

343. Geipel, G. *Bestehen korrelative Beziehungen zwischen den Fingerleistenmustern und den Blutgruppen?* Ztschr. f. Rassenphysiol., vol. 7, pp. 165–166, 1935.

344. Gercke, H., and H. Poll. *Untersuchungen über die Papillarmuster bei Asozialen.* Krim. Monatsh., vol. 6, no. 12, 1932.

345. Hahne, K. W., *Die Bedeutung der Blutgruppen und Tastfiguren in Vaterschaftsprozessen.* Dissertation, Bonn, 1929.

346. Hesch, M. *Papillarmuster bei Eingeborenen der Loyalty-Inseln. Beziehungen zwischen Papillarmustern und Blutgruppen bei diesen und einer deutschen Vergleichsgruppe.* Ztschr. f. Rassenphysiol., vol. 5, pp. 163–168, 1932.

347. Karl, E. *Systematische und erbbiologische Untersuchungen der Papillarmuster der menschlichen Fingerbeeren.* Dissertation, Leipzig, 1934.

348. Kirchmair, H. *Daktylographische Geschlechtsunterschiede des Ambimanuars.* Ztschr. f. Morphol. u. Anthropol., vol. 33, pp. 440–463, 1935.

349. ———. *Über relative und absolute Symmetrie der Papillarmuster bei gesunden und kranken Populationen.* Ztschr. f. Morphol. u. Anthropol., vol. 33, pp. 464–473, 1935.

350. Krieger, T. *Die Papillarleistenzeichnungen an Händen von Psoriatikern.* Ztschr. f. Anat. u. Entwicklungsgesch., vol. 102, pp. 389–401, 1934.

351. Leche, S. M. *Handedness and bimanual dermatoglyphic differences.* Am. J. Anat., vol. 53, pp. 1–53, 1933.

352. Locard, E. *Empreintes digitales et stigmates de dégénérescence.* Enfance anormale, New Series 13, pp. 515–519, 1913.

353. Møller, N. B. *Undersogelser over Fingeraftrykket som konstitutionelt Kendetegn ved Sinds-sygdomme.* Hospitalstidende, pp. 1085–1111, 1935.

354. ———. *Papillarmuster und Imbezillität.* Monatschr. f. Psychiat. u. Neurol., vol. 95, pp. 28–31, 1937.

355. Newman, H. H. *Dermatoglyphics and the problem of handedness.* Am. J. Anat., vol. 55, pp. 277–322, 1934.

356. Poll, H. *Dactylographische Geschlechtsunterschiede der Schizophrenen.* Monatschr. f. Psychiat. u. Neurol., vol. 91, pp. 65–71, 1935.

357. Rife, D. C. *Genetic interrelationships of dermatoglyphics and functional handedness.* Genetics, vol. 28, pp. 41–48, 1943.

358. ———. *Handedness and dermatoglyphics in twins.* Human Biol., vol. 15, pp. 46–54, 1943.

359. de Sanctis, S., and P. Toscano. *Le impronte digitali dei fanciulli normali frenastenici e sordomuti.* Atti. d. Soc. Rom. di Antropol., vol. 8, pp. 62–79, 1902.

360. Varela, F. B. *La dactiloscopia en las psicopatias.* Arq. de anat. e antropol., vol. 9, pp. 469–487, 1925–26.

361. Workman, G. *A study of the palmar dermatoglyphics of mongoloid idiots.* Thesis, Univ. of Toronto, 1939. [Microfilm, by courtesy of Dr. Norma Ford.]

INDEX

A CATALOGUE OF SELECTED DOVER BOOKS
IN ALL FIELDS OF INTEREST

A CATALOGUE OF SELECTED DOVER BOOKS
IN ALL FIELDS OF INTEREST

WHAT IS SCIENCE?, *N. Campbell*

The role of experiment and measurement, the function of mathematics, the nature of scientific laws, the difference between laws and theories, the limitations of science, and many similarly provocative topics are treated clearly and without technicalities by an eminent scientist. "Still an excellent introduction to scientific philosophy," H. Margenau in *Physics Today*. "A first-rate primer . . . deserves a wide audience," *Scientific American*. 192pp. 5⅜ x 8.

60043-2 Paperbound $1.25

THE NATURE OF LIGHT AND COLOUR IN THE OPEN AIR, *M. Minnaert*

Why are shadows sometimes blue, sometimes green, or other colors depending on the light and surroundings? What causes mirages? Why do multiple suns and moons appear in the sky? Professor Minnaert explains these unusual phenomena and hundreds of others in simple, easy-to-understand terms based on optical laws and the properties of light and color. No mathematics is required but artists, scientists, students, and everyone fascinated by these "tricks" of nature will find thousands of useful and amazing pieces of information. Hundreds of observational experiments are suggested which require no special equipment. 200 illustrations; 42 photos. xvi + 362pp. 5⅜ x 8.

20196-1 Paperbound $2.00

THE STRANGE STORY OF THE QUANTUM, AN ACCOUNT FOR THE GENERAL READER OF THE GROWTH OF IDEAS UNDERLYING OUR PRESENT ATOMIC KNOWLEDGE, *B. Hoffmann*

Presents lucidly and expertly, with barest amount of mathematics, the problems and theories which led to modern quantum physics. Dr. Hoffmann begins with the closing years of the 19th century, when certain trifling discrepancies were noticed, and with illuminating analogies and examples takes you through the brilliant concepts of Planck, Einstein, Pauli, Broglie, Bohr, Schroedinger, Heisenberg, Dirac, Sommerfeld, Feynman, etc. This edition includes a new, long postscript carrying the story through 1958. "Of the books attempting an account of the history and contents of our modern atomic physics which have come to my attention, this is the best," H. Margenau, Yale University, in *American Journal of Physics*. 32 tables and line illustrations. Index. 275pp. 5⅜ x 8.

20518-5 Paperbound $2.00

GREAT IDEAS OF MODERN MATHEMATICS: THEIR NATURE AND USE, *Jagjit Singh*

Reader with only high school math will understand main mathematical ideas of modern physics, astronomy, genetics, psychology, evolution, etc. better than many who use them as tools, but comprehend little of their basic structure. Author uses his wide knowledge of non-mathematical fields in brilliant exposition of differential equations, matrices, group theory, logic, statistics, problems of mathematical foundations, imaginary numbers, vectors, etc. Original publication. 2 appendixes. 2 indexes. 65 ills. 322pp. 5⅜ x 8.

20587-8 Paperbound $2.25

THE MUSIC OF THE SPHERES: THE MATERIAL UNIVERSE — FROM ATOM TO QUASAR, SIMPLY EXPLAINED, *Guy Murchie*
Vast compendium of fact, modern concept and theory, observed and calculated data, historical background guides intelligent layman through the material universe. Brilliant exposition of earth's construction, explanations for moon's craters, atmospheric components of Venus and Mars (with data from recent fly-by's), sun spots, sequences of star birth and death, neighboring galaxies, contributions of Galileo, Tycho Brahe, Kepler, etc.; and (Vol. 2) construction of the atom (describing newly discovered sigma and xi subatomic particles), theories of sound, color and light, space and time, including relativity theory, quantum theory, wave theory, probability theory, work of Newton, Maxwell, Faraday, Einstein, de Broglie, etc. "Best presentation yet offered to the intelligent general reader," *Saturday Review*. Revised (1967). Index. 319 illustrations by the author. Total of xx + 644pp. 5⅜ x 8½.
21809-0, 21810-4 Two volume set, paperbound $5.00

FOUR LECTURES ON RELATIVITY AND SPACE, *Charles Proteus Steinmetz*
Lecture series, given by great mathematician and electrical engineer, generally considered one of the best popular-level expositions of special and general relativity theories and related questions. Steinmetz translates complex mathematical reasoning into language accessible to laymen through analogy, example and comparison. Among topics covered are relativity of motion, location, time; of mass; acceleration; 4-dimensional time-space; geometry of the gravitational field; curvature and bending of space; non-Euclidean geometry. Index. 40 illustrations. x + 142pp. 5⅜ x 8½.   61771-8 Paperbound $1.35

HOW TO KNOW THE WILD FLOWERS, *Mrs. William Starr Dana*
Classic nature book that has introduced thousands to wonders of American wild flowers. Color-season principle of organization is easy to use, even by those with no botanical training, and the genial, refreshing discussions of history, folklore, uses of over 1,000 native and escape flowers, foliage plants are informative as well as fun to read. Over 170 full-page plates, collected from several editions, may be colored in to make permanent records of finds. Revised to conform with 1950 edition of Gray's Manual of Botany. xlii + 438pp. 5⅜ x 8½.   20332-8 Paperbound $2.50

MANUAL OF THE TREES OF NORTH AMERICA, *Charles Sprague Sargent*
Still unsurpassed as most comprehensive, reliable study of North American tree characteristics, precise locations and distribution. By dean of American dendrologists. Every tree native to U.S., Canada, Alaska; 185 genera, 717 species, described in detail—leaves, flowers, fruit, winterbuds, bark, wood, growth habits, etc. plus discussion of varieties and local variants, immaturity variations. Over 100 keys, including unusual 11-page analytical key to genera, aid in identification. 783 clear illustrations of flowers, fruit, leaves. An unmatched permanent reference work for all nature lovers. Second enlarged (1926) edition. Synopsis of families. Analytical key to genera. Glossary of technical terms. Index. 783 illustrations, 1 map. Total of 982pp. 5⅜ x 8.
20277-1, 20278-X Two volume set, paperbound $6.00

CATALOGUE OF DOVER BOOKS

IT'S FUN TO MAKE THINGS FROM SCRAP MATERIALS,
Evelyn Glantz Hershoff
What use are empty spools, tin cans, bottle tops? What can be made from rubber bands, clothes pins, paper clips, and buttons? This book provides simply worded instructions and large diagrams showing you how to make cookie cutters, toy trucks, paper turkeys, Halloween masks, telephone sets, aprons, linoleum block- and spatter prints — in all 399 projects! Many are easy enough for young children to figure out for themselves; some challenging enough to entertain adults; all are remarkably ingenious ways to make things from materials that cost pennies or less! Formerly "Scrap Fun for Everyone." Index. 214 illustrations. 373pp. 5⅜ x 8½.   21251-3 Paperbound $1.75

SYMBOLIC LOGIC and THE GAME OF LOGIC, *Lewis Carroll*
"Symbolic Logic" is not concerned with modern symbolic logic, but is instead a collection of over 380 problems posed with charm and imagination, using the syllogism and a fascinating diagrammatic method of drawing conclusions. In "The Game of Logic" Carroll's whimsical imagination devises a logical game played with 2 diagrams and counters (included) to manipulate hundreds of tricky syllogisms. The final section, "Hit or Miss" is a lagniappe of 101 additional puzzles in the delightful Carroll manner. Until this reprint edition, both of these books were rarities costing up to $15 each. Symbolic Logic: Index. xxxi + 199pp. The Game of Logic: 96pp. 2 vols. bound as one. 5⅜ x 8.
                    20492-8 Paperbound $2.50

MATHEMATICAL PUZZLES OF SAM LOYD, PART I
selected and edited by M. Gardner
Choice puzzles by the greatest American puzzle creator and innovator. Selected from his famous collection, "Cyclopedia of Puzzles," they retain the unique style and historical flavor of the originals. There are posers based on arithmetic, algebra, probability, game theory, route tracing, topology, counter and sliding block, operations research, geometrical dissection. Includes the famous "14-15" puzzle which was a national craze, and his "Horse of a Different Color" which sold millions of copies. 117 of his most ingenious puzzles in all. 120 line drawings and diagrams. Solutions. Selected references. xx + 167pp. 5⅜ x 8.
                    20498-7 Paperbound $1.35

STRING FIGURES AND HOW TO MAKE THEM, *Caroline Furness Jayne*
107 string figures plus variations selected from the best primitive and modern examples developed by Navajo, Apache, pygmies of Africa, Eskimo, in Europe, Australia, China, etc. The most readily understandable, easy-to-follow book in English on perennially popular recreation. Crystal-clear exposition; step-by-step diagrams. Everyone from kindergarten children to adults looking for unusual diversion will be endlessly amused. Index. Bibliography. Introduction by A. C. Haddon. 17 full-page plates, 960 illustrations. xxiii + 401pp. 5⅜ x 8½.
                    20152-X Paperbound $2.25

PAPER FOLDING FOR BEGINNERS, *W. D. Murray and F. J. Rigney*
A delightful introduction to the varied and entertaining Japanese art of origami (paper folding), with a full, crystal-clear text that anticipates every difficulty; over 275 clearly labeled diagrams of all important stages in creation. You get results at each stage, since complex figures are logically developed from simpler ones. 43 different pieces are explained: sailboats, frogs, roosters, etc. 6 photographic plates. 279 diagrams. 95pp. 5⅜ x 8⅜.
                    20713-7 Paperbound $1.00

PRINCIPLES OF ART HISTORY,
H. Wölfflin
Analyzing such terms as "baroque," "classic," "neoclassic," "primitive,"
"picturesque," and 164 different works by artists like Botticelli, van Cleve,
Dürer, Hobbema, Holbein, Hals, Rembrandt, Titian, Brueghel, Vermeer, and
many others, the author establishes the classifications of art history and style
on a firm, concrete basis. This classic of art criticism shows what really
occurred between the 14th-century primitives and the sophistication of the
18th century in terms of basic attitudes and philosophies. "A remarkable
lesson in the art of seeing," *Sat. Rev. of Literature.* Translated from the 7th
German edition. 150 illustrations. 254pp. 6⅛ x 9¼. 20276-3 Paperbound $2.25

PRIMITIVE ART,
Franz Boas
This authoritative and exhaustive work by a great American anthropologist
covers the entire gamut of primitive art. Pottery, leatherwork, metal work,
stone work, wood, basketry, are treated in detail. Theories of primitive art,
historical depth in art history, technical virtuosity, unconscious levels of patterning, symbolism, styles, literature, music, dance, etc. A must book for the
interested layman, the anthropologist, artist, handicrafter (hundreds of unusual motifs), and the historian. Over 900 illustrations (50 ceramic vessels,
12 totem poles, etc.). 376pp. 5⅜ x 8. 20025-6 Paperbound $2.50

THE GENTLEMAN AND CABINET MAKER'S DIRECTOR,
Thomas Chippendale
A reprint of the 1762 catalogue of furniture designs that went on to influence
generations of English and Colonial and Early Republic American furniture
makers. The 200 plates, most of them full-page sized, show Chippendale's
designs for French (Louis XV), Gothic, and Chinese-manner chairs, sofas,
canopy and dome beds, cornices, chamber organs, cabinets, shaving tables,
commodes, picture frames, frets, candle stands, chimney pieces, decorations, etc.
The drawings are all elegant and highly detailed; many include construction
diagrams and elevations. A supplement of 24 photographs shows surviving
pieces of original and Chippendale-style pieces of furniture. Brief biography
of Chippendale by N. I. Bienenstock, editor of *Furniture World.* Reproduced
from the 1762 edition. 200 plates, plus 19 photographic plates. vi + 249pp.
9⅛ x 12¼. 21601-2 Paperbound $3.50

AMERICAN ANTIQUE FURNITURE: A BOOK FOR AMATEURS,
Edgar G. Miller, Jr.
Standard introduction and practical guide to identification of valuable
American antique furniture. 2115 illustrations, mostly photographs taken by
the author in 148 private homes, are arranged in chronological order in extensive chapters on chairs, sofas, chests, desks, bedsteads, mirrors, tables, clocks,
and other articles. Focus is on furniture accessible to the collector, including
simpler pieces and a larger than usual coverage of Empire style. Introductory
chapters identify structural elements, characteristics of various styles, how to
avoid fakes, etc. "We are frequently asked to name some book on American
furniture that will meet the requirements of the novice collector, the beginning dealer, and . . . the general public. . . . We believe Mr. Miller's two
volumes more completely satisfy this specification than any other work,"
Antiques. Appendix. Index. Total of vi + 1106pp. 7⅞ x 10¾.
21599-7, 21600-4 Two volume set, paperbound $7.50

THE BAD CHILD'S BOOK OF BEASTS, MORE BEASTS FOR WORSE CHILDREN, and A MORAL ALPHABET, *H. Belloc*
Hardly and anthology of humorous verse has appeared in the last 50 years without at least a couple of these famous nonsense verses. But one must see the entire volumes — with all the delightful original illustrations by Sir Basil Blackwood — to appreciate fully Belloc's charming and witty verses that play so subacidly on the platitudes of life and morals that beset his day — and ours. A great humor classic. Three books in one. Total of 157pp. 5⅜ x 8.
20749-8 Paperbound $1.00

THE DEVIL'S DICTIONARY, *Ambrose Bierce*
Sardonic and irreverent barbs puncturing the pomposities and absurdities of American politics, business, religion, literature, and arts, by the country's greatest satirist in the classic tradition. Epigrammatic as Shaw, piercing as Swift, American as Mark Twain, Will Rogers, and Fred Allen, Bierce will always remain the favorite of a small coterie of enthusiasts, and of writers and speakers whom he supplies with "some of the most gorgeous witticisms of the English language" (H. L. Mencken). Over 1000 entries in alphabetical order. 144pp. 5⅜ x 8.
20487-1 Paperbound $1.00

THE COMPLETE NONSENSE OF EDWARD LEAR.
This is the only complete edition of this master of gentle madness available at a popular price. *A Book of Nonsense, Nonsense Songs, More Nonsense Songs and Stories* in their entirety with all the old favorites that have delighted children and adults for years. The Dong With A Luminous Nose, The Jumblies, The Owl and the Pussycat, and hundreds of other bits of wonderful nonsense: 214 limericks; 3 sets of Nonsense Botany, 5 Nonsense Alphabets, 546 drawings by Lear himself, and much more. 320pp. 5⅜ x 8. 20167-8 Paperbound $1.75

THE WIT AND HUMOR OF OSCAR WILDE, ed. by *Alvin Redman*
Wilde at his most brilliant, in 1000 epigrams exposing weaknesses and hypocrisies of "civilized" society. Divided into 49 categories—sin, wealth, women, America, etc.—to aid writers, speakers. Includes excerpts from his trials, books, plays, criticism. Formerly "The Epigrams of Oscar Wilde." Introduction by Vyvyan Holland, Wilde's only living son. Introductory essay by editor. 260pp. 5⅜ x 8.
20602-5 Paperbound $1.50

A CHILD'S PRIMER OF NATURAL HISTORY, *Oliver Herford*
Scarcely an anthology of whimsy and humor has appeared in the last 50 years without a contribution from Oliver Herford. Yet the works from which these examples are drawn have been almost impossible to obtain! Here at last are Herford's improbable definitions of a menagerie of familiar and weird animals, each verse illustrated by the author's own drawings. 24 drawings in 2 colors; 24 additional drawings. vii + 95pp. 6½ x 6. 21647-0 Paperbound $1.00

THE BROWNIES: THEIR BOOK, *Palmer Cox*
The book that made the Brownies a household word. Generations of readers have enjoyed the antics, predicaments and adventures of these jovial sprites, who emerge from the forest at night to play or to come to the aid of a deserving human. Delightful illustrations by the author decorate nearly every page. 24 short verse tales with 266 illustrations. 155pp. 6⅝ x 9¼.
21265-3 Paperbound $1.50

EASY-TO-DO ENTERTAINMENTS AND DIVERSIONS WITH COINS, CARDS, STRING, PAPER AND MATCHES, *R. M. Abraham*
Over 300 tricks, games and puzzles will provide young readers with absorbing fun. Sections on card games; paper-folding; tricks with coins, matches and pieces of string; games for the agile; toy-making from common household objects; mathematical recreations; and 50 miscellaneous pastimes. Anyone in charge of groups of youngsters, including hard-pressed parents, and in need of suggestions on how to keep children sensibly amused and quietly content will find this book indispensable. Clear, simple text, copious number of delightful line drawings and illustrative diagrams. Originally titled "Winter Nights' Entertainments." Introduction by Lord Baden Powell. 329 illustrations. v + 186pp. 5⅜ x 8½. 20921-0 Paperbound $1.00

AN INTRODUCTION TO CHESS MOVES AND TACTICS SIMPLY EXPLAINED, *Leonard Barden*
Beginner's introduction to the royal game. Names, possible moves of the pieces, definitions of essential terms; how games are won, etc. explained in 30-odd pages. With this background you'll be able to sit right down and play. Balance of book teaches strategy — openings, middle game, typical endgame play, and suggestions for improving your game. A sample game is fully analyzed. True middle-level introduction, teaching you all the essentials without oversimplifying or losing you in a maze of detail. 58 figures. 102pp. 5⅜ x 8½. 21210-6 Paperbound $1.25

LASKER'S MANUAL OF CHESS, *Dr. Emanuel Lasker*
Probably the greatest chess player of modern times, Dr. Emanuel Lasker held the world championship 28 years, independent of passing schools or fashions. This unmatched study of the game, chiefly for intermediate to skilled players, analyzes basic methods, combinations, position play, the aesthetics of chess, dozens of different openings, etc., with constant reference to great modern games. Contains a brilliant exposition of Steinitz's important theories. Introduction by Fred Reinfeld. Tables of Lasker's tournament record. 3 indices. 308 diagrams. 1 photograph. xxx + 349pp. 5⅜ x 8.20640-8 Paperbound $2.50

COMBINATIONS: THE HEART OF CHESS, *Irving Chernev*
Step-by-step from simple combinations to complex, this book, by a well-known chess writer, shows you the intricacies of pins, counter-pins, knight forks, and smothered mates. Other chapters show alternate lines of play to those taken in actual championship games; boomerang combinations; classic examples of brilliant combination play by Nimzovich, Rubinstein, Tarrasch, Botvinnik, Alekhine and Capablanca. Index. 356 diagrams. ix + 245pp. 5⅜ x 8½. 21744-2 Paperbound $2.00

HOW TO SOLVE CHESS PROBLEMS, *K. S. Howard*
Full of practical suggestions for the fan or the beginner — who knows only the moves of the chessmen. Contains preliminary section and 58 two-move, 46 three-move, and 8 four-move problems composed by 27 outstanding American problem creators in the last 30 years. Explanation of all terms and exhaustive index. "Just what is wanted for the student," Brian Harley. 112 problems, solutions. vi + 171pp. 5⅜ x 8. 20748-X Paperbound $1.50

FAIRY TALE COLLECTIONS, *edited by Andrew Lang*
Andrew Lang's fairy tale collections make up the richest shelf-full of traditional children's stories anywhere available. Lang supervised the translation of stories from all over the world—familiar European tales collected by Grimm, animal stories from Negro Africa, myths of primitive Australia, stories from Russia, Hungary, Iceland, Japan, and many other countries. Lang's selection of translations are unusually high; many authorities consider that the most familiar tales find their best versions in these volumes. All collections are richly decorated and illustrated by H. J. Ford and other artists.

THE BLUE FAIRY BOOK. 37 stories. 138 illustrations. ix + 390pp. 5⅜ x 8½.
21437-0 Paperbound $1.95

THE GREEN FAIRY BOOK. 42 stories. 100 illustrations. xiii + 366pp. 5⅜ x 8½.
21439-7 Paperbound $1.75

THE BROWN FAIRY BOOK. 32 stories. 50 illustrations, 8 in color. xii + 350pp. 5⅜ x 8½.
21438-9 Paperbound $1.95

THE BEST TALES OF HOFFMANN, *edited by E. F. Bleiler*
10 stories by E. T. A. Hoffmann, one of the greatest of all writers of fantasy. The tales include "The Golden Flower Pot," "Automata," "A New Year's Eve Adventure," "Nutcracker and the King of Mice," "Sand-Man," and others. Vigorous characterizations of highly eccentric personalities, remarkably imaginative situations, and intensely fast pacing has made these tales popular all over the world for 150 years. Editor's introduction. 7 drawings by Hoffmann. xxxiii + 419pp. 5⅜ x 8½.
21793-0 Paperbound $2.25

GHOST AND HORROR STORIES OF AMBROSE BIERCE, *edited by E. F. Bleiler*
Morbid, eerie, horrifying tales of possessed poets, shabby aristocrats, revived corpses, and haunted malefactors. Widely acknowledged as the best of their kind between Poe and the moderns, reflecting their author's inner torment and bitter view of life. Includes "Damned Thing," "The Middle Toe of the Right Foot," "The Eyes of the Panther," "Visions of the Night," "Moxon's Master," and over a dozen others. Editor's introduction. xxii + 199pp. 5⅜ x 8½.
20767-6 Paperbound $1.50

THREE GOTHIC NOVELS, *edited by E. F. Bleiler*
Originators of the still popular Gothic novel form, influential in ushering in early 19th-century Romanticism. Horace Walpole's *Castle of Otranto*, William Beckford's *Vathek*, John Polidori's *The Vampyre*, and a *Fragment* by Lord Byron are enjoyable as exciting reading or as documents in the history of English literature. Editor's introduction. xi + 291pp. 5⅜ x 8½.
21232-7 Paperbound $2.00

BEST GHOST STORIES OF LEFANU, *edited by E. F. Bleiler*
Though admired by such critics as V. S. Pritchett, Charles Dickens and Henry James, ghost stories by the Irish novelist Joseph Sheridan LeFanu have never become as widely known as his detective fiction. About half of the 16 stories in this collection have never before been available in America. Collection includes "Carmilla" (perhaps the best vampire story ever written), "The Haunted Baronet," "The Fortunes of Sir Robert Ardagh," and the classic "Green Tea." Editor's introduction. 7 contemporary illustrations. Portrait of LeFanu. xii + 467pp. 5⅜ x 8.
20415-4 Paperbound $2.50

EASY-TO-DO ENTERTAINMENTS AND DIVERSIONS WITH COINS, CARDS, STRING, PAPER AND MATCHES, *R. M. Abraham*

Over 300 tricks, games and puzzles will provide young readers with absorbing fun. Sections on card games; paper-folding; tricks with coins, matches and pieces of string; games for the agile; toy-making from common household objects; mathematical recreations; and 50 miscellaneous pastimes. Anyone in charge of groups of youngsters, including hard-pressed parents, and in need of suggestions on how to keep children sensibly amused and quietly content will find this book indispensable. Clear, simple text, copious number of delightful line drawings and illustrative diagrams. Originally titled "Winter Nights' Entertainments." Introduction by Lord Baden Powell. 329 illustrations. v + 186pp. 5⅜ x 8½.   20921-0 Paperbound $1.00

AN INTRODUCTION TO CHESS MOVES AND TACTICS SIMPLY EXPLAINED, *Leonard Barden*

Beginner's introduction to the royal game. Names, possible moves of the pieces, definitions of essential terms, how games are won, etc. explained in 30-odd pages. With this background you'll be able to sit right down and play. Balance of book teaches strategy — openings, middle game, typical endgame play, and suggestions for improving your game. A sample game is fully analyzed. True middle-level introduction, teaching you all the essentials without oversimplifying or losing you in a maze of detail. 58 figures. 102pp. 5⅜ x 8½.   21210-6 Paperbound $1.25

LASKER'S MANUAL OF CHESS, *Dr. Emanuel Lasker*

Probably the greatest chess player of modern times, Dr. Emanuel Lasker held the world championship 28 years, independent of passing schools or fashions. This unmatched study of the game, chiefly for intermediate to skilled players, analyzes basic methods, combinations, position play, the aesthetics of chess, dozens of different openings, etc., with constant reference to great modern games. Contains a brilliant exposition of Steinitz's important theories. Introduction by Fred Reinfeld. Tables of Lasker's tournament record. 3 indices. 308 diagrams. 1 photograph. xxx + 349pp. 5⅜ x 8.20640-8Paperbound $2.50

COMBINATIONS: THE HEART OF CHESS, *Irving Chernev*

Step-by-step from simple combinations to complex, this book, by a well-known chess writer, shows you the intricacies of pins, counter-pins, knight forks, and smothered mates. Other chapters show alternate lines of play to those taken in actual championship games; boomerang combinations; classic examples of brilliant combination play by Nimzovich, Rubinstein, Tarrasch, Botvinnik, Alekhine and Capablanca. Index. 356 diagrams. ix + 245pp. 5⅜ x 8½.   21744-2 Paperbound $2.00

HOW TO SOLVE CHESS PROBLEMS, *K. S. Howard*

Full of practical suggestions for the fan or the beginner — who knows only the moves of the chessmen. Contains preliminary section and 58 two-move, 46 three-move, and 8 four-move problems composed by 27 outstanding American problem creators in the last 30 years. Explanation of all terms and exhaustive index. "Just what is wanted for the student," Brian Harley. 112 problems, solutions. vi + 171pp. 5⅜ x 8.   20748-X Paperbound $1.50

SOCIAL THOUGHT FROM LORE TO SCIENCE,
H. E. Barnes and H. Becker
An immense survey of sociological thought and ways of viewing, studying, planning, and reforming society from earliest times to the present. Includes thought on society of preliterate peoples, ancient non-Western cultures, and every great movement in Europe, America, and modern Japan. Analyzes hundreds of great thinkers: Plato, Augustine, Bodin, Vico, Montesquieu, Herder, Comte, Marx, etc. Weighs the contributions of utopians, sophists, fascists and communists; economists, jurists, philosophers, ecclesiastics, and every 19th and 20th century school of scientific sociology, anthropology, and social psychology throughout the world. Combines topical, chronological, and regional approaches, treating the evolution of social thought as a process rather than as a series of mere topics. "Impressive accuracy, competence, and discrimination . . . easily the best single survey," *Nation.* Thoroughly revised, with new material up to 1960. 2 indexes. Over 2200 bibliographical notes. Three volume set. Total of 1586pp. 5⅜ x 8.

20901-6, 20902-4, 20903-2 Three volume set, paperbound $9.00

A HISTORY OF HISTORICAL WRITING, *Harry Elmer Barnes*
Virtually the only adequate survey of the whole course of historical writing in a single volume. Surveys developments from the beginnings of historiography in the ancient Near East and the Classical World, up through the Cold War. Covers major historians in detail, shows interrelationship with cultural background, makes clear individual contributions, evaluates and estimates importance; also enormously rich upon minor authors and thinkers who are usually passed over. Packed with scholarship and learning, clear, easily written. Indispensable to every student of history. Revised and enlarged up to 1961. Index and bibliography. xv + 442pp. 5⅜ x 8½.

20104-X Paperbound $2.75

JOHANN SEBASTIAN BACH, *Philipp Spitta*
The complete and unabridged text of the definitive study of Bach. Written some 70 years ago, it is still unsurpassed for its coverage of nearly all aspects of Bach's life and work. There could hardly be a finer non-technical introduction to Bach's music than the detailed, lucid analyses which Spitta provides for hundreds of individual pieces. 26 solid pages are devoted to the B minor mass, for example, and 30 pages to the glorious St. Matthew Passion. This monumental set also includes a major analysis of the music of the 18th century: Buxtehude, Pachelbel, etc. "Unchallenged as the last word on one of the supreme geniuses of music," John Barkham, *Saturday Review Syndicate.* Total of 1819pp. Heavy cloth binding. 5⅜ x 8.

22278-0, 22279-9 Two volume set, clothbound $15.00

BEETHOVEN AND HIS NINE SYMPHONIES, *George Grove*
In this modern middle-level classic of musicology Grove not only analyzes all nine of Beethoven's symphonies very thoroughly in terms of their musical structure, but also discusses the circumstances under which they were written, Beethoven's stylistic development, and much other background material. This is an extremely rich book, yet very easily followed; it is highly recommended to anyone seriously interested in music. Over 250 musical passages. Index. viii + 407pp. 5⅜ x 8.

20334-4 Paperbound $2.25

THREE SCIENCE FICTION NOVELS,
John Taine
Acknowledged by many as the best SF writer of the 1920's, Taine (under the
name Eric Temple Bell) was also a Professor of Mathematics of considerable
renown. Reprinted here are *The Time Stream*, generally considered Taine's
best, *The Greatest Game*, a biological-fiction novel, and *The Purple Sapphire*,
involving a supercivilization of the past. Taine's stories tie fantastic narratives
to frameworks of original and logical scientific concepts. Speculation is often
profound on such questions as the nature of time, concept of entropy, cyclical
universes, etc. 4 contemporary illustrations. v + 532pp. 5⅜ x 8⅜.
21180-0 Paperbound $2.50

SEVEN SCIENCE FICTION NOVELS,
H. G. Wells
Full unabridged texts of 7 science-fiction novels of the master. Ranging from
biology, physics, chemistry, astronomy, to sociology and other studies, Mr.
Wells extrapolates whole worlds of strange and intriguing character. "One
will have to go far to match this for entertainment, excitement, and sheer
pleasure . . ."*New York Times*. Contents: The Time Machine, The Island of
Dr. Moreau, The First Men in the Moon, The Invisible Man, The War of the
Worlds, The Food of the Gods, In The Days of the Comet. 1015pp. 5⅜ x 8.
20264-X Clothbound $5.00

28 SCIENCE FICTION STORIES OF H. G. WELLS.
Two full, unabridged novels, *Men Like Gods* and *Star Begotten*, plus 26 short
stories by the master science-fiction writer of all time! Stories of space, time,
invention, exploration, futuristic adventure. Partial contents: *The Country of
the Blind, In the Abyss, The Crystal Egg, The Man Who Could Work Miracles,
A Story of Days to Come, The Empire of the Ants, The Magic Shop, The
Valley of the Spiders, A Story of the Stone Age, Under the Knife, Sea Raiders*,
etc. An indispensable collection for the library of anyone interested in science
fiction adventure. 928pp. 5⅜ x 8. 20265-8 Clothbound $5.00

THREE MARTIAN NOVELS,
Edgar Rice Burroughs
Complete, unabridged reprinting, in one volume, of Thuvia, Maid of Mars;
Chessmen of Mars; The Master Mind of Mars. Hours of science-fiction adventure by a modern master storyteller. Reset in large clear type for easy reading.
16 illustrations by J. Allen St. John. vi + 490pp. 5⅜ x 8½.
20039-6 Paperbound $2.50

AN INTELLECTUAL AND CULTURAL HISTORY OF THE WESTERN WORLD,
Harry Elmer Barnes
Monumental 3-volume survey of intellectual development of Europe from
primitive cultures to the present day. Every significant product of human
intellect traced through history: art, literature, mathematics, physical sciences,
medicine, music, technology, social sciences, religions, jurisprudence, education,
etc. Presentation is lucid and specific, analyzing in detail specific discoveries,
theories, literary works, and so on. Revised (1965) by recognized scholars in
specialized fields under the direction of Prof. Barnes. Revised bibliography.
Indexes. 24 illustrations. Total of xxix + 1318pp.
21275-0, 21276-9, 21277-7 Three volume set, paperbound $8.25

LA BOHEME BY GIACOMO PUCCINI,
translated and introduced by Ellen H. Bleiler
Complete handbook for the operagoer, with everything needed for full enjoyment except the musical score itself. Complete Italian libretto, with new, modern English line-by-line translation—the only libretto printing all repeats; biography of Puccini; the librettists; background to the opera, Murger's La Boheme, etc.; circumstances of composition and performances; plot summary; and pictorial section of 73 illustrations showing Puccini, famous singers and performances, etc. Large clear type for easy reading. 124pp. 5⅜ x 8½.
20404-9 Paperbound $1.25

ANTONIO STRADIVARI: HIS LIFE AND WORK (1644-1737),
W. Henry Hill, Arthur F. Hill, and Alfred E. Hill
Still the only book that really delves into life and art of the incomparable Italian craftsman, maker of the finest musical instruments in the world today. The authors, expert violin-makers themselves, discuss Stradivari's ancestry, his construction and finishing techniques, distinguished characteristics of many of his instruments and their locations. Included, too, is story of introduction of his instruments into France, England, first revelation of their supreme merit, and information on his labels, number of instruments made, prices, mystery of ingredients of his varnish, tone of pre-1684 Stradivari violin and changes between 1684 and 1690. An extremely interesting, informative account for all music lovers, from craftsman to concert-goer. Republication of original (1902) edition. New introduction by Sydney Beck, Head of Rare Book and Manuscript Collections, Music Division, New York Public Library. Analytical index by Rembert Wurlitzer. Appendixes. 68 illustrations. 30 full-page plates. 4 in color. xxvi + 315pp. 5⅜ x 8½.
20425-1 Paperbound $2.25

MUSICAL AUTOGRAPHS FROM MONTEVERDI TO HINDEMITH,
Emanuel Winternitz
For beauty, for intrinsic interest, for perspective on the composer's personality, for subtleties of phrasing, shading, emphasis indicated in the autograph but suppressed in the printed score, the mss. of musical composition are fascinating documents which repay close study in many different ways. This 2-volume work reprints facsimiles of mss. by virtually every major composer, and many minor figures—196 examples in all. A full text points out what can be learned from mss., analyzes each sample. Index. Bibliography. 18 figures. 196 plates. Total of 170pp. of text. 7⅞ x 10¾.
21312-9, 21313-7 Two volume set, paperbound $5.00

J. S. BACH,
Albert Schweitzer
One of the few great full-length studies of Bach's life and work, and the study upon which Schweitzer's renown as a musicologist rests. On first appearance (1911), revolutionized Bach performance. The only writer on Bach to be musicologist, performing musician, and student of history, theology and philosophy, Schweitzer contributes particularly full sections on history of German Protestant church music, theories on motivic pictorial representations in vocal music, and practical suggestions for performance. Translated by Ernest Newman. Indexes. 5 illustrations. 650 musical examples. Total of xix + 928pp. 5⅜ x 8½.
21631-4, 21632-2 Two volume set, paperbound $4.50

THE METHODS OF ETHICS, *Henry Sidgwick*
Propounding no organized system of its own, study subjects every major
methodological approach to ethics to rigorous, objective analysis. Study discusses and relates ethical thought of Plato, Aristotle, Bentham, Clarke, Butler,
Hobbes, Hume, Mill, Spencer, Kant, and dozens of others. Sidgwick retains
conclusions from each system which follow from ethical premises, rejecting
the faulty. Considered by many in the field to be among the most important
treatises on ethical philosophy. Appendix. Index. xlvii + 528pp. 5⅜ x 8½.
21608-X Paperbound $2.50

TEUTONIC MYTHOLOGY, *Jakob Grimm*
A milestone in Western culture; the work which established on a modern
basis the study of history of religions and comparative religions. 4-volume
work assembles and interprets everything available on religious and folk-
loristic beliefs of Germanic people (including Scandinavians, Anglo-Saxons,
etc.). Assembling material from such sources as Tacitus, surviving Old Norse
and Icelandic texts, archeological remains, folktales, surviving superstitions,
comparative traditions, linguistic analysis, etc. Grimm explores pagan deities,
heroes, folklore of nature, religious practices, and every other area of pagan
German belief. To this day, the unrivaled, definitive, exhaustive study. Translated by J. S. Stallybrass from 4th (1883) German edition. Indexes. Total of
lxxvii + 1887pp. 5⅜ x 8½.
21602-0, 21603-9, 21604-7, 21605-5 Four volume set, paperbound $11.00

THE I CHING, *translated by James Legge*
Called "The Book of Changes" in English, this is one of the Five Classics
edited by Confucius, basic and central to Chinese thought. Explains perhaps
the most complex system of divination known, founded on the theory that all
things happening at any one time have characteristic features which can be
isolated and related. Significant in Oriental studies, in history of religions and
philosophy, and also to Jungian psychoanalysis and other areas of modern
European thought. Index. Appendixes. 6 plates. xxi + 448pp. 5⅜ x 8½.
21062-6 Paperbound $2.75

HISTORY OF ANCIENT PHILOSOPHY, *W. Windelband*
One of the clearest, most accurate comprehensive surveys of Greek and Roman
philosophy. Discusses ancient philosophy in general, intellectual life in Greece
in the 7th and 6th centuries B.C., Thales, Anaximander, Anaximenes, Herac-
litus, the Eleatics, Empedocles, Anaxagoras, Leucippus, the Pythagoreans,
the Sophists, Socrates, Democritus (20 pages), Plato (50 pages), Aristotle (70 pages),
the Peripatetics, Stoics, Epicureans, Sceptics, Neo-platonists, Christian Apolo-
gists, etc. 2nd German edition translated by H. E. Cushman. xv + 393pp.
5⅜ x 8. 20357-3 Paperbound $2.25

THE PALACE OF PLEASURE, *William Painter*
Elizabethan versions of Italian and French novels from *The Decameron*,
Cinthio, Straparola, Queen Margaret of Navarre, and other continental sources
— the very work that provided Shakespeare and dozens of his contemporaries
with many of their plots and sub-plots and, therefore, justly considered one of
the most influential books in all English literature. It is also a book that any
reader will still enjoy. Total of cviii + 1,224pp.
21691-8, 21692-6, 21693-4 Three volume set, paperbound $6.75

AN INTRODUCTION TO THE GEOMETRY OF N DIMENSIONS,
D. H. Y. Sommerville
An introduction presupposing no prior knowledge of the field, the only book in English devoted exclusively to higher dimensional geometry. Discusses fundamental ideas of incidence, parallelism, perpendicularity, angles between linear space; enumerative geometry; analytical geometry from projective and metric points of view; polytopes; elementary ideas in analysis situs; content of hyper-spacial figures. Bibliography. Index. 60 diagrams. 196pp. 5⅜ x 8.
60494-2 Paperbound $1.50

ELEMENTARY CONCEPTS OF TOPOLOGY, *P. Alexandroff*
First English translation of the famous brief introduction to topology for the beginner or for the mathematician not undertaking extensive study. This unusually useful intuitive approach deals primarily with the concepts of complex, cycle, and homology, and is wholly consistent with current investigations. Ranges from basic concepts of set-theoretic topology to the concept of Betti groups. "Glowing example of harmony between intuition and thought," David Hilbert. Translated by A. E. Farley. Introduction by D. Hilbert. Index. 25 figures. 73pp. 5⅜ x 8.
60747-X Paperbound $1.25

ELEMENTS OF NON-EUCLIDEAN GEOMETRY,
D. M. Y. Sommerville
Unique in proceeding step-by-step, in the manner of traditional geometry. Enables the student with only a good knowledge of high school algebra and geometry to grasp elementary hyperbolic, elliptic, analytic non-Euclidean geometries; space curvature and its philosophical implications; theory of radical axes; homothetic centres and systems of circles; parataxy and parallelism; absolute measure; Gauss' proof of the defect area theorem; geodesic representation; much more, all with exceptional clarity. 126 problems at chapter endings provide progressive practice and familiarity. 133 figures. Index. xvi + 274pp. 5⅜ x 8.
60460-8 Paperbound $2.00

INTRODUCTION TO THE THEORY OF NUMBERS, *L. E. Dickson*
Thorough, comprehensive approach with adequate coverage of classical literature, an introductory volume beginners can follow. Chapters on divisibility, congruences, quadratic residues & reciprocity. Diophantine equations, etc. Full treatment of binary quadratic forms without usual restriction to integral coefficients. Covers infinitude of primes, least residues. Fermat's theorem. Euler's phi function, Legendre's symbol, Gauss's lemma, automorphs, reduced forms, recent theorems of Thue & Siegel, many more. Much material not readily available elsewhere. 239 problems. Index. I figure. viii + 183pp. 5⅜ x 8.
60342-3 Paperbound $1.75

MATHEMATICAL TABLES AND FORMULAS,
compiled by Robert D. Carmichael and Edwin R. Smith
Valuable collection for students, etc. Contains all tables necessary in college algebra and trigonometry, such as five-place common logarithms, logarithmic sines and tangents of small angles, logarithmic trigonometric functions, natural trigonometric functions, four-place antilogarithms, tables for changing from sexagesimal to circular and from circular to sexagesimal measure of angles, etc. Also many tables and formulas not ordinarily accessible, including powers, roots, and reciprocals, exponential and hyperbolic functions, ten-place logarithms of prime numbers, and formulas and theorems from analytical and elementary geometry and from calculus. Explanatory introduction. viii + 269pp. 5⅜ x 8½.
60111-0 Paperbound $1.50

A Source Book in Mathematics,
D. E. Smith
Great discoveries in math, from Renaissance to end of 19th century, in English translation. Read announcements by Dedekind, Gauss, Delamain, Pascal, Fermat, Newton, Abel, Lobachevsky, Bolyai, Riemann, De Moivre, Legendre, Laplace, others of discoveries about imaginary numbers, number congruence, slide rule, equations, symbolism, cubic algebraic equations, non-Euclidean forms of geometry, calculus, function theory, quaternions, etc. Succinct selections from 125 different treatises, articles, most unavailable elsewhere in English. Each article preceded by biographical introduction. Vol. I: Fields of Number, Algebra. Index. 32 illus. 338pp. 5⅜ x 8. Vol. II: Fields of Geometry, Probability, Calculus, Functions, Quaternions. 83 illus. 432pp. 5⅜ x 8.
60552-3, 60553-1 Two volume set, paperbound $5.00

Foundations of Physics,
R. B. Lindsay & H. Margenau
Excellent bridge between semi-popular works & technical treatises. A discussion of methods of physical description, construction of theory; valuable for physicist with elementary calculus who is interested in ideas that give meaning to data, tools of modern physics. Contents include symbolism; mathematical equations; space & time foundations of mechanics; probability; physics & continua; electron theory; special & general relativity; quantum mechanics; causality. "Thorough and yet not overdetailed. Unreservedly recommended," *Nature* (London). Unabridged, corrected edition. List of recommended readings. 35 illustrations. xi + 537pp. 5⅜ x 8. 60377-6 Paperbound $3.50

Fundamental Formulas of Physics,
ed. by D. H. Menzel
High useful, full, inexpensive reference and study text, ranging from simple to highly sophisticated operations. Mathematics integrated into text—each chapter stands as short textbook of field represented. Vol. 1: Statistics, Physical Constants, Special Theory of Relativity, Hydrodynamics, Aerodynamics, Boundary Value Problems in Math, Physics, Viscosity, Electromagnetic Theory, etc. Vol. 2: Sound, Acoustics, Geometrical Optics, Electron Optics, High-Energy Phenomena, Magnetism, Biophysics, much more. Index. Total of 800pp. 5⅜ x 8.
60595-7, 60596-5 Two volume set, paperbound $4.75

Theoretical Physics,
A. S. Kompaneyets
One of the very few thorough studies of the subject in this price range. Provides advanced students with a comprehensive theoretical background. Especially strong on recent experimentation and developments in quantum theory. Contents: Mechanics (Generalized Coordinates, Lagrange's Equation, Collision of Particles, etc.), Electrodynamics (Vector Analysis, Maxwell's equations, Transmission of Signals, Theory of Relativity, etc.), Quantum Mechanics (the Inadequacy of Classical Mechanics, the Wave Equation, Motion in a Central Field, Quantum Theory of Radiation, Quantum Theories of Dispersion and Scattering, etc.), and Statistical Physics (Equilibrium Distribution of Molecules in an Ideal Gas, Boltzmann Statistics, Bose and Fermi Distribution. Thermodynamic Quantities, etc.). Revised to 1961. Translated by George Yankovsky, authorized by Kompaneyets. 137 exercises. 56 figures. 529pp. 5⅜ x 8½.
60972-3 Paperbound $3.50

MATHEMATICAL PHYSICS, *D. H. Menzel*
Thorough one-volume treatment of the mathematical techniques vital for classical mechanics, electromagnetic theory, quantum theory, and relativity. Written by the Harvard Professor of Astrophysics for junior, senior, and graduate courses, it gives clear explanations of all those aspects of function theory, vectors, matrices, dyadics, tensors, partial differential equations, etc., necessary for the understanding of the various physical theories. Electron theory, relativity, and other topics seldom presented appear here in considerable detail. Scores of definition, conversion factors, dimensional constants, etc. "More detailed than normal for an advanced text . . . excellent set of sections on Dyadics, Matrices, and Tensors," *Journal of the Franklin Institute.* Index. 193 problems, with answers. x + 412pp. 5⅜ x 8.   60056-4 Paperbound $2.50

THE THEORY OF SOUND, *Lord Rayleigh*
Most vibrating systems likely to be encountered in practice can be tackled successfully by the methods set forth by the great Nobel laureate, Lord Rayleigh. Complete coverage of experimental, mathematical aspects of sound theory. Partial contents: Harmonic motions, vibrating systems in general, lateral vibrations of bars, curved plates or shells, applications of Laplace's functions to acoustical problems, fluid friction, plane vortex-sheet, vibrations of solid bodies, etc. This is the first inexpensive edition of this great reference and study work. Bibliography, Historical introduction by R. B. Lindsay. Total of 1040pp. 97 figures. 5⅜ x 8.   60292-3, 60293-1 Two volume set, paperbound $6.00

HYDRODYNAMICS, *Horace Lamb*
Internationally famous complete coverage of standard reference work on dynamics of liquids & gases. Fundamental theorems, equations, methods, solutions, background, for classical hydrodynamics. Chapters include Equations of Motion, Integration of Equations in Special Gases, Irrotational Motion, Motion of Liquid in 2 Dimensions, Motion of Solids through Liquid-Dynamical Theory, Vortex Motion, Tidal Waves, Surface Waves, Waves of Expansion, Viscosity, Rotating Masses of Liquids. Excellently planned, arranged; clear, lucid presentation. 6th enlarged, revised edition. Index. Over 900 footnotes, mostly bibliographical. 119 figures. xv + 738pp. 6⅛ x 9¼.   60256-7 Paperbound $4.00

DYNAMICAL THEORY OF GASES, *James Jeans*
Divided into mathematical and physical chapters for the convenience of those not expert in mathematics, this volume discusses the mathematical theory of gas in a steady state, thermodynamics, Boltzmann and Maxwell, kinetic theory, quantum theory, exponentials, etc. 4th enlarged edition, with new material on quantum theory, quantum dynamics, etc. Indexes. 28 figures. 444pp. 6⅛ x 9¼.   60136-6 Paperbound $2.75

THERMODYNAMICS, *Enrico Fermi*
Unabridged reproduction of 1937 edition. Elementary in treatment; remarkable for clarity, organization. Requires no knowledge of advanced math beyond calculus, only familiarity with fundamentals of thermometry, calorimetry. Partial Contents: Thermodynamic systems; First & Second laws of thermodynamics; Entropy; Thermodynamic potentials: phase rule, reversible electric cell; Gaseous reactions: van't Hoff reaction box, principle of LeChatelier; Thermodynamics of dilute solutions: osmotic & vapor pressures, boiling & freezing points; Entropy constant. Index. 25 problems. 24 illustrations. x + 160pp. 5⅜ x 8.   60361-X Paperbound $2.00

CELESTIAL OBJECTS FOR COMMON TELESCOPES,
Rev. T. W. Webb
Classic handbook for the use and pleasure of the amateur astronomer. Of inestimable aid in locating and identifying thousands of celestial objects. Vol I, The Solar System: discussions of the principle and operation of the telescope, procedures of observations and telescope-photography, spectroscopy, etc., precise location information of sun, moon, planets, meteors. Vol. II, The Stars: alphabetical listing of constellations, information on double stars, clusters, stars with unusual spectra, variables, and nebulae, etc. Nearly 4,000 objects noted. Edited and extensively revised by Margaret W. Mayall, director of the American Assn. of Variable Star Observers. New Index by Mrs. Mayall giving the location of all objects mentioned in the text for Epoch 2000. New Precession Table added. New appendices on the planetary satellites, constellation names and abbreviations, and solar system data. Total of 46 illustrations. Total of xxxix + 606pp. 5⅜ x 8.   20917-2, 20918-0 Two volume set, paperbound $5.00

PLANETARY THEORY,
E. W. Brown and C. A. Shook
Provides a clear presentation of basic methods for calculating planetary orbits for today's astronomer. Begins with a careful exposition of specialized mathematical topics essential for handling perturbation theory and then goes on to indicate how most of the previous methods reduce ultimately to two general calculation methods: obtaining expressions either for the coordinates of planetary positions or for the elements which determine the perturbed paths. An example of each is given and worked in detail. Corrected edition. Preface. Appendix. Index. xii + 302pp. 5⅜ x 8½.   61133-7 Paperbound $2.25

STAR NAMES AND THEIR MEANINGS,
Richard Hinckley Allen
An unusual book documenting the various attributions of names to the individual stars over the centuries. Here is a treasure-house of information on a topic not normally delved into even by professional astronomers; provides a fascinating background to the stars in folk-lore, literary references, ancient writings, star catalogs and maps over the centuries. Constellation-by-constellation analysis covers hundreds of stars and other asterisms, including the Pleiades, Hyades, Andromedan Nebula, etc. Introduction. Indices. List of authors and authorities. xx + 563pp. 5⅜ x 8½.   21079-0 Paperbound $3.00

A SHORT HISTORY OF ASTRONOMY, *A. Berry*
Popular standard work for over 50 years, this thorough and accurate volume covers the science from primitive times to the end of the 19th century. After the Greeks and the Middle Ages, individual chapters analyze Copernicus, Brahe, Galileo, Kepler, and Newton, and the mixed reception of their discoveries. Post-Newtonian achievements are then discussed in unusual detail: Halley, Bradley, Lagrange, Laplace, Herschel, Bessel, etc. 2 Indexes. 104 illustrations, 9 portraits. xxxi + 440pp. 5⅜ x 8.   20210-0 Paperbound $2.75

SOME THEORY OF SAMPLING, *W. E. Deming*
The purpose of this book is to make sampling techniques understandable to and useable by social scientists, industrial managers, and natural scientists who are finding statistics increasingly part of their work. Over 200 exercises, plus dozens of actual applications. 61 tables. 90 figs. xix + 602pp. 5⅜ x 8½.
61755-6 Paperbound $3.50

HEAR ME TALKIN' TO YA, *edited by Nat Shapiro and Nat Hentoff*
In their own words, Louis Armstrong, King Oliver, Fletcher Henderson, Bunk Johnson, Bix Beiderbecke, Billy Holiday, Fats Waller, Jelly Roll Morton, Duke Ellington, and many others comment on the origins of jazz in New Orleans and its growth in Chicago's South Side, Kansas City's jam sessions, Depression Harlem, and the modernism of the West Coast schools. Taken from taped conversations, letters, magazine articles, other first-hand sources. Editors' introduction. xvi + 429pp. 5⅜ x 8½.   21726-4 Paperbound $2.00

THE JOURNAL OF HENRY D. THOREAU
A 25-year record by the great American observer and critic, as complete a record of a great man's inner life as is anywhere available. Thoreau's Journals served him as raw material for his formal pieces, as a place where he could develop his ideas, as an outlet for his interests in wild life and plants, in writing as an art, in classics of literature, Walt Whitman and other contemporaries, in politics, slavery, individual's relation to the State, etc. The Journals present a portrait of a remarkable man, and are an observant social history. Unabridged republication of 1906 edition, Bradford Torrey and Francis H. Allen, editors. Illustrations. Total of 1888pp. 8⅜ x 12¼.
20312-3, 20313-1 Two volume set. clothbound $30.00

A SHAKESPEARIAN GRAMMAR, E. A. *Abbott*
Basic reference to Shakespeare and his contemporaries, explaining through thousands of quotations from Shakespeare, Jonson, Beaumont and Fletcher, North's *Plutarch* and other sources the grammatical usage differing from the modern. First published in 1870 and written by a scholar who spent much of his life isolating principles of Elizabethan language, the book is unlikely ever to be superseded. Indexes. xxiv + 511pp. 5⅜ x 8½. 21582-2 Paperbound $3.00

FOLK-LORE OF SHAKESPEARE, T. F. *Thistelton Dyer*
Classic study, drawing from Shakespeare a large body of references to supernatural beliefs, terminology of falconry and hunting, games and sports, good luck charms, marriage customs, folk medicines, superstitions about plants, animals, birds, argot of the underworld, sexual slang of London, proverbs, drinking customs, weather lore, and much else. From full compilation comes a mirror of the 17th-century popular mind. Index. ix + 526pp. 5⅜ x 8½.
21614-4 Paperbound $2.75

THE NEW VARIORUM SHAKESPEARE, *edited by H. H. Furness*
By far the richest editions of the plays ever produced in any country or language. Each volume contains complete text (usually First Folio) of the play, all variants in Quarto and other Folio texts, editorial changes by every major editor to Furness's own time (1900), footnotes to obscure references or language, extensive quotes from literature of Shakespearian criticism, essays on plot sources (often reprinting sources in full), and much more.

HAMLET, *edited by H. H. Furness*
Total of xxvi + 905pp. 5⅜ x 8½.
21004-9, 21005-7 Two volume set, paperbound $5.25
TWELFTH NIGHT, *edited by H. H. Furness*
Index. xxii + 434pp. 5⅜ x 8½.   21189-4 Paperbound $2.75

THE WONDERFUL WIZARD OF OZ, *L. F. Baum*
All the original W. W. Denslow illustrations in full color—as much a part of "The Wizard" as Tenniel's drawings are of "Alice in Wonderland." "The Wizard" is still America's best-loved fairy tale, in which, as the author expresses it, "The wonderment and joy are retained and the heartaches and nightmares left out." Now today's young readers can enjoy every word and wonderful picture of the original book. New introduction by Martin Gardner. A Baum bibliography. 23 full-page color plates. viii + 268pp. 5⅜ x 8.
20691-2 Paperbound $1.95

THE MARVELOUS LAND OF OZ, *L. F. Baum*
This is the equally enchanting sequel to the "Wizard," continuing the adventures of the Scarecrow and the Tin Woodman. The hero this time is a little boy named Tip, and all the delightful Oz magic is still present. This is the Oz book with the Animated Saw-Horse, the Woggle-Bug, and Jack Pumpkinhead. All the original John R. Neill illustrations, 10 in full color. 287pp. 5⅜ x 8.
20692-0 Paperbound $1.75

ALICE'S ADVENTURES UNDER GROUND, *Lewis Carroll*
The original *Alice in Wonderland*, hand-lettered and illustrated by Carroll himself, and originally presented as a Christmas gift to a child-friend. Adults as well as children will enjoy this charming volume, reproduced faithfully in this Dover edition. While the story is essentially the same, there are slight changes, and Carroll's spritely drawings present an intriguing alternative to the famous Tenniel illustrations. One of the most popular books in Dover's catalogue. Introduction by Martin Gardner. 38 illustrations. 128pp. 5⅜ x 8½.
21482-6 Paperbound $1.00

THE NURSERY "ALICE," *Lewis Carroll*
While most of us consider *Alice in Wonderland* a story for children of all ages, Carroll himself felt it was beyond younger children. He therefore provided this simplified version, illustrated with the famous Tenniel drawings enlarged and colored in delicate tints, for children aged "from Nought to Five." Dover's edition of this now rare classic is a faithful copy of the 1889 printing, including 20 illustrations by Tenniel, and front and back covers reproduced in full color. Introduction by Martin Gardner. xxiii + 67pp. 6⅛ x 9¼.
21610-1 Paperbound $1.75

THE STORY OF KING ARTHUR AND HIS KNIGHTS, *Howard Pyle*
A fast-paced, exciting retelling of the best known Arthurian legends for young readers by one of America's best story tellers and illustrators. The sword Excalibur, wooing of Guinevere, Merlin and his downfall, adventures of Sir Pellias and Gawaine, and others. The pen and ink illustrations are vividly imagined and wonderfully drawn. 41 illustrations. xviii + 313pp. 6⅛ x 9¼.
21445-1 Paperbound $2.00